# Spinal Infections: Pathogenesis, Diagnosis, Management and Outcomes

# Spinal Infections: Pathogenesis, Diagnosis, Management and Outcomes

Editor

**Kalliopi Alpantaki**

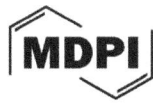

Basel • Beijing • Wuhan • Barcelona • Belgrade • Novi Sad • Cluj • Manchester

*Editor*
Kalliopi Alpantaki
"Venizeleion" General
Hospital of Crete
Heraklion
Greece

*Editorial Office*
MDPI
St. Alban-Anlage 66
4052 Basel, Switzerland

This is a reprint of articles from the Special Issue published online in the open access journal *Journal of Clinical Medicine* (ISSN 2077-0383) (available at: https://redmine.mdpi.cn/issues/4844302).

For citation purposes, cite each article independently as indicated on the article page online and as indicated below:

Lastname, A.A.; Lastname, B.B. Article Title. *Journal Name* **Year**, *Volume Number*, Page Range.

**ISBN 978-3-7258-0823-6 (Hbk)**
**ISBN 978-3-7258-0824-3 (PDF)**
doi.org/10.3390/books978-3-7258-0824-3

© 2024 by the authors. Articles in this book are Open Access and distributed under the Creative Commons Attribution (CC BY) license. The book as a whole is distributed by MDPI under the terms and conditions of the Creative Commons Attribution-NonCommercial-NoDerivs (CC BY-NC-ND) license.

# Contents

Nikolaos Spernovasilis, Apostolos Karantanas, Ioulia Markaki, Afroditi Konsoula, Zisis Ntontis, Christos Koutserimpas and Kalliopi Alpantaki  
*Brucella* Spondylitis: Current Knowledge and Recent Advances  
Reprinted from: *J. Clin. Med.* **2024**, *13*, 595, doi:10.3390/jcm13020595 . . . . . . . . . . . . . . . . 1

Lisa Klute, Marie Esser, Leopold Henssler, Moritz Riedl, Melanie Schindler, Markus Rupp, et al.  
Anterior Column Reconstruction of Destructive Vertebral Osteomyelitis at the Thoracolumbar Spine with an Expandable Vertebral Body Replacement Implant: A Retrospective, Monocentric Radiological Cohort Analysis of 24 Cases  
Reprinted from: *J. Clin. Med.* **2024**, *13*, 296, doi:10.3390/jcm13010296 . . . . . . . . . . . . . . . . 19

Mido Max Hijazi, Timo Siepmann, Ibrahim El-Battrawy, Assem Aweimer, Kay Engellandt, Dino Podlesek, et al.  
Diagnostics, Management, and Outcomes in Patients with Pyogenic Spinal Intra- or Epidural Abscess  
Reprinted from: *J. Clin. Med.* **2023**, *12*, 7691, doi:10.3390/jcm12247691 . . . . . . . . . . . . . . . . 30

Ann-Kathrin Joerger, Carolin Albrecht, Nicole Lange, Bernhard Meyer and Maria Wostrack  
In-Hospital Mortality from Spondylodiscitis: Insights from a Single-Center Retrospective Study  
Reprinted from: *J. Clin. Med.* **2023**, *12*, 7228, doi:10.3390/jcm12237228 . . . . . . . . . . . . . . . . 44

Mido Max Hijazi, Timo Siepmann, Ibrahim El-Battrawy, Percy Schröttner, Dino Podlesek, Kay Engellandt, et al.  
The Efficacy of Daily Local Antibiotic Lavage via an Epidural Suction–Irrigation Drainage Technique in Spondylodiscitis and Isolated Spinal Epidural Empyema: A 20-Year Experience of a Single Spine Center  
Reprinted from: *J. Clin. Med.* **2023**, *12*, 5078, doi:10.3390/jcm12155078 . . . . . . . . . . . . . . . . 57

Tomasz Piotr Ziarko, Nike Walter, Melanie Schindler, Volker Alt, Markus Rupp and Siegmund Lang  
Risk Factors for the In-Hospital Mortality in Pyogenic Vertebral Osteomyelitis: A Cross-Sectional Study on 9753 Patients  
Reprinted from: *J. Clin. Med.* **2023**, *12*, 4805, doi:10.3390/jcm12144805 . . . . . . . . . . . . . . . . 74

Stamatios A. Papadakis, Margarita-Michaela Ampadiotaki, Dimitrios Pallis, Konstantinos Tsivelekas, Petros Nikolakakos, Labrini Agapitou and George Sapkas  
Cervical Spinal Epidural Abscess: Diagnosis, Treatment, and Outcomes: A Case Series and a Literature Review  
Reprinted from: *J. Clin. Med.* **2023**, *12*, 4509, doi:10.3390/jcm12134509 . . . . . . . . . . . . . . . . 84

Mido Max Hijazi, Timo Siepmann, Alexander Carl Disch, Uwe Platz, Tareq A. Juratli, Ilker Y. Eyüpoglu and Dino Podlesek  
Diagnostic Sensitivity of Blood Culture, Intraoperative Specimen, and Computed Tomography-Guided Biopsy in Patients with Spondylodiscitis and Isolated Spinal Epidural Empyema Requiring Surgical Treatment  
Reprinted from: *J. Clin. Med.* **2023**, *12*, 3693, doi:10.3390/jcm12113693 . . . . . . . . . . . . . . . . 104

Siegmund Lang, Nike Walter, Melanie Schindler, Susanne Baertl, Dominik Szymski, Markus Loibl, et al.  
The Epidemiology of Spondylodiscitis in Germany: A Descriptive Report of Incidence Rates, Pathogens, In-Hospital Mortality, and Hospital Stays between 2010 and 2020  
Reprinted from: *J. Clin. Med.* **2023**, *12*, 3373, doi:10.3390/jcm12103373 . . . . . . . . . . . . . . . . 119

**Redwan Jabbar, Bartosz Szmyd, Jakub Jankowski, Weronika Lusa, Agnieszka Pawełczyk, Grzegorz Wysiadecki, et al.**
Intramedullary Spinal Cord Abscess with Concomitant Spinal Degenerative Diseases: A Case Report and Systematic Literature Review
Reprinted from: *J. Clin. Med.* **2022**, *11*, 5148, doi:10.3390/jcm11175148 . . . . . . . . . . . . . . . . **129**

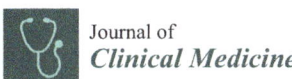
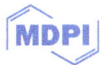

*Review*

# *Brucella* Spondylitis: Current Knowledge and Recent Advances

**Nikolaos Spernovasilis** [1,*], **Apostolos Karantanas** [2,3,4], **Ioulia Markaki** [5], **Afroditi Konsoula** [6], **Zisis Ntontis** [7], **Christos Koutserimpas** [8] **and Kalliopi Alpantaki** [7,*]

1. Department of Infectious Diseases, German Oncology Center, 4108 Limassol, Cyprus
2. Department of Medical Imaging, University Hospital of Heraklion, 71500 Heraklion, Greece; akarantanas@gmail.com
3. Advanced Hybrid Imaging Systems, Institute of Computer Science, FORTH, 71500 Heraklion, Greece
4. Department of Radiology, School of Medicine, University of Crete, 71003 Heraklion, Greece
5. Internal Medicine Department, Thoracic Diseases General Hospital Sotiria, 11527 Athens, Greece; tzouliamar95@gmail.com
6. Department of Pediatrics, General Hospital of Sitia, 72300 Sitia, Greece; aphrodite.konsoula@gmail.com
7. Department of Orthopaedics and Trauma Surgery, Venizeleio General Hospital of Heraklion, 71409 Heraklion, Greece; ntontis1997@gmail.com
8. Department of Orthopaedics and Traumatology, "251" Hellenic Air Force General Hospital of Athens, 11525 Athens, Greece; chrisku91@hotmail.com
* Correspondence: nikspe@hotmail.com (N.S.); apopaki@yahoo.gr (K.A.)

**Abstract:** The most prevalent zoonotic disease is brucellosis, which poses a significant threat for worldwide public health. Particularly in endemic areas, spinal involvement is a major source of morbidity and mortality and can complicate the course of the disease. The diagnosis of *Brucella* spondylitis is challenging and should be suspected in the appropriate epidemiological and clinical context, in correlation with microbiological and radiological findings. Treatment depends largely on the affected parts of the body. Available treatment options include antibiotic administration for an adequate period of time and, when appropriate, surgical intervention. In this article, we examined the most recent data on the pathophysiology, clinical manifestation, diagnosis, and management of spinal brucellosis in adults.

**Keywords:** *Brucella*; brucellosis; spine; spondylitis; spondylodiscitis; imaging

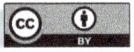

## 1. Introduction

Brucellosis is a zoonotic infection caused by the bacterial genus *Brucella*. Humans represent occasional hosts, but brucellosis remains a major public health problem globally and is the most common zoonotic infection. Spinal involvement may complicate the course of the disease and is a significant cause of morbidity and mortality, especially in endemic areas [1].

In this article, we reviewed the current literature on the epidemiology, pathophysiology, clinical presentation, diagnosis, and treatment of a spinal infection due to *Brucella* spp.

## 2. Epidemiology

Brucellosis is caused by a group of small (diameter: 0.5–0.7; length: 0.6–1.5 µm), non-motile, non-spore-forming, slow-growing, facultative intracellular, Gram-negative coccobacilli [2]. It is an ancient disease known by various names, including Mediterranean fever, Malta fever, and undulant fever. The genus *Brucella* was named after David Bruce in 1887. He isolated and identified the causative bacterium from the spleen of a British soldier who had died of a febrile illness that was common among military personnel stationed in Malta [3]. Twelve species are known to date [4], and each has its preferred animal host, although it can also infect other hosts [5]. The major *Brucella* species known to cause disease in humans are *B. melitensis* (sheep and goats), *B. abortus* (cattle, including the vaccine strain

RB51), *B. suis* (pigs), and *B. canis* (dogs) [5]. The vast majority of human cases worldwide are associated with *B. melitensis* [6].

The disease can be transmitted to humans through the consumption of unpasteurized animal products (especially raw milk, soft cheese, butter, and ice cream), direct skin or mucous membrane contact with infected animal tissue, or inhalation of infected aerosol particles [6]. The risk of transmission is generally greater for people working with the bacteria in laboratories, slaughterhouses, veterinarians, hunters, shepherds, and meat-packing plant workers. In rare cases, human-to-human transmission has been documented through sexual contact, breastfeeding, congenital transmission, bone marrow transplantation, blood transfusion, and aerosol from an infected patient [7].

Although accurate epidemiologic data are not available for many endemic areas, it is estimated that more than 500,000 new human cases are reported worldwide each year [8]. The disease is most common in people who have travelled to or live in areas where the disease is endemic in animals along the Mediterranean basin (Portugal, Spain, Southern France, Italy, Greece, Turkey, and North Africa), Mexico, South and Central America, Eastern Europe, Asia, Africa, and the Middle East [9,10]. Even though it is a nationally notifiable disease in most countries and must be reported to the local health authorities, this is not always the case, and official numbers represent only a fraction of the actual incidence of the disease [10].

Osteoarticular involvement is one of the most common complications of brucellosis and varies in the literature from 10% to 85% of patients [11–15]. The wide range between reports in the literature may be due to the characteristics of the study populations, the radio-diagnostic methods used, and the different diagnostic criteria [13]. It may present as sacroiliitis, spondylitis, osteomyelitis, peripheral arthritis, bursitis, and tenosynovitis [14]. The type of skeletal involvement depends in part on the age of the patient [1]. The most common osteoarticular finding in children is monoarticular arthritis (usually of the knees and hips) [16], whereas in adults, the sacroiliac (up to 80%) and spinal (up to 54%) joints are most commonly involved [17]. According to one study, patients with osteoarticular brucellosis have a longer duration of illness before diagnosis [11].

*Brucella* spondylitis is among the most serious manifestations of the disease and is associated with complications such as epidural, paravertebral, and psoas abscesses, and possible resultant nerve compression [17]. The incidence of spondylitis among the cases of brucellosis varies in the literature between 2 and 60% [18]. In a review study regarding spinal brucellosis, the predominant radiologic finding was spondylitis or spondylodiscitis, which was documented in 92% of cases, followed by a pre- or paravertebral abscess at a rate of 18% [18]. According to several studies, spondylitis is more common in men and in patients aged between 50 and 60 years [11,19,20]. It mainly affects the lumbar spine, followed by the thoracic, sacral, and cervical areas [21]. The most frequently involved site of infection is the L5–S1 level [15,21]. One study showed that although the lumbar spine is most commonly affected, the involvement of the thoracic spine was more frequent in severely complicated cases [19]. Notably, multilevel vertebral involvement has been reported to occur in 2–36% of cases of *Brucella* spondylitis [11,18–23].

### 3. Pathogenesis

Brucellosis may present as a multisystemic disease. Infectious organisms have been described to reach the spine by hematogenous or non-hematogenous routes, such as direct external bacterial inoculation or contiguous spread from an adjacent infectious site [24]. As for *Brucella* species, they mainly spread to the spine hematogenously through the nutrient arterioles of the vertebral bodies [25] or, rarely, by retrograde flow through the venous plexus of Batson, which was first described in an attempt to explain the preference of metastatic disease for the posterior aspect of the vertebral body [26,27]. As the vascularization of the vertebral bodies has been meticulously studied, the natural history of *Brucella* spondylitis can be explained sufficiently. Early *Brucella* spondylitis involves the anterior portion of the vertebral rim as the arterial vascularization of the vertebral bodies is anatomically denser on that surface [28]. Later, the infection progresses to the remainder of the vertebral body using the medullary spaces, eventually reaching the disc annulus and the nucleus pulposus [1,25]. It is worth noting that in adult life intra-osseous arteries are end arteries and therefore, in the event of septic emboli entrapment, extensive destruction of the vertebral body cannot be prevented by the presence of an anastomotic network [29]. The most commonly affected sites are the lumbar spine, followed by the thoracic and cervical spine, while multilevel involvement has also been described [21,30].

Before diving deeper into the pathophysiological mechanisms that orchestrate the deleterious effects of a *Brucella* infection on joints and bones, we will first analyze the key aspects of normal bone physiology. Bone is primarily comprised of cells and an extracellular matrix, the osteoid, which becomes mineralized after the deposition of calcium and phosphate in the form of hydroxyapatite, a process essential for the structural integrity of the bone. There are three types of bone cells: osteoblasts, osteoclasts, and osteocytes [31]. Osteoblasts are bone-forming cells responsible for bone mineralization and the production of the receptor activator of nuclear factor kappa-B ligand (RANKL) and osteoprotegerin, which induce and suppress osteoclastogenesis, respectively [32]. Osteocytes are terminally differentiated osteoblasts that become entrapped in the mineralized matrix [31]. Finally, osteoclasts are bone-resorbing cells with the unique ability to digest the calcified bone matrix. Until recently, it was established that the formation of osteoclasts can be accomplished either by the fusion of osteoclast progenitor cells that originate from the monocyte/macrophage lineage of the bone marrow or through the differentiation of osteal macrophages, which are the bone marrow resident macrophages [33,34]. Nonetheless, the latest research has demonstrated that peripheral blood mononuclear cells can also fuse and become mature multinucleated osteoblasts and that these may significantly contribute to the bone damage seen during inflammatory conditions such as rheumatoid arthritis [35,36].

Bone is often regarded as a metabolically inert structure with an innate resistance to infection. Nevertheless, osteoarticular brucellosis is the most frequent complication of a *Brucella* infection in humans [11,12]. The underlying mechanisms involved in this process have only recently been elucidated (Figure 1). The available data are mainly derived from research regarding *B. abortus* but can be safely used for the understanding of the pathogenesis of *Brucella* spondylitis in general. By now, it is evident that *Brucella*'s success as a pathogen relies on its ability to maintain an intracellular lifestyle, primarily by invading and replicating within macrophages. However, macrophages are not the only intracellular niche that *Brucella* can penetrate [37]. Firstly, it has been established that *B. abortus* can infect and replicate within osteoblasts in vitro [38,39]. Once inside osteoblasts, *Brucella* interferes with the physiological functions of these cells via, principally, three mechanisms: the induction of osteoblast apoptosis and the hampering of their differentiation; the inhibition of mineralization and organic matrix deposition; and the upregulation of RANKL [39]. These changes are the result of the direct effect of *Brucella* on osteoblasts, but also the result of *Brucella*-infected macrophages, the ones that already reside in the bone and the ones that are attracted to the site of infection. The induction of apoptosis is largely dependent upon the phosphorylation of p38 and extracellular signal-regulated kinase 1 and 2 (ERK1/2), which is activated in *Brucella*-infected osteoblasts. P38 and ERK1/2 are mitogen-activated protein kinases (MAPK) that regulate a plethora of functions in terms of cell growth, development, and survival [40]. Another critical function of these pathways is the production of monocyte chemotactic protein 1 (MCP-1) by osteoblasts, which is responsible for the attraction of monocytes and macrophages to the site of infection. In turn, these cells secrete tumor necrosis factor alpha (TNF-a) that results in osteoblast apoptosis, decreased bone mineralization, and upregulation of RANKL [39].

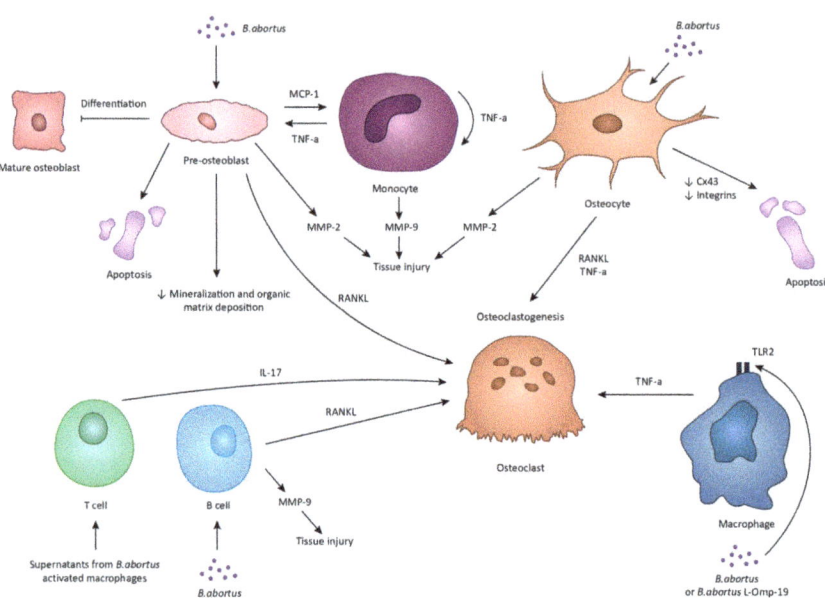

**Figure 1.** The underlying mechanisms of *Brucella*-induced osteoarticular disease are multiple, complex, and largely rely on experimental data from *B. abortus* studies. *B. abortus* can infect and replicate within osteoblasts and interfere with the physiological functions of these cells via three mechanisms: the induction of osteoblast apoptosis and the hampering of their differentiation; the inhibition of mineralization and organic matrix deposition; and the upregulation of receptor activator of nuclear factor kappa-B ligand (RANKL). *Brucella*-infected osteoblasts also secrete monocyte chemotactic protein 1 (MCP-1) that attracts monocytes and macrophages to the site of infection. In turn, these cells secrete tumor necrosis factor alpha (TNF-a) that, similarly, results in osteoblast apoptosis, decreased bone mineralization, and upregulation of RANKL. *Brucella*-infected osteoblasts and monocytes can also secrete matrix metalloproteinases, MMP-2 and MMP-9, respectively. Specifically, MMP-9 production is the result of the autocrine function of TNF-a produced by monocytes. Additionally, *Brucella* can multiply within osteocytes and lead to the production of MMP-2, RANKL, TNF-a, and proinflammatory cytokines. Moreover, *Brucella* and supernatants from *Brucella*-infected macrophages inhibit the expression of connexin 43 along with the expression of integrins, ultimately leading to osteocyte apoptotic cell death. Upon *Brucella* infection or in response to *B. abortus*, lipidated outer membrane protein 19 macrophages release inflammatory mediators such as TNF-a, eventually enhancing osteoclastogenesis. Moreover, supernatants from *B. abortus*-activated macrophages stimulate T cells to produce interleukin-17 which promotes osteoclast differentiation through the induction of proinflammatory cytokines. Finally, *B. abortus*-infected B cells produce MMP-9 and RANKL.

Matrix metalloproteinases (MMPs) also contribute to the osteoarticular damage in the context of brucellosis. Specifically, two types of MMPs, MMP-2 and MMP-9, which aid in the degradation of type I collagen present in bones and type II collagen present in cartilage, have been demonstrated to be involved in *Brucella*-induced tissue injury [41,42]. In particular, in vitro studies have shown that *B. abortus*-infected osteoblasts produce MMP-2 in a process that is largely mediated by the production of granulocyte-macrophage colony-stimulating factor (GM-CSF) by the same cells [42]. In addition, as mentioned above, *Brucella*-infected osteoblasts produce MCP-1 that attracts monocytes, which then secrete MMP-9 [42]. MMP-9 production is the result of the autocrine function of TNF-a produced by monocytes in response to GM-CSF [42].

*Brucella* can also infect and multiply within osteocytes in vitro [43]. Infected osteocytes then secrete MMP-2, RANKL, TNF-a, and proinflammatory cytokines [43]. This response ultimately leads bone marrow-derived monocytes (BMM) to undergo osteoclastogenesis. At this point it should be mentioned that one of the ways by which coordinated communication among osteocytes and between osteocytes and osteoblasts is achieved is via gap junctions, and the most abundant protein in these gap junctions is connexin 43 (Cx43) [44]. Interestingly, the *B. abortus* infection has been found to reduce the expression of Cx43 [43]. Moreover, the interaction between osteocytes and supernatants from *Brucella*-infected macrophages inhibits the expression of Cx43 along with the expression of integrins [43], which also participate in osteocyte adhesion and signaling [45]. The outcome of these changes is osteocyte apoptotic cell death [43]. Based on these findings, it can be safely deducted that *Brucella* harms osteocyte activity and viability, directly and indirectly, thus contributing to the tissue damage observed in an osteoarticular infection.

The role of macrophages and monocytes in the pathophysiology of tissue damage noted in *Brucella* infections is not limited to their interaction with osteoblasts and osteocytes. Upon infection with *Brucella* or in response to *Brucella* lipoproteins, such as the lipidated outer membrane protein 19 (L-Omp19), macrophages release inflammatory mediators such as TNF-a, interleukin-6 (IL-6), and IL-1β in a toll-like receptor 2-dependent manner (TLR2) [46]. In turn, TNF-a production results in the differentiation of BMM into osteoclasts [46]. Another intriguing observation is that supernatants from *B. abortus*-infected monocytes or L-Omp19-stimulated monocytes are able to induce, again, through TNF-a production, the differentiation of human monocytes to osteoclasts [46]. It should be pointed out that osteoclastogenesis associated with *B. abortus* does not require bacterial viability but is equally elicited by structural bacterial components. It is established that these components are the *Brucella* lipoproteins but not the *Brucella* lipopolysaccharide [46,47].

*Brucella* affects the bone tissue not only through macrophages and monocytes but also through T cells and B cells by exploiting them to induce bone loss. Specifically, stimulation of activated T cells with supernatants from *B. abortus*-activated macrophages results in the production of RANKL and IL-17 which promote osteoclastogenesis in vitro [48]. In addition, it appears that IL-17 is the main driving force for osteoclast differentiation through the induction of proinflammatory cytokines, primarily TNF-a, by osteoclast precursors [48]. This phenomenon has also been replicated in vivo when injection of mice tibiae with T cells that were treated with supernatants from *Brucella*-infected macrophages induced extensive osteoclastogenesis [48]. Similarly, *B. abortus*-infected B cells produce MMP-9, proinflammatory cytokines, and RANKL, the latter being the main mediator of B cell-induced osteoclastogenesis in vitro [49].

Finally, the role of several cytokines, their receptors, and single-nucleotide polymorphisms for cytokine-encoded genes in the inflammatory damaged observed during *Brucella* spondylitis is still unclear and demands further research [50–52].

In summary, the osteoarticular damage observed in a *Brucella* infection is the aftereffect of the direct changes that the bacterium causes on bone cells and also the result of the intricate interactions between *Brucella*, bone cells, and the immune system.

## 4. Clinical Features

Brucellosis in humans affects numerous systems and manifests with a wide range of symptoms, in both acute and chronic forms, but it can also be asymptomatic [53]. Fever, chills, headaches, malaise, and fatigue are some of the most prevalent, nonspecific symptoms of both uncomplicated and complicated forms of the disease. Other symptoms and signs are abdominal pain, splenomegaly, and hepatomegaly [54]. Apart from all the aforementioned symptoms, brucellosis should also be considered in the differential diagnosis of a fever of unknown origin, especially in non-endemic areas [55]. Complicated forms of the disease include osteoarticular, genitourinary, neurologic, cardiovascular, and pulmonary involvement [56,57].

In a recent systematic review, it has been shown that in approximately one third of adult patients, brucellosis manifests as spondylitis or sacroiliitis [58]. In a set of different studies, the percentage of osteoarticular involvement ranged between 20% and 60%, and the percentage of spondylitis between 8% and 13% [59]. When it comes to the musculoskeletal manifestations of the infection, sacroiliitis and hip joint involvement are more common in young individuals in the acute form of the disease, whereas spondylitis and spondylodiscitis are more common in the elderly and in chronic forms of the disease [60]. The most commonly afflicted vertebrae in spondylitis are the lumbar (60%), sacral (19%), and cervical (12%) [21]. Lumbar (60–70%), thoracic (20%), and cervical (6–13%) segments are usually implicated in spondylodiscitis [17].

There are two forms of spinal brucellosis: localized and diffuse. In localized involvement, osteomyelitis is restricted to the anterior region of an endplate at the discovertebral junction, while in extensive involvement it affects the whole vertebral endplate or the entire vertebral body [17].

Arthralgias are present in the majority of adults affected by brucellosis, and approximately half of them suffer from myalgia and back pain [58]. Nevertheless, axial back pain remains a non-specific clinical sign of spinal brucellosis. As a result, many patients presenting with lower back pain combined with sciatic radiculopathy are misdiagnosed or are diagnosed belatedly [17,61].

Because of its association with epidural, paravertebral, and psoas abscesses, and probable nerve compression, spondylitis is a significant brucellosis complication. These types of abscesses are present in a minority of patients suffering from *Brucella* spondylitis and manifest as episodes of high-grade fever, lower back pain, and inability to bear weight, possibly leading to permanent neurological deficits or even death in cases of delayed or inappropriate treatment [17]. Lastly, it is important to keep in mind that tuberculous spondylodiscitis can greatly resemble spinal brucellosis in terms of clinical presentation. However, it appears that systemic symptoms such as fatigue and fever are more common in a *Brucella* infection, whereas back pain, local tenderness, and spinal complications are observed with a higher frequency in tuberculous spondylodiscitis [62].

## 5. Diagnosis
### 5.1. Microbiological Diagnosis

Because brucellosis in humans presents with nonspecific clinical and laboratory findings, a microbiological analysis is crucial for a definite diagnosis. A *Brucella* infection should be suspected in the appropriate clinical context and with relevant epidemiologic exposure (consumption of unpasteurized dairy products, animal exposure in an endemic area, and/or occupational exposure).

Laboratory findings of brucellosis may include mildly elevated erythrocyte sedimentation rate and liver function enzyme levels, as well as hematologic abnormalities such as anemia, leukopenia or leukocytosis with relative lymphocytosis, and thrombocytopenia [1,63]. Rarely, pancytopenia is observed in patients with a *Brucella* infection and is attributed to hypersplenism, hemophagocytic syndrome, diffuse intravascular coagulation, or immune-mediated cellular destruction [6,64–66].

According to the CDC and the Council of State and Territorial Epidemiologists, a definitive diagnosis is established by direct detection of *Brucella* species by a culture from a clinical specimen or indirectly by a fourfold or greater increase in *Brucella* antibody titer between serum specimens from the acute and convalescent phases obtained at least 2 weeks apart [67]. However, a presumptive diagnosis is made by a *Brucella* total antibody titer of at least 1:160 in the serum agglutination test (SAT) or *Brucella* microagglutination test (BMAT) in one or more serum specimens obtained after the onset of symptoms or by detection of *Brucella* DNA in a clinical specimen by a polymerase chain reaction (PCR) [67].

A positive blood culture or a positive culture from other specimens (e.g., bone marrow, bone, synovial fluid, cerebrospinal fluid, urine) is the cornerstone of diagnosis [68]. Brucellosis is characterized by initial bacteremia that is followed by a macrophage invasion resulting in a reduction of blood-circulating bacteria [69]. Therefore, at least two or three separate peripheral blood culture sets should be drawn as soon as the disease is suspected [70]. The sensitivity of blood cultures ranges from 10% to 90% [69]. Because of slow growth in culture media, the physician should inform the microbiology laboratory to extend the incubation period up to 4 weeks, although the new BACTEC system has higher reliability and can detect the bacterium within 5 to 7 days. Because of the high rate of transmission to laboratory personnel, biosafety measures should be taken when isolating this organism [71].

Bone marrow culture is more sensitive than blood and is considered the gold standard for the diagnosis of brucellosis, but the invasiveness of the procedure should be considered [72]. In a study of 50 patients diagnosed with brucellosis, the bone marrow culture was positive in 92% of cases. The bone marrow culture has a shorter time of detection than blood culture does, and its sensitivity is not affected by prior antibiotic use. Individuals with chronic infections are less likely to have a positive culture [73]. If focal disease is suspected, such as in cases of spondylitis, samples should be obtained from the infected area (e.g., bone, joint aspirate, cerebrospinal fluid) [8]. Rapid identification of *Brucella* species recovered from cultures is essential to making a timely diagnosis, avoiding biological risk to laboratory personnel, confirming the presence of the disease in its early stages when antibody titers are negative or low/borderline, distinguishing between wild and vaccine *Brucella* strains, and identifying the source of transmission, since the individual species and their naturally occurring hosts are highly interrelated [68].

In patients with a clinically compatible illness, serologic testing is the most commonly used diagnostic method, especially in endemic areas, because they are inexpensive, user-friendly, and have high negative predictive value [68]. The most common serologic tests for detecting specific antibodies in the serum of infected patients are the SAT and the enzyme-linked immunosorbent assay (ELISA). The Rose Bengal agglutination test (RBT) is a rapid, accurate method in the acute phases of the disease and can be used as a screening tool [74]. Other tests that are most useful in chronic or/and complicated cases are the 2-mercaptoethanol (2-ME) agglutination test, the immunocapture agglutination (BrucellaCapt) test, and the indirect Coombs test [68].

The SAT, which measures total IgM, IgA, and IgG antibodies against smooth lipopolysaccharide (S-LPS), remains the most popular method. Although a single titer is not diagnostic, SAT titers > 1:160 outside endemic areas and >1:320 within endemic areas are considered highly suggestive of an infection [6]. Seroconversion and a fourfold or greater increase in titers measured at least 2 weeks apart indicate a definitive diagnosis [6]. SAT can detect antibodies against *B. abortus*, *B. suis*, and *B. melitensis* but not *B. canis* or the vaccine strain RB51 [6,72]. In a study that included patients with a blood culture-proven *Brucella* infection, the initial titer of SAT was $\geq$1:320 in 96% of patients [75].

When interpreting positive SAT results, the possibility of cross-reactions of IgM antibodies of *Brucella* with other Gram-negative bacteria such as *Yersinia enterocolitica*, *Escherichia coli* O:116 and O:157, *Moraxella phenylpyruvica*, *Francisella tularensis*, certain *Salmonella* serotypes, and from individuals vaccinated against *Vibrio cholerae* should be considered [71,72]. Early, chronic, or complicated disease is associated with high rates of false-negative antibody titers [68].

ELISA is a sensitive quantitative method for measuring specific IgA, IgM, and IgG anti-*Brucella* antibody titers that allows for a better interpretation of the clinical situation. IgM antibodies are predominant in acute infection but decrease within a few weeks. Low IgM titers may persist for months or years after the initial infection. Relapses are accompanied by transient increases in IgG and IgA antibodies, but not IgM [71]. However, until better standardization is established, ELISA should be used in cases of strong clinical suspicion when SAT is negative to confirm the diagnosis or in chronic, focal, or complicated cases [68].

PCR tests can be performed on serum or any tissue samples, such as bone, and allow for a diagnosis within a few hours with high sensitivity and specificity, but are not a routine diagnostic tool. Caution should be taken when interpreting results, as a false positive result could be due to low bacterial inoculum in frequently exposed healthy individuals in endemic areas, DNA from dead bacteria, or a patient who has recovered [76]. In one study, real-time PCR demonstrated high sensitivity (93.5%) and specificity (100%) in formalin-fixed, paraffin-embedded samples from patients with *Brucella* vertebral osteomyelitis who required surgical treatment for neurologic deficits. In terms of sensitivity, real-time PCR proved to be better than blood culture (35.5%), SAT test (80.6%), and Giemsa stain (51.6%) [77].

Lastly, a special mention must be made regarding the pathological features of *Brucella* spondylitis, although these are not routinely used as a diagnostic tool. Firstly, chronic inflammation along with in-acute-phase chronic inflammation are the most commonly encountered pathological changes of spinal brucellosis [78]. Furthermore, histopathology can potentially aid in the differentiation between brucellar and tuberculous spondylitis through specific findings like caseous necrosis, which is typically identified in tuberculous lesions, and through staining markers like Angiopoietin-like protein 4 [79].

## 5.2. Radiological Diagnosis

The focal form of the disease is confined to the anterior portion of the endplate, typically in the anterior superior of a lumbar vertebra, often at the L4–L5 level [6]. The diffuse form involves the entire vertebral body and extends to the adjacent disc and the paravertebral and epidural space. Multifocal involvement has been described in sporadic cases [80]. Plain radiographs show no findings initially. At about 3–5 weeks after the onset of symptoms, osteolysis demonstrated with loss of the osteosclerotic epiphyseal plate is shown (Figure 2). Focal erosions of the superior or inferior vertebral body are characteristic [30].

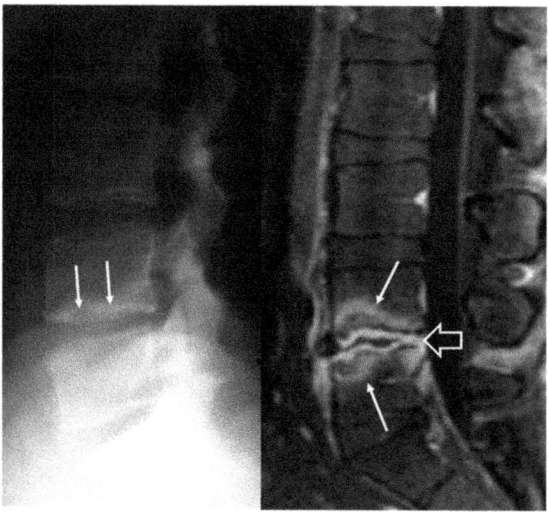

**Figure 2.** A 34-year-old man with *Brucella* spondylodiscitis. The initial lateral radiograph (**left**) shows a cortical disruption at the inferior epiphyseal plate of L4 vertebral body (arrows). The sagittal fat suppressed contrast enhanced T1-w MR image (**right**) shows septic discitis (open arrow) and bone barrow edema on both L4 and L5 vertebral bodies (arrows), suggesting spondylitis.

A gas vacuum may be observed in the anterior part of the disc, either due to disc ischemia and necrosis or due to focal instability [81]. Osteophytosis at the anterior vertebral endplate is shown in long-standing or poorly treated cases. It has to be pointed out that osseous remodeling may progress slowly, and radiographic findings may simulate degenerative spinal disease. Computed tomography (CT) depicts the changes earlier in the course of the disease, and due to lack of overlapping tissues, gas within the disc can be depicted in 25–30% of the cases. Post-contrast CT may show abscess formation either in the paravertebral spaces or in the spinal canal [82].

Magnetic resonance imaging (MRI) findings are not specific and follow the typical infection pattern, including a hypointense signal on T1-w images, hyperintensity on T2-w and STIR images, and enhancement of the disc and bone marrow edema foci (Figures 2–4) [14,30]. The presence of intracanalicular abscess formation is confirmed with wall enhancement and is an indication for surgical decompression (Figure 3). Similarly, paravertebral abscesses are observed in approximately 30% of cases and are typically demonstrated with wall enhancement [30].

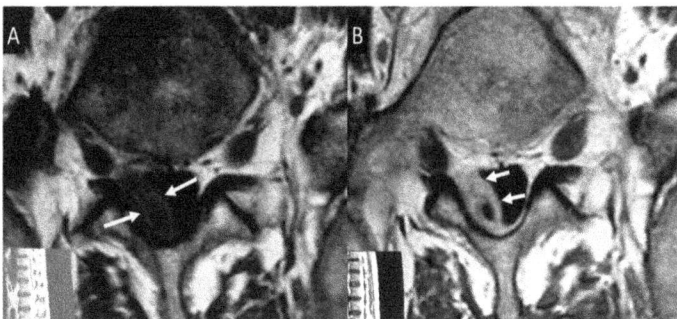

**Figure 3.** Axial plain (**A**) and contrast-enhanced (**B**) T1-w MR images, showing the epidural abscess formation on the right side (arrows in **A**), with wall enhancement (arrows in **B**), and displacement of the dural sac to the left.

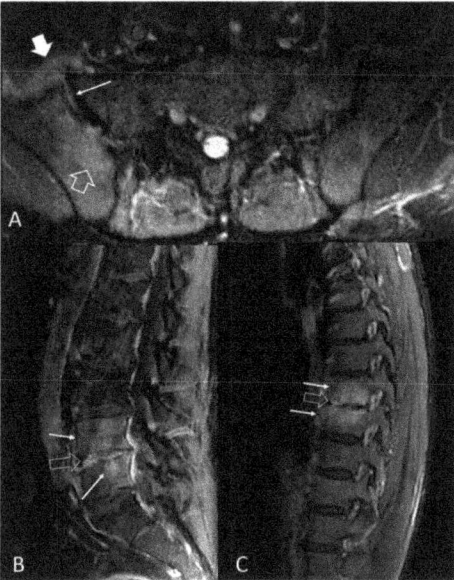

**Figure 4.** Noncontiguous multifocal musculoskeletal brucellosis. (**A**) Axial STIR MR image, showing bone marrow edema (open arrow), joint effusion (thin arrow), and capsular thickening (thick arrow) in keeping with sacroiliac joint involvement. Sagittal fat-suppressed contrast-enhanced MR images of the lumbar spine (**B**) and thoracic spine (**C**) showing discitis (open arrows) with spondylitis (thin white arrows).

Extraspinal involvement occurs primarily in the sacroiliac joints and the knee. In most of the cases (>80%), *Brucella* sacroiliitis is unilateral [82]. Radiographic findings of sacroiliitis 3 weeks after the onset of symptoms include disruption of the subchondral sclerotic line and later narrowing or widening of the joint space. Erosions, subchondral sclerosis, and ankylosis of the joint may be seen in chronic cases. Early in the course of the disease, MRI findings are not specific and include bone marrow edema, joint effusion, and capsular thickening (Figures 4 and 5).

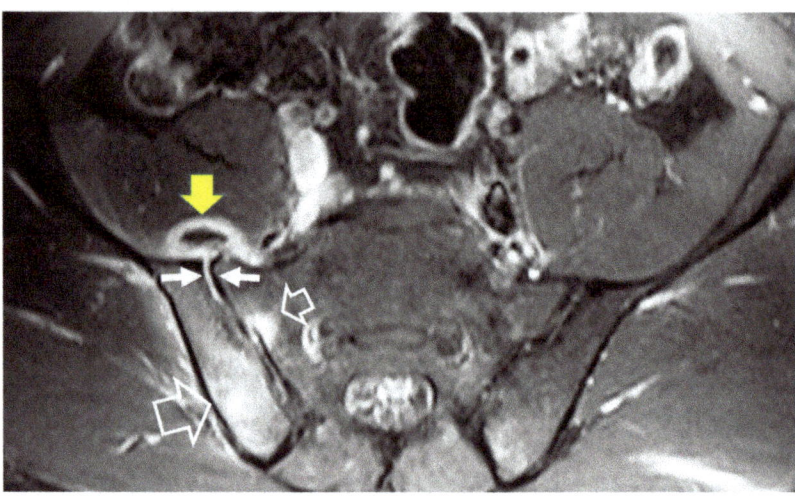

**Figure 5.** A 23-year-old male with a serologically proven diagnosis of brucellosis 9 months prior to current imaging. The patient received treatment for 3 months and now presents with recurrent symptoms. Axial fat-suppressed T1-w MR image showing enhancing bone marrow edema on both sides of the sacroiliac joints (open arrows), joint effusion (arrows), and anterior capsular thickening and enhancement (yellow arrow) in keeping with septic sacroiliitis.

The main differential diagnosis of spinal brucellosis is spinal tuberculosis. As a rule, radiographic findings occur later in the course of the disease. In spinal tuberculosis, CT appears to be superior to plain radiographs in identifying endplate irregularity and osseous destruction and can guide a percutaneous biopsy. CT and MRI findings in tuberculosis include contiguous on non-contiguous vertebral involvement with preservation of the disc spaces until later in the course of the disease, prevertebral and paravertebral collections, often in the psoas muscles, with an extension beneath the anterior longitudinal ligament, and epidural abscess formation. A straightforward diagnosis may be difficult in atypical cases, and the differential diagnosis should also be supported by clinical and serological findings [83,84].

## 6. Treatment

### 6.1. Conservative Management

Brucellosis treatment depends largely on the affected parts of the body. Available treatment options include antibiotic administration for an adequate period of time and, when appropriate, surgical intervention. Antibiotics agents which accumulate into phagocytes may be pivotal for the successful treatment of brucellosis. Combinations of tetracyclines, rifampicin, aminoglycosides, trimethoprim-sulfamethoxazole (TMP-SMX), and quinolones have been used [85]. The most commonly used combination regimens in the absence of focal disease are doxycycline (100 mg BID) for 6 weeks plus an aminoglycoside (streptomycin 1 gr OD for 2–3 weeks or gentamicin 5 mg/kg/day OD for 7–10 days) or doxycycline (100 mg bid) plus rifampicin (600–900 mg OD) both for 6 weeks [6,86]. Resistance of *Brucella* species to tetracyclines or aminoglycosides does not occur [87,88], while decreased susceptibility or even resistance to rifampicin has been described [89,90]. Relapses occur usually within the first 6 months of treatment completion and are only rarely due to antibiotic resistance if a combination treatment has been used. Inadequate antimicrobial choice, short treatment duration, undiagnosed focal disease, and lack of compliance are the main reasons for relapse [91]. Most of the relapsed cases respond favorably to a repeated course of the antimicrobial regimen that was administrated during the first episode [92].

While sacroiliitis does not appear to require special treatment, *Brucella* spondylitis requires a longer course of antibiotics than uncomplicated brucellosis, and surgical intervention might be required [85,93,94], while delayed initiation of treatment can result in long-term disability, as is usually the case in spondylodiscitis in general irrespective of the cause [95]. Regrettably, the optimal approach in terms of treatment duration and antibiotic combination has yet to be defined [61,96,97]. A combination of two or three antibiotics is commonly used for 3–6 months and in many cases for even longer [91,98].

In an open, controlled, nonrandomized study which involved only 31 patients with spinal brucellosis treated for a median time of 12 weeks, clinical response did not differ between patients who received ciprofloxacin plus rifampicin and patients who received doxycycline plus streptomycin [99]. In another retrospective observational study there were no significant differences between patients receiving doxycycline-streptomycin and those receiving doxycycline-rifampicin for 3 months but it should be underlined that treatment failure rate ranged between 15–18% [100]. In a large multicenter retrospective comparative study including 293 patients with spinal brucellosis, five major treatment regimens were used for at least 12 weeks: doxycycline plus rifampicin plus streptomycin; doxycycline plus rifampicin plus gentamicin; doxycycline plus rifampicin plus ciprofloxacin; doxycycline plus streptomycin; and doxycycline plus rifampicin [19]. There were no significant differences among these antibiotic groups regarding outcomes [19]. On the contrary, in a recent retrospective cohort study on 100 patients with *Brucella* spondylitis, the triple antibiotic regimen of doxycycline, compound sulfamethoxazole, and rifampicin was more successful in treating *Brucella* spondylitis compared to the dual antibiotic regimen of compound sulfamethoxazole and rifampicin [101].

Many clinicians, including us, favor a triple-regimen antibiotic treatment for *Brucella* spondylitis. The combination of doxycycline (100 mg BID for at least 12 weeks) plus rifampicin (600–900 mg OD for at least 12 weeks) plus streptomycin (1 gr OD for 2–3 weeks) or gentamycin (5 mg/kg/d OD for 5–7 days) is commonly used in adults and is associated with high rates of favorable outcomes and reduced relapse rates [102]. Other treatment regimens are derived from the substitution of the aminoglycoside with a quinolone (e.g., ciprofloxacin 500 mg BID for at least 12 weeks) or TMP-SMX (TMP 10 mg/kg/day and SMX 50 mg/kg/day, both divided in 2 doses for at least 12 weeks) [19,103,104]. Pregnant women can be treated with a combination of two or three of the following antibiotics: rifampicin (600–900 mg OD for at least 12 weeks), TMP-SMX (160 mg TMP/800 mg SMX OD for at least 12 weeks), and ceftriaxone (2 g OD for 4–6 weeks). For pregnant patients $\geq$36 weeks of gestation, only rifampicin and ceftriaxone are prudent to be administered until delivery, due to the risk of neonatal kernicterus with the use of TMP-SMX in the last 4 weeks of pregnancy [105,106].

*6.2. Surgical Management*

As mentioned, long term administration of antimicrobial agents is the mainstay of treatment of *Brucella* spondylodiscitis [104]. According to Lozano et al., surgery is required in 3% to 29% of patients [107]. Surgical treatment is indicated for patients with neurological symptoms caused by bone deformities and purulent epidural abscesses due to possible irreversible neural damage [108]. Patients with partial or temporary response to antimicrobial therapy, such as patients with large paravertebral abscesses, might also require surgical intervention [107]. There are limited data regarding the surgical treatment of *Brucella* spondylitis. The role of surgical intervention, particularly in patients without neurological symptoms, remains to be determined [108,109]. In the past, the use of spinal implants in the presence of infection was highly controversial. Nowadays, there is sufficient evidence to support the claim that the use of spinal instrumentation in patients with infections is safe since it does not compromise the eradication of the pathogen [110].

6.2.1. Open Surgery

In patients with spinal instability, symptomatic neural compression, or progressive kyphotic deformity, decompression of the spinal canal and stabilization are mandatory. The main surgical approaches include anterior debridement, traditional posterior decompressive procedures with or without instrumentation surgery, and combined anterior and posterior approaches. However, there is no consensus on the optimal surgical approach [111,112]. The surgical approach should be chosen according to the location of the spinal lesion, the degree of vertebral destruction and nerve compression, and the surgeon's experience and technical skills [113].

In the past, anterior decompression combined with posterior internal fixation was commonly used. The current development of spinal surgery implants and techniques has facilitated the treatment of lumbar brucellosis with abscesses only by the posterior approach [114]. Posterior surgery is considered suitable for intraspinal granulation and abscess removal, especially for patients with nerve compression caused by posterior column lesions, whereas combined surgery is recommended for patients with perivertebral abscess, psoas abscess, or severe anterior column destruction [113,114].

Anterior standalone approach with reconstruction of the spinal column has been described by several authors as safe and effective in the treatment of spinal infections, including cases of *Brucella* spondylitis. This approach remains the only way to obtain direct and adequate neural decompression as well as optimal spine reconstruction and fixation through a single surgical procedure [115]. Katonis et al. have recommended anterior decompression with corpectomy, reconstruction with a titanium cage filled with autograft, and stabilization with an anterior plate in cases of kyphotic deformity with cord compression caused by *Brucella* spondylitis in the lower thoracic spine, whereas when the infection was localized in the lumbar spine, a posterior approach and laminectomy were chosen [108]. Yin et al. more recently reported their results on treating 16 patients with lumbar *Brucella* spondylitis with one-stage anterior internal fixation, debridement, and bone fusion. The mean follow-up was $35.3 \pm 8.1$ months (range, 24–48 months). All patients were considered completely cured, with bone fusion achieved in $4.8 \pm 1.3$ months. Pain and neurological function were significantly improved between the preoperative and last follow-up visits, as well as kyphotic deformity, as the Cobb angle was $20.7 \pm 9.8°$ preoperatively and measured $8.1 \pm 1.3°$ at the last follow-up visit. The authors concluded that one-stage surgical treatment with anterior debridement, fusion, and instrumentation can be an effective and feasible treatment method for lumbar *Brucella* spondylitis [116].

However, the opponents of the anterior standalone approach in the treatment of vertebral osteomyelitis consider this approach inadequate to restore and to ensure stability of the infected spine and to correct kyphosis and, therefore, believe that supplemented posterior fixation is mandatory [117]. In order to determine the optimal surgical approach, Na et al. compared 2 groups of patients undergoing surgical treatment for lumbar *Brucella* spondylitis. The clinical and surgical outcomes were compared in terms of operative time, intraoperative blood loss, hospitalizations, bony fusion time, complications, visual analog scale score, recovery of neurological function, and deformity correction. Both anterior and posterior approaches were successful, and fusion was achieved within 11 months in all cases. Yet, the posterior approach resulted in better kyphotic deformity correction, less surgical invasiveness, and fewer complications [112]. Similar results have been reported by Jiang et al. in 62 patients with lumbar *Brucella* spondylitis who underwent either one-stage posterior pedicle fixation, debridement, and interbody fusion or anterior debridement, bone grafting, and posterior instrumentation. Both surgical interventions were equally effective in the treatment of lumbar *Brucella* spondylitis. However, the posterior approach demonstrates advantages such as reduced surgical time, less blood loss and hospital stays, and fewer perioperative complications. Therefore, the one-stage posterior pedicle fixation, debridement, and interbody fusion represent a superior treatment option [118]. Significant shorter operation time, hospitalization time, and intraoperative blood loss has also been reported in patients with thoracolumbar *Brucella* spondylitis who were treated with posterior debridement and instrumented fusion compared to patients treated with one-stage anterior radical debridement combined with bone grafting and fusion and posterior internal fixation (360° surgery). No significant difference has been found between the two groups in terms of pain control, neurological improvement and deformity correction [119].

### 6.2.2. Minimally Invasive Surgical Techniques

Spinal brucellosis is less destructive compared to other infectious spinal diseases such as pyogenic spondylitis or spinal tuberculosis, and therefore, minimally invasive procedures should be preferred as much as possible in patients undergoing surgical treatment, especially in cases with poor general health and comorbidities [120]. Hadjipavlou et al. have reported their technique of percutaneous transpedicular discectomy and drainage of purulent material in patients with pyogenic spondylodiscitis [121,122], including patients with *Brucella* spondylitis [108]. In a series of 10 patients receiving surgical treatment for spinal brucellosis, 3 patients with spondylodiscitis without epidural abscesses underwent transpedicular discectomy and drainage with good and sustained results [108]. According to the authors this minimally invasive technique has high diagnostic and therapeutic effectiveness when applied in the early stages of uncomplicated spondylodiscitis because it promotes pain relief and healing by stimulating granulation tissue to enter the avascular disc space from the subchondral bone, but is contraindicated in the presence of instability, kyphosis from bone destruction, and neurological deficit [122]. This technique is also ideal for collecting samples for microbiological diagnosis with greater sensitivity compared to CT-guided biopsies [123].

Recently, *Wang* et al. retrospectively analyzed 13 patients with lumbar *Brucella* spondylitis who underwent bi-portal endoscopic decompression, debridement, and interbody fusion, combined with percutaneous screw fixation, with 92.3% of the patients reporting good to excellent outcomes [109]. Indications for this procedure are similar to those of open surgery and include severe disc or vertebral destruction resulting in intractable low back pain refractory to medication treatment, severe or progressive neurological dysfunction due to compression of the spinal cord or cauda equina by inflammatory tissue in the spinal canal or epidural abscesses, spinal instability, and ineffective medical therapy. However, this operation is contraindicated in cases with severe destruction of the anterior column requiring anterior debridement and interbody fusion through a retroperitoneal approach or in cases with massive paravertebral abscesses [124].

Other minimally invasive procedures, such as percutaneous endoscopic discectomy and drainage [125,126], percutaneous endoscopic debridement with dilute Betadine solution irrigation [123], and thoracoscopic debridement and stabilization [127], have been described for the management of bacterial spondylodiscitis, including cases of spinal tuberculosis, and could potentially be recruited for the surgical treatment of *Brucella* spondylitis.

## 7. Conclusions

Brucellosis is the most common zoonosis worldwide, posing a significant public health problem. Spinal involvement presenting as spondylitis, spondylodiscitis, and epidural, paravertebral, and psoas abscesses is a frequent and serious complication of the disease, often with post-treatment residual damage. The therapeutic approach of spinal brucellosis should always be multidisciplinary with a team of infectious disease specialists, microbiologists, radiologists, neurosurgeons, and orthopedics in order to achieve a favorable outcome.

**Author Contributions:** Conceptualization, N.S. and K.A.; methodology, N.S. and A.K. (Apostolos Karantanas); data curation, I.M., A.K. (Afroditi Konsoula) and Z.N.; writing—original draft preparation I.M., A.K. (Afroditi Konsoula), Z.N. and C.K.; writing—review and editing, N.S., A.K. (Apostolos Karantanas), C.K. and A.K. (Afroditi Konsoula); supervision N.S., A.K. (Apostolos Karantanas) and K.A. All authors have read and agreed to the published version of the manuscript.

**Funding:** This research received no external funding.

**Institutional Review Board Statement:** Not applicable.

**Informed Consent Statement:** Not applicable.

**Data Availability Statement:** The data presented in this study are available on request from the corresponding author.

**Conflicts of Interest:** The authors declare no conflicts of interest.

## References

1. Tali, E.T.; Koc, A.M.; Oner, A.Y. Spinal brucellosis. *Neuroimaging Clin. N. Am.* **2015**, *25*, 233–245. [CrossRef] [PubMed]
2. Percin, D. Microbiology of Brucella. *Recent. Pat. Antiinfect. Drug Discov.* **2013**, *8*, 13–17. [CrossRef] [PubMed]
3. Bruce, D. Note on Discovery of a Micrococcus in Malta Fever. *Practicioner* **1887**, *39*, 161–170.
4. El-Sayed, A.; Awad, W. Brucellosis: Evolution and expected comeback. *Int. J. Vet. Sci. Med.* **2018**, *6*, S31–S35. [CrossRef] [PubMed]
5. Rajendhran, J. Genomic insights into *Brucella*. *Infect. Genet. Evol.* **2021**, *87*, 104635. [CrossRef]
6. Pappas, G.; Akritidis, N.; Bosilkovski, M.; Tsianos, E. Brucellosis. *N. Engl. J. Med.* **2005**, *352*, 2325–2336. [CrossRef] [PubMed]
7. Tuon, F.F.; Gondolfo, R.B.; Cerchiari, N. Human-to-human transmission of *Brucella*—A systematic review. *Trop. Med. Int. Health* **2017**, *22*, 539–546. [CrossRef] [PubMed]
8. CDC. *CDC Yellow Book 2024: Health Information for International Travel*; Oxford University Press: Oxford, UK, 2023.
9. Pappas, G.; Papadimitriou, P.; Akritidis, N.; Christou, L.; Tsianos, E.V. The new global map of human brucellosis. *Lancet Infect. Dis.* **2006**, *6*, 91–99. [CrossRef]
10. Seleem, M.N.; Boyle, S.M.; Sriranganathan, N. Brucellosis: A re-emerging zoonosis. *Vet. Microbiol.* **2010**, *140*, 392–398. [CrossRef]
11. Bosilkovski, M.; Krteva, L.; Caparoska, S.; Dimzova, M. Osteoarticular involvement in brucellosis: Study of 196 cases in the Republic of Macedonia. *Croat. Med. J.* **2004**, *45*, 727–733.
12. Geyik, M.F.; Gur, A.; Nas, K.; Cevik, R.; Sarac, J.; Dikici, B.; Ayaz, C. Musculoskeletal involvement of brucellosis in different age groups: A study of 195 cases. *Swiss Med. Wkly.* **2002**, *132*, 98–105. [CrossRef] [PubMed]
13. Buzgan, T.; Karahocagil, M.K.; Irmak, H.; Baran, A.I.; Karsen, H.; Evirgen, O.; Akdeniz, H. Clinical manifestations and complications in 1028 cases of brucellosis: A retrospective evaluation and review of the literature. *Int. J. Infect. Dis.* **2010**, *14*, e469–e478. [CrossRef] [PubMed]
14. Arkun, R.; Mete, B.D. Musculoskeletal brucellosis. *Semin. Musculoskelet. Radiol.* **2011**, *15*, 470–479. [CrossRef] [PubMed]
15. Turan, H.; Serefhanoglu, K.; Karadeli, E.; Togan, T.; Arslan, H. Osteoarticular involvement among 202 brucellosis cases identified in Central Anatolia region of Turkey. *Intern. Med.* **2011**, *50*, 421–428. [CrossRef] [PubMed]
16. Bosilkovski, M.; Kirova-Urosevic, V.; Cekovska, Z.; Labacevski, N.; Cvetanovska, M.; Rangelov, G.; Cana, F.; Bogoeva-Tasevska, S. Osteoarticular involvement in childhood brucellosis: Experience with 133 cases in an endemic region. *Pediatr. Infect. Dis. J.* **2013**, *32*, 815–819. [CrossRef] [PubMed]
17. Esmaeilnejad-Ganji, S.M.; Esmaeilnejad-Ganji, S.M.R. Osteoarticular manifestations of human brucellosis: A review. *World J. Orthop.* **2019**, *10*, 54–62. [CrossRef] [PubMed]
18. Turgut, M.; Turgut, A.T.; Kosar, U. Spinal brucellosis: Turkish experience based on 452 cases published during the last century. *Acta Neurochir.* **2006**, *148*, 1033–1044, discussion 1044. [CrossRef]
19. Ulu-Kilic, A.; Karakas, A.; Erdem, H.; Turker, T.; Inal, A.S.; Ak, O.; Turan, H.; Kazak, E.; Inan, A.; Duygu, F.; et al. Update on treatment options for spinal brucellosis. *Clin. Microbiol. Infect.* **2014**, *20*, O75–O82. [CrossRef]
20. Bozgeyik, Z.; Ozdemir, H.; Demirdag, K.; Ozden, M.; Sonmezgoz, F.; Ozgocmen, S. Clinical and MRI findings of brucellar spondylodiscitis. *Eur. J. Radiol.* **2008**, *67*, 153–158. [CrossRef]
21. Bozgeyik, Z.; Aglamis, S.; Bozdag, P.G.; Denk, A. Magnetic resonance imaging findings of musculoskeletal brucellosis. *Clin. Imaging* **2014**, *38*, 719–723. [CrossRef]
22. Ozaksoy, D.; Yucesoy, K.; Yucesoy, M.; Kovanlikaya, I.; Yuce, A.; Naderi, S. Brucellar spondylitis: MRI findings. *Eur. Spine J.* **2001**, *10*, 529–533. [CrossRef] [PubMed]
23. Harman, M.; Unal, O.; Onbasi, K.T.; Kiymaz, N.; Arslan, H. Brucellar spondylodiscitis: MRI diagnosis. *Clin. Imaging* **2001**, *25*, 421–427. [CrossRef] [PubMed]
24. Mavrogenis, A.F.; Megaloikonomos, P.D.; Igoumenou, V.G.; Panagopoulos, G.N.; Giannitsioti, E.; Papadopoulos, A.; Papagelopoulos, P.J. Spondylodiscitis revisited. *EFORT Open Rev.* **2017**, *2*, 447–461. [CrossRef] [PubMed]
25. Morales, H. Infectious Spondylitis Mimics: Mechanisms of Disease and Imaging Findings. *Semin. Ultrasound CT MR* **2018**, *39*, 587–604. [CrossRef] [PubMed]
26. Batson, O.V. The Function of the Vertebral Veins and Their Role in the Spread of Metastases. *Ann. Surg.* **1940**, *112*, 138–149. [CrossRef] [PubMed]
27. Turunc, T.; Demiroglu, Y.Z.; Uncu, H.; Colakoglu, S.; Arslan, H. A comparative analysis of tuberculous, brucellar and pyogenic spontaneous spondylodiscitis patients. *J. Infect.* **2007**, *55*, 158–163. [CrossRef]
28. Ratcliffe, J.F. Anatomic basis for the pathogenesis and radiologic features of vertebral osteomyelitis and its differentiation from childhood discitis. A microarteriographic investigation. *Acta Radiol. Diagn.* **1985**, *26*, 137–143. [CrossRef] [PubMed]

29. Ratcliffe, J.F. An evaluation of the intra-osseous arterial anastomoses in the human vertebral body at different ages. A microarteriographic study. *J. Anat.* **1982**, *134*, 373–382.
30. Chelli Bouaziz, M.; Ladeb, M.F.; Chakroun, M.; Chaabane, S. Spinal brucellosis: A review. *Skelet. Radiol.* **2008**, *37*, 785–790. [CrossRef]
31. Lopes, D.; Martins-Cruz, C.; Oliveira, M.B.; Mano, J.F. Bone physiology as inspiration for tissue regenerative therapies. *Biomaterials* **2018**, *185*, 240–275. [CrossRef]
32. Neve, A.; Corrado, A.; Cantatore, F.P. Osteoblast physiology in normal and pathological conditions. *Cell Tissue Res.* **2011**, *343*, 289–302. [CrossRef] [PubMed]
33. Sun, Y.; Li, J.; Xie, X.; Gu, F.; Sui, Z.; Zhang, K.; Yu, T. Recent Advances in Osteoclast Biological Behavior. *Front. Cell Dev. Biol.* **2021**, *9*, 788680. [CrossRef] [PubMed]
34. Yao, Y.; Cai, X.; Ren, F.; Ye, Y.; Wang, F.; Zheng, C.; Qian, Y.; Zhang, M. The Macrophage-Osteoclast Axis in Osteoimmunity and Osteo-Related Diseases. *Front. Immunol.* **2021**, *12*, 664871. [CrossRef] [PubMed]
35. Sprangers, S.; Schoenmaker, T.; Cao, Y.; Everts, V.; de Vries, T.J. Different Blood-Borne Human Osteoclast Precursors Respond in Distinct Ways to IL-17A. *J. Cell Physiol.* **2016**, *231*, 1249–1260. [CrossRef] [PubMed]
36. Iwamoto, N.; Kawakami, A. The monocyte-to-osteoclast transition in rheumatoid arthritis: Recent findings. *Front. Immunol.* **2022**, *13*, 998554. [CrossRef] [PubMed]
37. Roop, R.M., 2nd; Barton, I.S.; Hopersberger, D.; Martin, D.W. Uncovering the Hidden Credentials of *Brucella* Virulence. *Microbiol. Mol. Biol. Rev.* **2021**, *85*, e00021-19. [CrossRef] [PubMed]
38. Delpino, M.V.; Fossati, C.A.; Baldi, P.C. Proinflammatory response of human osteoblastic cell lines and osteoblast-monocyte interaction upon infection with *Brucella* spp. *Infect. Immun.* **2009**, *77*, 984–995. [CrossRef]
39. Scian, R.; Barrionuevo, P.; Fossati, C.A.; Giambartolomei, G.H.; Delpino, M.V. *Brucella abortus* invasion of osteoblasts inhibits bone formation. *Infect. Immun.* **2012**, *80*, 2333–2345. [CrossRef]
40. Roskoski, R., Jr. ERK1/2 MAP kinases: Structure, function, and regulation. *Pharmacol. Res.* **2012**, *66*, 105–143. [CrossRef]
41. Burrage, P.S.; Mix, K.S.; Brinckerhoff, C.E. Matrix metalloproteinases: Role in arthritis. *Front. Biosci.* **2006**, *11*, 529–543. [CrossRef]
42. Scian, R.; Barrionuevo, P.; Giambartolomei, G.H.; Fossati, C.A.; Baldi, P.C.; Delpino, M.V. Granulocyte-macrophage colony-stimulating factor- and tumor necrosis factor alpha-mediated matrix metalloproteinase production by human osteoblasts and monocytes after infection with *Brucella abortus*. *Infect. Immun.* **2011**, *79*, 192–202. [CrossRef]
43. Pesce Vigliettii, A.I.; Arriola Benitez, P.C.; Gentilini, M.V.; Velasquez, L.N.; Fossati, C.A.; Giambartolomei, G.H.; Delpino, M.V. *Brucella abortus* Invasion of Osteocytes Modulates Connexin 43 and Integrin Expression and Induces Osteoclastogenesis via Receptor Activator of NF-kappaB Ligand and Tumor Necrosis Factor Alpha Secretion. *Infect. Immun.* **2016**, *84*, 11–20. [CrossRef]
44. Civitelli, R. Cell-cell communication in the osteoblast/osteocyte lineage. *Arch. Biochem. Biophys.* **2008**, *473*, 188–192. [CrossRef]
45. Geoghegan, I.P.; Hoey, D.A.; McNamara, L.M. Integrins in Osteocyte Biology and Mechanotransduction. *Curr. Osteoporos. Rep.* **2019**, *17*, 195–206. [CrossRef]
46. Delpino, M.V.; Barrionuevo, P.; Macedo, G.C.; Oliveira, S.C.; Genaro, S.D.; Scian, R.; Miraglia, M.C.; Fossati, C.A.; Baldi, P.C.; Giambartolomei, G.H. Macrophage-elicited osteoclastogenesis in response to *Brucella abortus* infection requires TLR2/MyD88-dependent TNF-alpha production. *J. Leukoc. Biol.* **2012**, *91*, 285–298. [CrossRef]
47. Giambartolomei, G.H.; Zwerdling, A.; Cassataro, J.; Bruno, L.; Fossati, C.A.; Philipp, M.T. Lipoproteins, not lipopolysaccharide, are the key mediators of the proinflammatory response elicited by heat-killed *Brucella abortus*. *J. Immunol.* **2004**, *173*, 4635–4642. [CrossRef]
48. Giambartolomei, G.H.; Scian, R.; Acosta-Rodriguez, E.; Fossati, C.A.; Delpino, M.V. *Brucella abortus*-infected macrophages modulate T lymphocytes to promote osteoclastogenesis via IL-17. *Am. J. Pathol.* **2012**, *181*, 887–896. [CrossRef]
49. Pesce Viglietti, A.I.; Arriola Benitez, P.C.; Giambartolomei, G.H.; Delpino, M.V. *Brucella abortus*-infected B cells induce osteoclastogenesis. *Microbes Infect.* **2016**, *18*, 529–535. [CrossRef]
50. Hu, X.; Shang, X.; Wang, L.; Fan, J.; Wang, Y.; Lv, J.; Nazierhan, S.; Wang, H.; Wang, J.; Ma, X. The role of CXCR3 and its ligands expression in Brucellar spondylitis. *BMC Immunol.* **2020**, *21*, 59. [CrossRef]
51. Fu, J.; He, H.Y.; Ojha, S.C.; Shi, H.; Sun, C.F.; Deng, C.L.; Sheng, Y.J. Association of IL-6, IL-10 and TGF-beta1 gene polymorphisms with brucellosis: A systematic review with meta-analysis. *Microb. Pathog.* **2019**, *135*, 103640. [CrossRef]
52. Zafari, P.; Zarifian, A.; Alizadeh-Navaei, R.; Taghadosi, M.; Rafiei, A. Association between polymorphisms of cytokine genes and brucellosis: A comprehensive systematic review and meta-analysis. *Cytokine* **2020**, *127*, 154949. [CrossRef] [PubMed]
53. Li, F.; Du, L.; Zhen, H.; Li, M.; An, S.; Fan, W.; Yan, Y.; Zhao, M.; Han, X.; Li, Z.; et al. Follow-up outcomes of asymptomatic brucellosis: A systematic review and meta-analysis. *Emerg. Microbes Infect.* **2023**, *12*, 2185464. [CrossRef] [PubMed]
54. Cama, B.A.V.; Ceccarelli, M.; Venanzi Rullo, E.; Ferraiolo, F.; Paolucci, I.A.; Maranto, D.; Mondello, P.; Lo Presti Costantino, M.R.; Marano, F.; D'Andrea, G.; et al. Outbreak of *Brucella melitensis* infection in Eastern Sicily: Risk factors, clinical characteristics and complication rate. *New Microbiol.* **2019**, *42*, 43–48. [PubMed]
55. Wu, Z.G.; Song, Z.Y.; Wang, W.X.; Xi, W.N.; Jin, D.; Ai, M.X.; Wu, Y.C.; Lan, Y.; Song, S.F.; Zhang, G.C.; et al. Human brucellosis and fever of unknown origin. *BMC Infect. Dis.* **2022**, *22*, 868. [CrossRef] [PubMed]
56. Solera, J.; Solis Garcia Del Pozo, J. Treatment of pulmonary brucellosis: A systematic review. *Expert. Rev. Anti Infect. Ther.* **2017**, *15*, 33–42. [CrossRef] [PubMed]

57. Qiangsheng, F.; Xiaoqin, H.; Tong, L.; Wenyun, G.; Yuejuan, S. Brucella cultures characteristics, clinical characteristics, and infection biomarkers of human Brucellosis. *J. Infect. Public Health* **2023**, *16*, 303–309. [CrossRef] [PubMed]
58. Dean, A.S.; Crump, L.; Greter, H.; Hattendorf, J.; Schelling, E.; Zinsstag, J. Clinical manifestations of human brucellosis: A systematic review and meta-analysis. *PLoS Negl. Trop. Dis.* **2012**, *6*, e1929. [CrossRef] [PubMed]
59. Namiduru, M.; Karaoglan, I.; Gursoy, S.; Bayazit, N.; Sirikci, A. Brucellosis of the spine: Evaluation of the clinical, laboratory, and radiological findings of 14 patients. *Rheumatol. Int.* **2004**, *24*, 125–129. [CrossRef]
60. Colmenero, J.D.; Jimenez-Mejias, M.E.; Sanchez-Lora, F.J.; Reguera, J.M.; Palomino-Nicas, J.; Martos, F.; Garcia de las Heras, J.; Pachon, J. Pyogenic, tuberculous, and brucellar vertebral osteomyelitis: A descriptive and comparative study of 219 cases. *Ann. Rheum. Dis.* **1997**, *56*, 709–715. [CrossRef]
61. Giannitsioti, E.; Papadopoulos, A.; Nikou, P.; Athanasia, S.; Kelekis, A.; Economopoulos, N.; Drakou, A.; Papagelopoulos, P.; Papakonstantinou, O.; Sakka, V.; et al. Long-term triple-antibiotic treatment against brucellar vertebral osteomyelitis. *Int. J. Antimicrob. Agents* **2012**, *40*, 91–93. [CrossRef]
62. Erdem, H.; Elaldi, N.; Batirel, A.; Aliyu, S.; Sengoz, G.; Pehlivanoglu, F.; Ramosaco, E.; Gulsun, S.; Tekin, R.; Mete, B.; et al. Comparison of brucellar and tuberculous spondylodiscitis patients: Results of the multicenter "Backbone-1 Study". *Spine J.* **2015**, *15*, 2509–2517. [CrossRef]
63. Bosilkovski, M.; Krteva, L.; Dimzova, M.; Vidinic, I.; Sopova, Z.; Spasovska, K. Human brucellosis in Macedonia-10 years of clinical experience in endemic region. *Croat. Med. J.* **2010**, *51*, 327–336. [CrossRef]
64. Martin-Moreno, S.; Soto-Guzman, O.; Bernaldo-de-Quiros, J.; Reverte-Cejudo, D.; Bascones-Casas, C. Pancytopenia due to hemophagocytosis in patients with brucellosis: A report of four cases. *J. Infect. Dis.* **1983**, *147*, 445–449. [CrossRef]
65. Young, E.J.; Tarry, A.; Genta, R.M.; Ayden, N.; Gotuzzo, E. Thrombocytopenic purpura associated with brucellosis: Report of 2 cases and literature review. *Clin. Infect. Dis.* **2000**, *31*, 904–909. [CrossRef]
66. Pappas, G.; Kitsanou, M.; Christou, L.; Tsianos, E. Immune thrombocytopenia attributed to brucellosis and other mechanisms of *Brucella*-induced thrombocytopenia. *Am. J. Hematol.* **2004**, *75*, 139–141. [CrossRef]
67. CDC. Brucellosis (Brucella spp.) 2010 Case Definition. Available online: https://ndc.services.cdc.gov/case-definitions/brucellosis-2010/ (accessed on 16 June 2023).
68. Di Bonaventura, G.; Angeletti, S.; Ianni, A.; Petitti, T.; Gherardi, G. Microbiological Laboratory Diagnosis of Human Brucellosis: An Overview. *Pathogens* **2021**, *10*, 1623. [CrossRef]
69. Pappas, G.; Papadimitriou, P. Challenges in Brucella bacteraemia. *Int. J. Antimicrob. Agents* **2007**, *30* (Suppl. S1), S29–S31. [CrossRef]
70. Lee, A.; Mirrett, S.; Reller, L.B.; Weinstein, M.P. Detection of bloodstream infections in adults: How many blood cultures are needed? *J. Clin. Microbiol.* **2007**, *45*, 3546–3548. [CrossRef]
71. Kimberlin, D.W.; Barnett, E.D.; Lynfield, R.; Sawyer, M.H. *Red Book: 2021–2024 Report of the Committee on Infectious Diseases*, 32nd ed.; American Academy of Pediatrics: Elk Grove, IL, USA, 2021.
72. CDC. Brucellosis Reference Guide 2017. Available online: https://www.cdc.gov/brucellosis/pdf/brucellosi-reference-guide.pdf (accessed on 16 June 2023).
73. Gotuzzo, E.; Carrillo, C.; Guerra, J.; Llosa, L. An evaluation of diagnostic methods for brucellosis—The value of bone marrow culture. *J. Infect. Dis.* **1986**, *153*, 122–125. [CrossRef]
74. Diaz, R.; Casanova, A.; Ariza, J.; Moriyon, I. The Rose Bengal Test in human brucellosis: A neglected test for the diagnosis of a neglected disease. *PLoS Negl. Trop. Dis.* **2011**, *5*, e950. [CrossRef] [PubMed]
75. Memish, Z.A.; Almuneef, M.; Mah, M.W.; Qassem, L.A.; Osoba, A.O. Comparison of the Brucella Standard Agglutination Test with the ELISA IgG and IgM in patients with Brucella bacteremia. *Diagn. Microbiol. Infect. Dis.* **2002**, *44*, 129–132. [CrossRef] [PubMed]
76. Yagupsky, P.; Morata, P.; Colmenero, J.D. Laboratory Diagnosis of Human Brucellosis. *Clin. Microbiol. Rev.* **2019**, *33*. [CrossRef] [PubMed]
77. Li, M.; Zhou, X.; Li, J.; Sun, L.; Chen, X.; Wang, P. Real-time PCR assays for diagnosing brucellar spondylitis using formalin-fixed paraffin-embedded tissues. *Medicine* **2018**, *97*, e0062. [CrossRef] [PubMed]
78. Ma, H.; Zhang, N.; Liu, J.; Wang, X.; Yang, Z.; Lou, C.; Ji, J.; Zhai, X.; Niu, N. Pathological features of Brucella spondylitis: A single-center study. *Ann. Diagn. Pathol.* **2022**, *58*, 151910. [CrossRef] [PubMed]
79. Lan, S.; He, Y.; Tiheiran, M.; Liu, W.; Guo, H. The Angiopoietin-like protein 4: A promising biomarker to distinguish brucella spondylitis from tuberculous spondylitis. *Clin. Rheumatol.* **2021**, *40*, 4289–4294. [CrossRef]
80. Raptopoulou, A.; Karantanas, A.H.; Poumboulidis, K.; Grollios, G.; Raptopoulou-Gigi, M.; Garyfallos, A. Brucellar spondylodiscitis: Noncontiguous multifocal involvement of the cervical, thoracic, and lumbar spine. *Clin. Imaging* **2006**, *30*, 214–217. [CrossRef] [PubMed]
81. Sharif, H.S.; Clark, D.C.; Aabed, M.Y.; Haddad, M.C.; al Deeb, S.M.; Yaqub, B.; al Moutaery, K.R. Granulomatous spinal infections: MR imaging. *Radiology* **1990**, *177*, 101–107. [CrossRef]
82. al-Shahed, M.S.; Sharif, H.S.; Haddad, M.C.; Aabed, M.Y.; Sammak, B.M.; Mutairi, M.A. Imaging features of musculoskeletal brucellosis. *Radiographics* **1994**, *14*, 333–348. [CrossRef]
83. Guo, H.; Lan, S.; He, Y.; Tiheiran, M.; Liu, W. Differentiating brucella spondylitis from tuberculous spondylitis by the conventional MRI and MR T2 mapping: A prospective study. *Eur. J. Med. Res.* **2021**, *26*, 125. [CrossRef]

84. Li, W.; Zhao, Y.H.; Liu, J.; Duan, Y.W.; Gao, M.; Lu, Y.T.; Yao, L.; Li, S.L. Imaging diagnosis of brucella spondylitis and tuberculous spondylitis. *Zhonghua Yi Xue Za Zhi* **2018**, *98*, 2341–2345. [CrossRef]
85. Resorlu, H.; Sacar, S.; Inceer, B.S.; Akbal, A.; Gokmen, F.; Zateri, C.; Savas, Y. Cervical Spondylitis and Epidural Abscess Caused by Brucellosis: A Case Report and Literature Review. *Folia Medica* **2016**, *58*, 289–292. [CrossRef]
86. Yousefi-Nooraie, R.; Mortaz-Hejri, S.; Mehrani, M.; Sadeghipour, P. Antibiotics for treating human brucellosis. *Cochrane Database Syst. Rev.* **2012**, *10*, CD007179. [CrossRef]
87. Marianelli, C.; Graziani, C.; Santangelo, C.; Xibilia, M.T.; Imbriani, A.; Amato, R.; Neri, D.; Cuccia, M.; Rinnone, S.; Di Marco, V.; et al. Molecular epidemiological and antibiotic susceptibility characterization of *Brucella* isolates from humans in Sicily, Italy. *J. Clin. Microbiol.* **2007**, *45*, 2923–2928. [CrossRef]
88. Maves, R.C.; Castillo, R.; Guillen, A.; Espinosa, B.; Meza, R.; Espinoza, N.; Nunez, G.; Sanchez, L.; Chacaltana, J.; Cepeda, D.; et al. Antimicrobial susceptibility of *Brucella melitensis* isolates in Peru. *Antimicrob. Agents Chemother.* **2011**, *55*, 1279–1281. [CrossRef]
89. Shevtsov, A.; Syzdykov, M.; Kuznetsov, A.; Shustov, A.; Shevtsova, E.; Berdimuratova, K.; Mukanov, K.; Ramankulov, Y. Antimicrobial susceptibility of *Brucella melitensis* in Kazakhstan. *Antimicrob. Resist. Infect. Control* **2017**, *6*, 130. [CrossRef]
90. Torkaman Asadi, F.; Hashemi, S.H.; Alikhani, M.Y.; Moghimbeigi, A.; Naseri, Z. Clinical and Diagnostic Aspects of Brucellosis and Antimicrobial Susceptibility of *Brucella* Isolates in Hamedan, Iran. *Jpn. J. Infect. Dis.* **2017**, *70*, 235–238. [CrossRef]
91. Bosilkovski, M.; Keramat, F.; Arapovic, J. The current therapeutical strategies in human brucellosis. *Infection* **2021**, *49*, 823–832. [CrossRef]
92. Solera, J. Update on brucellosis: Therapeutic challenges. *Int. J. Antimicrob. Agents* **2010**, *36* (Suppl. S1), S18–S20. [CrossRef]
93. Ariza, J.; Gudiol, F.; Pallares, R.; Viladrich, P.F.; Rufi, G.; Corredoira, J.; Miravitlles, M.R. Treatment of human brucellosis with doxycycline plus rifampin or doxycycline plus streptomycin. A randomized, double-blind study. *Ann. Intern. Med.* **1992**, *117*, 25–30. [CrossRef]
94. Ariza, J.; Bosilkovski, M.; Cascio, A.; Colmenero, J.D.; Corbel, M.J.; Falagas, M.E.; Memish, Z.A.; Roushan, M.R.; Rubinstein, E.; Sipsas, N.V.; et al. Perspectives for the treatment of brucellosis in the 21st century: The Ioannina recommendations. *PLoS Med.* **2007**, *4*, e317. [CrossRef] [PubMed]
95. Solis Garcia del Pozo, J.; Vives Soto, M.; Solera, J. Vertebral osteomyelitis: Long-term disability assessment and prognostic factors. *J. Infect.* **2007**, *54*, 129–134. [CrossRef] [PubMed]
96. Ranjbar, M.; Keramat, F.; Mamani, M.; Kia, A.R.; Khalilian, F.O.; Hashemi, S.H.; Nojomi, M. Comparison between doxycycline-rifampin-amikacin and doxycycline-rifampin regimens in the treatment of brucellosis. *Int. J. Infect. Dis.* **2007**, *11*, 152–156. [CrossRef] [PubMed]
97. Ioannou, S.; Karadima, D.; Pneumaticos, S.; Athanasiou, H.; Pontikis, J.; Zormpala, A.; Sipsas, N.V. Efficacy of prolonged antimicrobial chemotherapy for brucellar spondylodiscitis. *Clin. Microbiol. Infect.* **2011**, *17*, 756–762. [CrossRef] [PubMed]
98. Unuvar, G.K.; Kilic, A.U.; Doganay, M. Current therapeutic strategy in osteoarticular brucellosis. *North. Clin. Istanb.* **2019**, *6*, 415–420. [CrossRef]
99. Alp, E.; Koc, R.K.; Durak, A.C.; Yildiz, O.; Aygen, B.; Sumerkan, B.; Doganay, M. Doxycycline plus streptomycin versus ciprofloxacin plus rifampicin in spinal brucellosis [ISRCTN31053647]. *BMC Infect. Dis.* **2006**, *6*, 72. [CrossRef]
100. Colmenero, J.D.; Ruiz-Mesa, J.D.; Plata, A.; Bermudez, P.; Martin-Rico, P.; Queipo-Ortuno, M.I.; Reguera, J.M. Clinical findings, therapeutic approach, and outcome of brucellar vertebral osteomyelitis. *Clin. Infect. Dis.* **2008**, *46*, 426–433. [CrossRef]
101. Yang, X.M.; Jia, Y.L.; Zhang, Y.; Zhang, P.N.; Yao, Y.; Yin, Y.L.; Tian, Y. Clinical Effect of Doxycycline Combined with Compound Sulfamethoxazole and Rifampicin in the Treatment of Brucellosis Spondylitis. *Drug Des. Devel Ther.* **2021**, *15*, 4733–4740. [CrossRef]
102. Bayindir, Y.; Sonmez, E.; Aladag, A.; Buyukberber, N. Comparison of five antimicrobial regimens for the treatment of brucellar spondylitis: A prospective, randomized study. *J. Chemother.* **2003**, *15*, 466–471. [CrossRef]
103. Smailnejad Gangi, S.M.; Hasanjani Roushan, M.R.; Janmohammadi, N.; Mehraeen, R.; Soleimani Amiri, M.J.; Khalilian, E. Outcomes of treatment in 50 cases with spinal brucellosis in Babol, Northern Iran. *J. Infect. Dev. Ctries.* **2012**, *6*, 654–659. [CrossRef]
104. Koubaa, M.; Maaloul, I.; Marrakchi, C.; Lahiani, D.; Hammami, B.; Mnif, Z.; Ben Mahfoudh, K.; Hammami, A.; Ben Jemaa, M. Spinal brucellosis in South of Tunisia: Review of 32 cases. *Spine J.* **2014**, *14*, 1538–1544. [CrossRef]
105. Gulsun, S.; Aslan, S.; Satici, O.; Gul, T. Brucellosis in pregnancy. *Trop. Doct* **2011**, *41*, 82–84. [CrossRef] [PubMed]
106. Cebesoy, F.B.; Balat, O.; Mete, A. An extraordinary cause of vertebral fracture in pregnant woman: Brucellosis. *Arch. Gynecol. Obs.* **2009**, *280*, 301–303. [CrossRef]
107. Solera, J.; Lozano, E.; Martinez-Alfaro, E.; Espinosa, A.; Castillejos, M.L.; Abad, L. Brucellar spondylitis: Review of 35 cases and literature survey. *Clin. Infect. Dis.* **1999**, *29*, 1440–1449. [CrossRef] [PubMed]
108. Katonis, P.; Tzermiadianos, M.; Gikas, A.; Papagelopoulos, P.; Hadjipavlou, A. Surgical treatment of spinal brucellosis. *Clin. Orthop. Relat. Res.* **2006**, *444*, 66–72. [CrossRef] [PubMed]
109. Wang, X.; Long, Y.; Li, Y.; Guo, Y.; Mansuerjiang, M.; Tian, Z.; Younusi, A.; Cao, L.; Wang, C. Biportal endoscopic decompression, debridement, and interbody fusion, combined with percutaneous screw fixation for lumbar brucellosis spondylitis. *Front. Surg.* **2022**, *9*, 1024510. [CrossRef] [PubMed]
110. Faraj, A.A.; Webb, J.K. Spinal instrumentation for primary pyogenic infection report of 31 patients. *Acta Orthop. Belg.* **2000**, *66*, 242–247. [PubMed]
111. Alp, E.; Doganay, M. Current therapeutic strategy in spinal brucellosis. *Int. J. Infect. Dis.* **2008**, *12*, 573–577. [CrossRef]

112. Na, P.; Mingzhi, Y.; Yin, X.; Chen, Y. Surgical management for lumbar brucella spondylitis: Posterior versus anterior approaches. *Medicine* **2021**, *100*, e26076. [CrossRef]
113. Luan, H.; Liu, K.; Deng, X.; Sheng, W.; Mamat, M.; Guo, H.; Li, H.; Deng, Q. One-stage posterior surgery combined with anti-Brucella therapy in the management of lumbosacral brucellosis spondylitis: A retrospective study. *BMC Surg.* **2022**, *22*, 394. [CrossRef]
114. Feng, Z.; Wang, X.; Yin, X.; Han, J.; Tang, W. Analysis of the Curative Effect of Posterior Approach on Lumbar Brucellar Spondylitis with Abscess through Magnetic Resonance Imaging under Improved Watershed Algorithm. *Contrast Media Mol. Imaging* **2021**, *2021*, 1933706. [CrossRef]
115. D'Aliberti, G.; Talamonti, G.; Villa, F.; Debernardi, A. The anterior stand-alone approach (ASAA) during the acute phase of spondylodiscitis: Results in 40 consecutively treated patients. *Eur. Spine J.* **2012**, *21* (Suppl. S1), S75–S82. [CrossRef] [PubMed]
116. Yin, X.H.; Liu, Z.K.; He, B.R.; Hao, D.J. One-stage surgical management for lumber brucella spondylitis with anterior debridement, autogenous graft, and instrumentation. *Medicine* **2018**, *97*, e11704. [CrossRef] [PubMed]
117. Safran, O.; Rand, N.; Kaplan, L.; Sagiv, S.; Floman, Y. Sequential or simultaneous, same-day anterior decompression and posterior stabilization in the management of vertebral osteomyelitis of the lumbar spine. *Spine* **1998**, *23*, 1885–1890. [CrossRef]
118. Jiang, D.; Ma, L.; Wang, X.; Xu, Z.; Sun, G.; Jia, R.; Wu, Y.; Zhang, Y. Comparison of two surgical interventions for lumbar brucella spondylitis in adults: A retrospective analysis. *Sci. Rep.* **2023**, *13*, 16684. [CrossRef] [PubMed]
119. Yang, X.; Zuo, X.; Jia, Y.; Chang, Y.; Zhang, P.; Ren, Y. Comparison of effectiveness between two surgical methods in treatment of thoracolumbar brucella spondylitis. *Zhongguo Xiu Fu Chong Jian Wai Ke Za Zhi* **2014**, *28*, 1241–1247. [PubMed]
120. Cingoz, I.D. Role of Surgery in Brucella Spondylodiscitis: An Evaluation of 28 Patients. *Cureus* **2023**, *15*, e33542. [CrossRef] [PubMed]
121. Hadjipavlou, A.G.; Crow, W.N.; Borowski, A.; Mader, J.T.; Adesokan, A.; Jensen, R.E. Percutaneous transpedicular discectomy and drainage in pyogenic spondylodiscitis. *Am. J. Orthop.* **1998**, *27*, 188–197. [CrossRef]
122. Hadjipavlou, A.G.; Katonis, P.K.; Gaitanis, I.N.; Muffoletto, A.J.; Tzermiadianos, M.N.; Crow, W. Percutaneous transpedicular discectomy and drainage in pyogenic spondylodiscitis. *Eur. Spine J.* **2004**, *13*, 707–713. [CrossRef]
123. Pola, E.; Pambianco, V.; Autore, G.; Cipolloni, V.; Fantoni, M. Minimally invasive surgery for the treatment of thoraco lumbar pyogenic spondylodiscitis: Indications and outcomes. *Eur. Rev. Med. Pharmacol. Sci.* **2019**, *23*, 94–100. [CrossRef]
124. Choi, D.J.; Kim, J.E.; Jung, J.T.; Kim, Y.S.; Jang, H.J.; Yoo, B.; Kang, I.H. Biportal Endoscopic Spine Surgery for Various Foraminal Lesions at the Lumbosacral Lesion. *Asian Spine J.* **2018**, *12*, 569–573. [CrossRef]
125. Yang, S.C.; Fu, T.S.; Chen, L.H.; Niu, C.C.; Lai, P.L.; Chen, W.J. Percutaneous endoscopic discectomy and drainage for infectious spondylitis. *Int. Orthop.* **2007**, *31*, 367–373. [CrossRef] [PubMed]
126. Fu, T.S.; Chen, L.H.; Chen, W.J. Minimally invasive percutaneous endoscopic discectomy and drainage for infectious spondylodiscitis. *Biomed. J.* **2013**, *36*, 168–174. [CrossRef] [PubMed]
127. Amini, A.; Beisse, R.; Schmidt, M.H. Thoracoscopic debridement and stabilization of pyogenic vertebral osteomyelitis. *Surg. Laparosc. Endosc. Percutan Tech.* **2007**, *17*, 354–357. [CrossRef] [PubMed]

**Disclaimer/Publisher's Note:** The statements, opinions and data contained in all publications are solely those of the individual author(s) and contributor(s) and not of MDPI and/or the editor(s). MDPI and/or the editor(s) disclaim responsibility for any injury to people or property resulting from any ideas, methods, instructions or products referred to in the content.

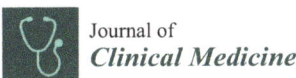 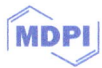

Article

# Anterior Column Reconstruction of Destructive Vertebral Osteomyelitis at the Thoracolumbar Spine with an Expandable Vertebral Body Replacement Implant: A Retrospective, Monocentric Radiological Cohort Analysis of 24 Cases

Lisa Klute, Marie Esser, Leopold Henssler, Moritz Riedl, Melanie Schindler, Markus Rupp, Volker Alt, Maximilian Kerschbaum and Siegmund Lang *

Clinic of Trauma Surgery, University Medical Center Regensburg, Franz-Josef-Strauss-Allee 11, 93053 Regensburg, Germany
* Correspondence: siegmund.lang@ukr.de; Tel.: +49-941-944-6841

**Abstract:** Background: Vertebral osteomyelitis (VO) often necessitates surgical intervention due to bone loss-induced spinal instability. Anterior column reconstruction, utilizing expandable vertebral body replacement (VBR) implants, is a recognized approach to restore stability and prevent neurological compromise. Despite various techniques, clinical evidence regarding the safety and efficacy of these implants in VO remains limited. Methods: A retrospective cohort analysis, spanning 2000 to 2020, was conducted on 24 destructive VO cases at a Level 1 orthopedic trauma center. Diagnosis relied on clinical, radiological, and microbiological criteria. Patient demographics, clinical presentation, surgical interventions, and radiological outcomes were assessed. Results: The study included 24 patients (62.5% male; mean age 65.6 ± 35.0 years), with 58% having healthcare-associated infections (HAVO). The mean radiological follow-up was 137.2 ± 161.7 weeks. Surgical intervention significantly improved the bi-segmental kyphotic endplate angle (BKA) postoperatively (mean −1.4° ± 13.6°). However, a noticeable loss of correction was observed over time. The study reported a mortality rate of 1/24. Conclusions: Anterior column reconstruction using expandable VBR effectively improved local spinal alignment in destructive VO. However, the study underscores the necessity for prolonged follow-up and continuous research to refine surgical techniques and postoperative care. Addressing long-term complications and refining surgical approaches will be pivotal as the field progresses.

**Keywords:** expandable vertebral body replacement; vertebral osteomyelitis; bony fusion rate; anterior column reconstruction; spondylodiscitis

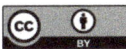

## 1. Introduction

Vertebral osteomyelitis (VO) is the most common manifestation of osteomyelitis in the adult population with an increasing incidence rate [1,2]. A feared complication is spinal instability due to progressive bone loss of the infected vertebral bodies (VB) [3]. However, VO requires complete surgical debridement only in chosen, severe cases [4]. In most other cases, conservative treatment, or a limited surgical regime is sufficient. In cases in which surgery is indicated, it has been suggested to significantly reduce pain, enhance neurologic function, and result in a high percentage of patients going back to their previous functional/work status [5]. In these cases, segmental stabilization with dorsal instrumentation and the option of interbody fusion, combined with systemic antibiotic therapy, usually is the therapy of choice [6,7]. Indications for surgical treatment of pyogenic spondylodiscitis are sepsis, an epidural abscess, neurological deficits/complications, and instabilities/deformities in the affected motion segment, which are also included in current classification systems [8]. Preservation of vertebral body integrity, development of spinal deformities, refractory back pain, inadequate patient compliance, and failure of conservative therapy are considered relative surgical indications. Segmental kyphosis >15°, vertebral body loss >50%, and/or translation >5 mm are considered instability criteria [9,10]. Combined posterior–anterior surgery is considered in cases of large anterior defects. It has been demonstrated that a better reconstruction of the sagittal profile could be achieved with posterior–anterior stabilization in comparison to posterior only constructs [11]. The indication for the posterior–anterior stabilization [12] mainly depends on the clinical course, radiological parameters for segmental instability, and on the experience of the treating surgeons [13,14]. An autologous iliac bone crest can be used to restore the ventral load-bearing column. This has the disadvantage of donor site morbidity and the risk of subsequent graft failure due to collapse of the bone chip. Alternatively, cages filled with autologous bone or, in the case of larger defects, (expandable) vertebral body replacement implants can be used. The titanium cage is considered the gold standard, although polyetheretherketone (PEEK) cages show comparable results in the medium term [15]. Expandable vertebral body replacement (VBR) implants have been shown to be an effective alternative for bone blocks and cages [16–19]. Data on restoring the bi-segmental kyphotic endplate angle (BKA) in VO patients are scarce, despite the fact that it has been demonstrated that they are effective in supplying primary stability. It is noteworthy that reports have been made of cage subsidence and loss of ventral support over time [20,21]. The ensuing kyphotic malalignment may also cause subsequent neurological signs and diseases, impairing spinal function [22,23].

This study aimed to examine the safety and radiological outcome of posterior–anterior treatment with anterior column reconstruction of destructive vertebral osteomyelitis at the thoracolumbar spine with an expandable VBR (ObeliscTM, Ulrich Medical, Ulm, Germany).

## 2. Materials and Methods

This retrospective study conducted at a Level 1 orthopedic trauma center in Germany focused on patients with spondylodiscitis who underwent vertebral body replacement (VBR) between 1 January 2000 and 31 December 2020. The evaluation considered three time points: pre-operation, post-operation, and the final follow-up, ensuring a minimum follow-up period of 6 weeks.

### 2.1. Patient Selection and Characterization

Patients eligible for this study were those aged 18 years or older diagnosed with vertebral osteomyelitis (VO) per ICD-10 codes: M46.2 (osteomyelitis of vertebra), M46.3 (infection of the intervertebral disc, pyogenic), M46.4 (discitis, unspecified), and M46.5 (other infective spondylopathies). The cases were meticulously screened, and the diagnosis was confirmed by compatible clinical features, radiological evidence in CT and/or MRI, and microbiologic demonstration of bacterial pathogens.

The study differentiated between healthcare-associated vertebral osteomyelitis (HAVO) and community-acquired vertebral osteomyelitis (CAVO) [24,25]. HAVO was identified if symptoms developed a month after hospitalization without prior evidence of VO, or if there was a hospital admission or outpatient diagnostic or therapeutic manipulation six months before symptom onset. If none of these criteria were met, VO cases were classified as CAVO.

The inclusion criterion was patients with vertebral osteomyelitis in the thoracolumbar spine who were treated with a VBR implant and had at least two radiological follow-ups after surgery, with the latter one after a minimum follow-up period of 6 weeks. Exclusion criteria were patients under 18, those with non-operative treatment or surgical treatment other than an expandable VBR, and those with incomplete radiological follow-up. Given the retrospective nature of the data-set, VO patients with heterogeneous infection courses were indicated for ventral column reconstruction. In general, we consider vertebral body replacement for defects encompassing 50% or more of the vertebral body, progressive osteolysis, persistent symptoms despite dorsal instrumentation and antibiotic therapy, and cases with severe local sagittal deformity. The indication primarily depended on the individual patient's situation.

## 2.2. Data Collection and Ethics

Data were retrospectively collected, focusing on patient demographics, injury mechanism, neurological status, treatment details, and microbiological details on the causative pathogens and treatments. Septic patients admitted to the Intensive Care Unit were classified according to the Sequential Organ Failure Assessment score. The study adhered to the Declaration of Helsinki and was approved by the University of Regensburg's ethics committee (Number: 12-218_2-101 09/2021).

## 2.3. Radiological Assessment

Radiological assessment involved pre- and postoperative CT scans and X-rays for surgical planning and implant verification, with subsequent X-rays conducted at least 6 weeks post-surgery. The evaluation utilized the bi-segmental kyphotic endplate angle (BKA), visualized in Figure 1, to measure medio-lateral X-rays. In the assessment, BKA values below zero denote kyphosis, while values above zero denote lordosis. In a subset analysis, we separately evaluated the BKA at the thoracic spine (T1-T10), thoracolumbar transition (T11-L2), and the lumbar spine (L3-L5). Fusion at the final follow-up was assessed using the Bridwell [26] classification system. Briefly, the evaluation of fusion rates was conducted via lateral X-ray examination, where the absence of radiolucency, lack of bone sclerosis, and presence of bridging trabecular bone within the fusion area were assessed. Additionally, the observation of screw loosening or implant displacement indicated the presumption of insufficient fusion.

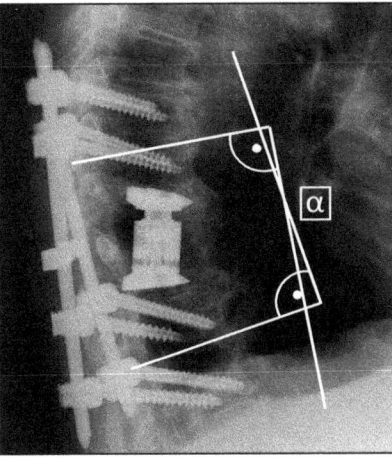

**Figure 1.** Measurement of the bi-segmental kyphotic endplate angle (BKA) in medio-lateral X-rays.

## 2.4. Statistical Analysis

Statistical analysis was conducted using SPSS software, version 28. Tests, including Mann–Whitney U, Kruskal–Wallis, and independent $t$-tests, were performed as appropriate. The associations between implant specifications and the loss of correction were assessed using Pearson correlation analysis. $p$-values < 0.05 were deemed statistically significant. Continuous variables are presented as mean ± standard deviation, and categorical data as frequencies.

## 3. Results

The study included 24 patients (Figure 2), with a male predominance (62.5%) and a mean age of 65.6 ± 35.0 years. The average BMI was 29.5 ± 6.3. Symptoms had been present for 71.0 ± 46.3 days on average before hospitalization. Healthcare-associated infections (HAVO) were identified in 58% of cases (Table 1), with 54.2% potentially being iatrogenic. The mean hospital stay was 33.2 ± 22.3 days, and 75.0% (18/24) of patients required ICU (Intensive Care Unit) admission, with an average ICU (Intensive Care Unit) stay of 3.3 ± 3.4 days. A third of the patients (33.3%) developed sepsis during their hospitalization, according to the reviewed diagnoses in the patient charts. Initial CRP levels upon admission were high at 149.3 ± 11.2 mg/L, decreasing to a mean of 83.6 ± 9.7 mg/L by the end of the hospitalization. Leukocyte counts increased slightly from an initial mean of $9.4 \pm 3.5 \times 10^9/L$ to a final mean of $10.0 \pm 7.5 \times 10^9/L$.

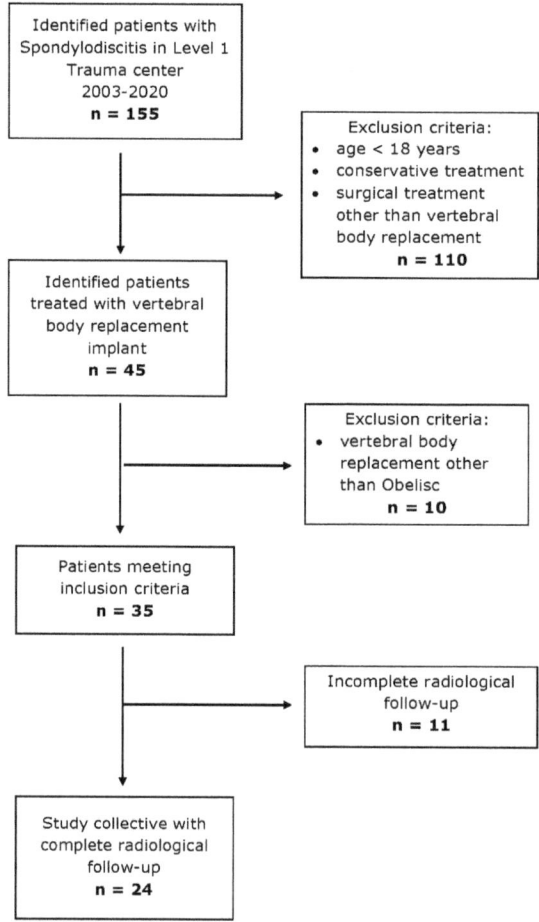

**Figure 2.** Inclusion and exclusion criteria of study cohort.

Six (25.0%) patients had a paravertebral abscess, eight (33.3%) had a psoas abscess, and three (12.5%) had an epidural abscess. Neurological complications were also present: eight (33.3%) patients had paresis, two (8.3%) had hyposensitivity, and two (8.3%) had paresthesia. Six (25.0%) patients experienced a spinal cord injury. Additionally, 19 patients (79.2%) reported back pain.

Table 1. Baseline statistics of study cohort.

|  |  | Percentage [n] |
|---|---|---|
| n |  | 100.0% [24] |
| age [years] |  | 65.9 ± 11.9 |
| sex |  | ♂ = 62.5% [15]<br>♀ = 37.5% [9] |
| BMI |  | 29.5 ± 6.3 |
| HAVO/CAVO [n] |  | HAVO = 58.4% [14]<br>CAVO = 41.7% [10] |
| hospital stay duration [days] |  | 33.2 ± 22.3 |
| intensive care unit stay |  | 75.0% [18] |
| intensive care unit stay duration [days] |  | 3.3 ± 3.4 |
| duration of symptoms [days] |  | 71 ± 46.3 |
| mortality (in-hospital) |  | 4.2% [1] |
| localisation | thoracic spine<br>thoracolumbal junction<br>lumbar spine | 45.9% [11]<br>29.2% [7]<br>25.0% [6] |
| abscess | no abscess<br>total<br>paravertebral<br>psoas<br>epidural | 37.5% [9]<br>62.5% [15]<br>25.0% [6]<br>33.4% [8]<br>12.5% [3] |

An acute fulminant septic course was observed in eight cases (33.4%). With *Staphylococcus aureus* being the most isolated pathogen ($n = 10$, 41.7%), *Streptococcus* species ($n = 1$, 4.2%) and *Enterococcus* ($n = 1$, 4.2%) were detected in patients' microbiological samples. In 12 cases, no pathogen could be isolated. The most frequent comorbidity was diabetes mellitus ($n = 10$, 41.7%), followed by congestive heart failure ($n = 7$, 29.2%). Perioperative abscess formation occurred in 15 cases (62.5%), with percutaneous drainage performed in 11 cases. All patients received empirical broad-spectrum antibiotic therapy, which was subsequently adjusted according to antibiotic susceptibility testing in cases where pathogens were identified. Nine patients were treated with antibiotic monotherapy, while the remaining patients received combination antibiotic regimens, including the addition of rifampicin in five cases, among other variations. The mean duration of antibiotic therapy was 62.4 ± 28 days.

Among the cohort, 22 (91.6%) cases underwent dorsal instrumentation. The reconstruction of the anterior column and implantation of the VBR was conducted using a thoracoscopic approach in $n = 11$ cases (45.8%) and a lumbotomy in $n = 4$ (16.7%) cases, whereas in $n = 9$ (37.5%) cases an isolated dorsal approach was used. In 20 cases (83.3%), implants with 0° angulation base- and endplates were used, while in two cases (8.3%) 5° and 10° angulations were utilized, respectively. A total of seven different VBR sizes were utilized, ranging from 17–23 mm to 40–62 mm.

A total of 17 patients underwent a one-staged procedure, and in seven cases a two-staged procedure was performed. The mean surgical duration for the reconstruction of the anterior column was calculated at 155.5 ± 65 min. Complications were observed in six patients (25.0%), encompassing a dislocation of the VBR implant in one case (4.2%), material irritation in three cases (12.5%), postoperative hematoma in one case (4.2%), and screw dislocation in one case (4.2%). Among these cases, five (20.8%) required subsequent revision surgeries to address the identified complications. In the study population, material irritation manifested as localized discomfort and pain at the site of the implanted dorsal instrumentation material, while VBR dislocation, observed radiographically during follow-up, did not exhibit any clinical symptoms. However, it necessitated implant removal due to a high risk of potential further damage. The time to failure, defined as the need for revision surgery, was recorded at an average of 280.5 ± 386.8 days (as shown in Table 2). The in-hospital mortality rate was observed to be 4.2% ($n = 1$). Recurrent infection related to the VBR was not recorded during the follow-up period.

**Table 2.** Complications and revisions after surgical implantation of VBR.

|  |  | Percentage [n] |
|---|---|---|
| n |  | 100.0% [24] |
| revision surgery |  | 20.8% [5] |
| time to failure [days] |  | 280.5 ± 386.8 |
| consolidation |  | 75.0% [18] |
| Bridwell classification | I | 4.2% [1] |
|  | II | 58.4% [14] |
|  | III | 8.4% [2] |
|  | IV | 4.2% [1] |
| complications | no complications | 75.0% [18] |
|  | total | 25.0% [6] |
|  | VBR dislocation | 4.2% [1] |
|  | material irritation | 12.5% [3] |
|  | bleeding | 4.2% [1] |
|  | screw dislocation | 4.2% [1] |

*Radiological Outcome*

The mean radiological follow-up was after 137.2 ± 161.7 weeks with a minimum follow-up of 6 weeks. Examining the entire cohort initially, we found a mean preoperative BKA of −7.3° (±17.9°). Post-surgery, a significant correction in the BKA was observed, demonstrated by a postoperative mean of −1.4° (±13.6°; $p = 0.023$). At the follow-up, we observed a decrease of the BKA to a mean of −8.3° (±14.4°), indicating a significant loss of surgical correction over time by 8.7 ± 7.7° ($p < 0.000$, Figure 3).

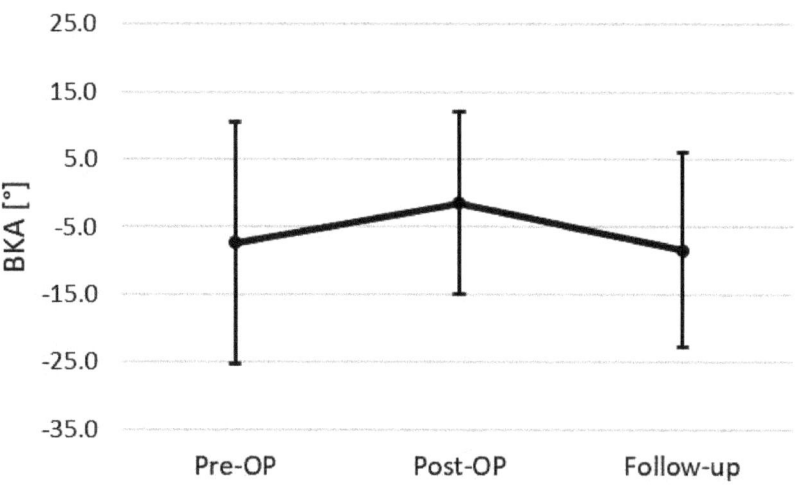

**Figure 3.** BKA changes of the total cohort ($n = 24$).

For the thoracic spine subset of patients, the preoperative mean BKA was −19.3 ± 12.7°, showing a more pronounced kyphotic deformity than the overall cohort.

Post-surgery, a correction was noted with a postoperative mean BKA of $-10.8 \pm 8.6°$ ($p = 0.123$). By the time of follow-up, the mean BKA had decreased to $-17.8 \pm 11.4°$, reflecting a significant loss of correction by $8.3 \pm 7.1°$ ($p = 0.021$; Figure 4A).

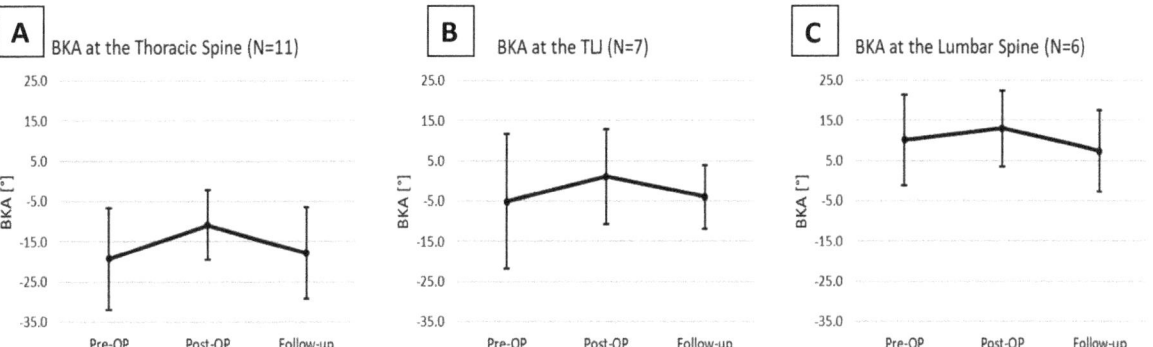

**Figure 4.** Changes in the BKA in the Thoracic Spine (**A**), the Thoracolumbar junction (**B**), and the Lumbar Spine (**C**).

At the thoracolumbar junction the preoperative mean BKA was $-5.1 \pm 16.7°$. Postoperative measurements indicated a corrected mean of $1.1 \pm 11.7°$, yet the change did not reach statistical significance ($p = 0.245$). By the time of follow-up, the mean BKA was $-4.0 \pm 7.8°$, implying loss of correction by $11.1 \pm 10.1°$ ($p = 0.067$, Figure 4B).

At the lumbar spine, the preoperative mean BKA was $10.1° \pm 11.2°$. Postoperatively, there was an observed correction to a postoperative mean of $12.9 \pm 9.4°$, showing a correction by $4.1 \pm 3.4°$ ($p = 0.210$). At follow-up, the mean BKA decreased to $7.4 \pm 10.2°$, demonstrating a loss of correction by $6.8 \pm 6.1°$ ($p = 0.109$; Figure 4C).

We did not detect a correlation between the VBR size and the amount of loss of correction ($r = 0.178$; $p = 0.400$). There was a medium positive correlation between the used VBR base-and endplate angulation and the loss of correction at the final follow-up ($r = 0.513$; $p < 0.05$). A subsidence rate of 5/24 was documented in patients but did not exhibit a significant correlation with changes in the BKA.

In 18 of 24 patients, we were able to assess the bony consolidation progress using the Bridwell classification [26]. Among those 18 patients, we observed varying progress in fusion at the follow-up period. Specifically, 4.2% of the patients were classified as Bridwell stage 1, 58.4% as Bridwell stage 2, 8.4% as Bridwell stage 3 and 4.2% as stage 4 (as shown in Table 2).

## 4. Discussion

The present study provides a comprehensive analysis of the surgical treatment and vertebral body replacement in patients with VO, focusing on the thoracolumbar spine. Our findings suggest that surgical intervention, specifically posterior–anterior treatment with anterior column reconstruction using an expandable VBR (ObeliscTM, Ulrich Medical, Ulm, Germany), can significantly improve the bi-segmental kyphotic endplate angle (BKA) postoperatively. However, a significant loss of this surgical correction was observed over time, indicating the potential for long-term complications, cage subsidence and the need for further research and improvement in surgical techniques and postoperative care.

Our findings align with previous studies that have highlighted the effectiveness of surgical intervention in spondylodiscitis cases. For instance, a study by Kehrer et al. reported that surgical intervention could significantly reduce pain, enhance neurological function, and enable a high percentage of patients to return to their previous functional or work status [27]. Similarly, our study found that surgical intervention could significantly improve the BKA postoperatively, suggesting an improvement in spinal alignment and potentially reducing pain and enhancing neurological function. However, this study did not include a detailed clinical follow-up. It has been recently demonstrated that spondylodiscitis patients show acceptable but impaired patient-reported outcome measurements, regardless the therapy strategy [15]. A recent study by Neuhoff et al. demonstrated a sagittal correction of 10° (range 0–54°) in a cohort of 100 patients with spinal infections treated via vertebral body replacements. This aligns with our study's results, which indicated an approximate average 6° correction in the BKA [28].

Our study also revealed a significant loss of surgical correction over time, as evidenced by the decrease in the BKA at follow-up. This finding is consistent with previous reports of cage subsidence and loss of ventral support over time in thoracolumbar vertebral body replacement [19,29]. The ensuing kyphotic malalignment may also cause subsequent neurological impairment, limiting spinal function [22,23]. This suggests that while surgical intervention can provide immediate relief and improvement, long-term complications may arise.

In the cohort studied by Neuhoff et al., 31 patients were followed up for more than one year. They found that the main causes for revision surgery were wound healing disorders (12%) and implant failure (11%), with specific complications including posterior pedicle screw loosening (8%) and anterior cage subsidence (3%) [28]. Aseptic mechanical complications were more common in longer pedicle-screw constructs, occurring significantly less in shorter constructs (0–4 levels). In comparison, 6/24 patients in our study experienced complications, including VBR implant dislocation ($n = 1$), material irritation ($n = 3$), postoperative hematoma ($n = 1$), and screw dislocation ($n = 1$), leading to revision surgeries in five cases. The average time until the unplanned revision surgery was 280.5 days. A subsidence rate of 5/24 was documented in patients but did not exhibit a significant correlation with changes in the BKA. A subsidence rate of 5 out of 24 was noted, but this did not show a significant association with alterations in the BKA during the overall follow-up period. The study's findings underscore the complexity of managing VO, particularly within the thoracolumbar region, and depending on the complexity of the surgical intervention, due to the intricate interplay of anatomical, biomechanical, and infectious factors.

The choice of surgical intervention for anterior column reconstruction using an expandable VBR represents a strategic approach to address the multifaceted challenges posed by VO. However, it is important to acknowledge that surgical management in this context demands meticulous patient selection, thorough preoperative planning, and a nuanced assessment of risk factors to ensure optimal outcomes [2].

Furthermore, the noted decrease in the BKA over time highlights the ongoing biomechanical challenges associated with vertebral body replacement. Darwich et al. showed overall low complication rates and a good functional outcome within their cohort treated with VBR, but also that significant height gain was associated with higher complication rates [30]. While immediate improvements in spinal alignment are evident, the long-term biomechanical implications require continuous scrutiny. The interplay between surgical correction, fusion, and load distribution underscores the importance of biomechanical studies that provide insights into the longevity and sustainability of surgical outcomes.

Additionally, a reported mortality rate of 4.2% and septic complications in one third of the cohort indicate the potential severity of VO and its associated challenges. This underlines the importance of early diagnosis, timely intervention, and comprehensive management to mitigate adverse outcomes [2,31].

In analyzing our results, the study revealed a statistically significant improvement in the bi-segmental kyphotic endplate angle (BKA) postoperatively across the entire cohort, emphasizing the effectiveness of posterior–anterior treatment with anterior column reconstruction using an expandable VBR. However, the observed long-term loss of surgical correction underscores the need for continuous scrutiny and further research to address potential complications such as cage subsidence, contributing to the ongoing biomechanical challenges associated with vertebral body replacement [32,33].

*Limitations*

An important limitation of our study is the unavailability of longstanding X-rays for all the cases to assess global spinal alignment. In our study, follow-up X-rays were conducted with the patient standing upright. However, we did not apply X-rays of the whole spine because global deformity correction was not the main surgical goal for the mostly severely ill patients, but rather local reconstruction and stabilization. It is worth noting that comparison between the pre- and postoperative kyphotic angle might partially be influenced by the difference of patient positioning [34]. While the preoperative CT was conducted with the patient in supine position, the postoperative follow-up X-rays were taken with the patient standing upright. Additionally, beyond these considerations, 11 patients were excluded from the analysis because of incomplete radiological follow-up. The reported follow-up time of 137 $\pm$ 161.7 weeks exhibits a notably uneven distribution. This asymmetry in follow-up duration is a relevant consideration that may have influenced the interpretation of the radiographic results. Another limitation is that our retrospective design restricts our study's capability to thoroughly analyze the multifaceted factors, including heterogeneous infection courses in VO patients, that influenced the decision for patients to undergo either one- or two-staged procedures. Generally, the two-staged procedure is selected for patients with multimorbidity, as it allows for a more cautious surgical approach, minimizing operative time and blood loss. Furthermore, it is worth emphasizing that a more comprehensive understanding of the reasons behind the loss of correction is desirable, for example through a comparison with another patient group. This could be achieved through the implementation of a prospectively designed study, which might also include an evaluation of the height of the VBR in correlation to postoperative outcomes. Such an approach could provide valuable insights into optimizing patient care and surgical strategies in the future. Additionally, the evaluation of the role of osteoporosis, with VBR combined allo- or autografts as well as local antibiotics, should be taken into consideration.

In light of the retrospective design and limited sample size acknowledged in our study, it is imperative to recognize that our findings offer a valuable mid-term analysis of surgical interventions for vertebral osteomyelitis in the thoracolumbar spine. While the study's limitations necessitate careful consideration, the observed biomechanical challenges and long-term complications underscore the importance of ongoing research and refinement in surgical techniques and postoperative care to optimize patient outcomes in this complex clinical scenario. Also, due to the retrospective design of our study, a notable limitation is the absence of an assessment of functional outcomes or other patient-associated symptoms, which could have provided a more comprehensive understanding of the clinical impact of the procedures. The potential influence of patient positioning on the comparison between pre- and postoperative kyphotic angles emphasizes the importance of standardized imaging protocols in future studies, with a recommendation for consistent positioning, such as standing lateral radiographs, to ensure more accurate and reliable measurements.

While the study has certain limitations inherent to its retrospective design and small sample size, its comprehensive analysis, clinical relevance, and focus on mid-term considerations contribute valuable insights into the outcomes of surgical interventions for VO. The findings provide a foundation for further research and optimization of treatment strategies to improve patient outcomes in this challenging clinical scenario.

## 5. Conclusions

In conclusion, the study's radiological outcomes highlight the promising potential of surgical interventions in the management of spondylodiscitis, specifically within the thoracolumbar spine. The immediate benefits in spinal alignment improvement need to be balanced with a keen awareness of potential long-term complications and the imperative for ongoing research to refine surgical techniques and postoperative care. As the field advances, collaborative efforts that integrate biomechanical, clinical, and microbiological insights will be essential in optimizing treatment strategies and enhancing patient outcomes in this complex clinical scenario.

**Author Contributions:** L.K.: Conceptualization, resources, supervision, investigation, data curation, writing. M.E.: Formal analysis, writing—original draft preparation, writing—review and editing. L.H.: Supervision, writing—original draft preparation, writing—review and editing. M.R. (Moritz Riedl): Investigation, data curation, writing—original draft preparation, writing. M.S.: Formal analysis, writing—original draft preparation, writing—review and editing. M.R. (Markus Rupp): Writing—original draft preparation, writing—review and editing. V.A.: supervision, writing—original draft preparation, writing—review and editing. M.K.: Conceptualization, methodology, supervision, statistical analysis. S.L.: Conceptualization, resources, supervision, investigation, data curation, writing. All authors have read and agreed to the published version of the manuscript.

**Funding:** This research received no external funding.

**Institutional Review Board Statement:** The study adhered to the Declaration of Helsinki and was approved by the University of Regensburg's ethics committee (Number: 12-218_2-101 09/2021).

**Informed Consent Statement:** Not applicable.

**Data Availability Statement:** The data presented in this study are available on request from the corresponding author. The data are not publicly available due to privacy.

**Conflicts of Interest:** The authors declare no conflicts of interest.

# References

1. Conan, Y.; Laurent, E.; Belin, Y.; Lacasse, M.; Amelot, A.; Mulleman, D.; Rosset, P.; Bernard, L.; Grammatico-Guillon, L. Large increase of vertebral osteomyelitis in France: A 2010–2019 cross-sectional study. *Epidemiol. Infect.* **2021**, *149*, e227. [CrossRef] [PubMed]
2. Lang, S.; Walter, N.; Schindler, M.; Baertl, S.; Szymski, D.; Loibl, M.; Alt, V.; Rupp, M. The Epidemiology of Spondylodiscitis in Germany: A Descriptive Report of Incidence Rates, Pathogens, In-Hospital Mortality, and Hospital Stays between 2010 and 2020. *J. Clin. Med.* **2023**, *12*, 3373. [CrossRef] [PubMed]
3. Schömig, F.; Li, Z.; Perka, L.; Vu-Han, T.-L.; Diekhoff, T.; Fisher, C.G.; Pumberger, M. Georg schmorl prize of the German spine society (DWG) 2021: Spinal Instability Spondylodiscitis Score (SISS)—A novel classification system for spinal instability in spontaneous spondylodiscitis. *Eur. Spine J.* **2022**, *31*, 1099–1106. [CrossRef] [PubMed]
4. Pola, E.; Pambianco, V.; Autore, G.; Cipolloni, V.; Fantoni, M. Minimally invasive surgery for the treatment of thoraco lumbar pyogenic spondylodiscitis: Indications and outcomes. *Eur. Rev. Med. Pharmacol. Sci.* **2019**, *23*, 94–100. [CrossRef] [PubMed]
5. Taylor, D.G.; Buchholz, A.L.; Sure, D.R.; Buell, T.J.; Nguyen, J.H.; Chen, C.-J.; Diamond, J.M.; Washburn, P.A.; Harrop, J.; Shaffrey, C.I.; et al. Presentation and Outcomes After Medical and Surgical Treatment Versus Medical Treatment Alone of Spontaneous Infectious Spondylodiscitis: A Systematic Literature Review and Meta-Analysis. *Glob. Spine J.* **2018**, *8*, 49S–58S. [CrossRef] [PubMed]
6. Nasto, L.A.; Colangelo, D.; Mazzotta, V.; Di Meco, E.; Neri, V.; Nasto, R.A.; Fantoni, M.; Pola, E. Is posterior percutaneous screw-rod instrumentation a safe and effective alternative approach to TLSO rigid bracing for single-level pyogenic spondylodiscitis? Results of a retrospective cohort analysis. *Spine J.* **2014**, *14*, 1139–1146. [CrossRef]
7. Rutges, J.P.H.J.; Kempen, D.H.; van Dijk, M.; Oner, F.C. Outcome of conservative and surgical treatment of pyogenic spondylodiscitis: A systematic literature review. *Eur. Spine J.* **2015**, *25*, 983–999. [CrossRef]
8. Almansour, H.; Pepke, W.; Akbar, M. Pyogenic spondylodiscitis. *Orthopäde* **2019**, *49*, 482–493. [CrossRef]
9. Dietze, D.D.; Fessler, R.G.; Jacob, R.P. Primary reconstruction for spinal infections. *J. Neurosurg.* **1997**, *86*, 981–989. [CrossRef]
10. Fleege, C.; Wichelhaus, T.; Rauschmann, M. Systemische und lokale Antibiotikatherapie bei konservativ und operativ behandelten Spondylodiszitiden. *Orthopäde* **2012**, *41*, 727–735. [CrossRef]
11. von der Hoeh, N.H.; Voelker, A.; Hofmann, A.; Zajonz, D.; Spiegl, U.A.; Jarvers, J.-S.; Heyde, C.-E. Pyogenic Spondylodiscitis of the Thoracic Spine: Outcome of 1-Stage Posterior Versus 2-Stage Posterior and Anterior Spinal Reconstruction in Adults. *World Neurosurg.* **2018**, *120*, e297–e303. [CrossRef] [PubMed]
12. Lang, S.; Loibl, M.; Neumann, C.; Alt, V. Einsatz der videoassistierten Thorakoskopie bei der dorsoventralen Stabilisierung einer osteodestruktiven pyogenen Spondylodiszitis der Brustwirbelsäule. *Unfallchirurg* **2021**, *124*, 505–511. [CrossRef] [PubMed]
13. Lang, S.; Rupp, M.; Hanses, F.; Neumann, C.; Loibl, M.; Alt, V. Infektionen der Wirbelsäule. *Unfallchirurg* **2021**, *124*, 489–504. [CrossRef] [PubMed]
14. Blecher, R.; Frieler, S.; Qutteineh, B.; Pierre, C.A.; Yilmaz, E.; Ishak, B.; Von Glinski, A.; Oskouian, R.J.; Kramer, M.; Drexler, M.; et al. Who Needs Surgical Stabilization for Pyogenic Spondylodiscitis? Retrospective Analysis of Non-Surgically Treated Patients. *Glob. Spine J.* **2021**, *13*, 1550–1557. [CrossRef] [PubMed]

15. Lang, S.; Walter, N.; Froemming, A.; Baertl, S.; Szymski, D.; Alt, V.; Rupp, M. Long-term patient-related quality of life outcomes and ICD-10 symptom rating (ISR) of patients with pyogenic vertebral osteomyelitis: What is the psychological impact of this life-threatening disease? *Eur. Spine J.* **2023**, *32*, 1810–1817. [CrossRef] [PubMed]
16. Schnake, K.J.; Stavridis, S.I.; Kandziora, F. Five-year clinical and radiological results of combined anteroposterior stabilization of thoracolumbar fractures. *J. Neurosurg. Spine* **2014**, *20*, 497–504. [CrossRef] [PubMed]
17. Knop, C.; Blauth, M.; Bühren, V.; Arand, M.; Egbers, H.J.; Hax, P.M.; Wentzensen, A. Surgical treatment of injuries of the thoracolumbar tran-sition—3: Follow-up examination. Results of a prospective multi-center study by the "Spinal" Study Group of the German Society of Trauma Surgery. *Unfallchirurg* **2001**, *104*, 583–600. [CrossRef]
18. Kreinest, M.; Schmahl, D.; Grützner, P.A.; Matschke, S. Radiological Results and Clinical Patient Outcome After Implantation of a Hydraulic Expandable Vertebral Body Replacement following Traumatic Vertebral Fractures in the Thoracic and Lumbar Spine: A 3-Year Follow-Up. *Spine* **2017**, *42*, E482–E489. [CrossRef]
19. Lang, S.; Neumann, C.; Schwaiger, C.; Voss, A.; Alt, V.; Loibl, M.; Kerschbaum, M. Radiological and mid- to long-term patient-reported outcome after stabilization of traumatic thoraco-lumbar spinal fractures using an expandable vertebral body replacement implant. *BMC Musculoskelet. Disord.* **2021**, *22*, 744. [CrossRef]
20. Schmieder, K.; Wolzik-Grossmann, M.; Pechlivanis, I.; Engelhardt, M.; Scholz, M.; Harders, A. Subsidence of the Wing titanium cage after anterior cervical interbody fusion: 2-year follow-up study. *J. Neurosurg. Spine* **2006**, *4*, 447–453. [CrossRef]
21. Briem, D.; Lehmann, W.; Ruecker, A.; Windolf, J.; Rueger, J.; Linhart, W. Factors influencing the quality of life after burst fractures of the thoracolumbar transition. *Arch. Orthop. Trauma Surg.* **2004**, *124*, 461–468. [CrossRef] [PubMed]
22. McLain, R.F. Functional Outcomes After Surgery for Spinal Fractures: Return to Work and Activity. *Spine* **2004**, *29*, 470–477. [CrossRef] [PubMed]
23. Gertzbein, S.D. Neurologic Deterioration in Patients with Thoracic and Lumbar Fractures After Admission to the Hospital. *Spine* **1994**, *19*, 1723–1725. [CrossRef] [PubMed]
24. Lang, S.; Frömming, A.; Walter, N.; Freigang, V.; Neumann, C.; Loibl, M.; Ehrenschwender, M.; Alt, V.; Rupp, M. Is There a Difference in Clinical Features, Microbiological Epidemiology and Effective Empiric Antimicrobial Therapy Comparing Healthcare-Associated and Community-Acquired Vertebral Osteomyelitis? *Antibiotics* **2021**, *10*, 1410. [CrossRef] [PubMed]
25. Park, K.-H.; Kim, D.Y.; Lee, Y.-M.; Lee, M.S.; Kang, K.-C.; Lee, J.-H.; Park, S.Y.; Moon, C.; Chong, Y.P.; Kim, S.-H.; et al. Selection of an appropriate empiric antibiotic regimen in hematogenous vertebral osteomyelitis. *PLoS ONE* **2019**, *14*, e0211888. [CrossRef] [PubMed]
26. Bridwell, K.H.; Lenke, L.G.; McEnery, K.W.; Baldus, C.; Blanke, K. Anterior fresh frozen structural allografts in the thoracic and lumbar spine. Do they work if combined with posterior fusion and instrumentation in adult patients with kyphosis or anterior column defects? *Spine* **1995**, *20*, 1410–1418. [CrossRef]
27. Kehrer, M.; Pedersen, C.; Jensen, T.G.; Lassen, A.T. Increasing incidence of pyogenic spondylodiscitis: A 14-year population-based study. *J. Infect.* **2014**, *68*, 313–320. [CrossRef]
28. Neuhoff, J.; Berkulian, O.; Kramer, A.; Thavarajasingam, S.; Wengert, A.; Schleicher, P.; Pingel, A.; Kandziora, F. Single- and Multilevel Corpectomy and Vertebral body replacement for treatment of spinal infections. A retrospective single-center study of 100 cases. *Brain Spine* **2024**, *4*, 102721. [CrossRef]
29. Thaker, R.A.; Gautam, V.K. Study of Vertebral Body Replacement with Reconstruction Spinal Cages in Dorsolumbar Traumatic and Koch's Spine. *Asian Spine J.* **2014**, *8*, 786–792. [CrossRef]
30. Darwich, A.; Vogel, J.; Dally, F.-J.; Hetjens, S.; Gravius, S.; Faymonville, C.; Bludau, F. Cervical vertebral body replacement using a modern *in situ* expandable and angulable corpectomy cage system: Early clinical and radiological outcome. *Br. J. Neurosurg.* **2022**, *37*, 1101–1111. [CrossRef]
31. Pluemer, J.; Freyvert, Y.; Pratt, N.; E Robinson, J.; Cooke, J.A.; Tataryn, Z.L.; Godolias, P.; Daher, Z.A.; Oskouian, R.J.; Chapman, J.R. An Assessment of the Safety of Surgery and Hardware Placement in de-novo Spinal Infections. A Systematic Review and Meta-Analysis of the Literature. *Glob. Spine J.* **2022**, *13*, 1418–1428. [CrossRef] [PubMed]
32. Liebsch, C.; Kocak, T.; Aleinikov, V.; Kerimbayev, T.; Akshulakov, S.; Jansen, J.U.; Vogt, M.; Wilke, H.-J. Thoracic Spinal Stability and Motion Behavior Are Affected by the Length of Posterior Instrumentation After Vertebral Body Replacement, but Not by the Surgical Approach Type: An in vitro Study with Entire Rib Cage Specimens. *Front. Bioeng. Biotechnol.* **2020**, *8*, 572. [CrossRef] [PubMed]
33. Viswanathan, A.; Abd-El-Barr, M.M.; Doppenberg, E.; Suki, D.; Gokaslan, Z.; Mendel, E.; Rao, G.; Rhines, L.D. Initial experience with the use of an expandable titanium cage as a vertebral body replacement in patients with tumors of the spinal column: A report of 95 patients. *Eur. Spine J.* **2011**, *21*, 84–92. [CrossRef] [PubMed]
34. Lee, E.S.; Ko, C.W.; Suh, S.W.; Kumar, S.; Kang, I.K.; Yang, J.H. The effect of age on sagittal plane profile of the lumbar spine according to standing, supine, and various sitting positions. *J. Orthop. Surg. Res.* **2014**, *9*, 11. [CrossRef]

**Disclaimer/Publisher's Note:** The statements, opinions and data contained in all publications are solely those of the individual author(s) and contributor(s) and not of MDPI and/or the editor(s). MDPI and/or the editor(s) disclaim responsibility for any injury to people or property resulting from any ideas, methods, instructions or products referred to in the content.

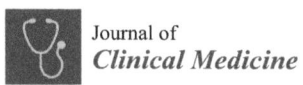 

Article

# Diagnostics, Management, and Outcomes in Patients with Pyogenic Spinal Intra- or Epidural Abscess

Mido Max Hijazi [1,*], Timo Siepmann [2], Ibrahim El-Battrawy [3], Assem Aweimer [3], Kay Engellandt [4], Dino Podlesek [1], Gabriele Schackert [1], Tareq A. Juratli [1], Ilker Y. Eyüpoglu [1] and Andreas Filis [1]

[1] Department of Neurosurgery, Division of Spine Surgery, Faculty of Medicine, Technische Universität Dresden, University Hospital Carl Gustav Carus, Fetscherstrasse 74, 01307 Dresden, Germany; dino.podlesek@ukdd.de (D.P.); gabriele.schackert@ukdd.de (G.S.); tareq.juratli@ukdd.de (T.A.J.); ilker.eyuepoglu@ukdd.de (I.Y.E.); afilis@neuromaster.gr (A.F.)

[2] Department of Neurology, Faculty of Medicine, Technische Universität Dresden, University Hospital Carl Gustav Carus, Fetscherstrasse 74, 01307 Dresden, Germany; timo.siepmann@ukdd.de

[3] Department of Cardiology, Bergmannsheil University Hospital, Ruhr University Bochum, Bürkle De La Camp-Platz 1, 44789 Bochum, Germany; ibrahim.elbattrawy2006@gmail.com (I.E.-B.); assem.aweimer@bergmannsheil.de (A.A.)

[4] Institute of Diagnostic and Interventional Neuroradiology, Faculty of Medicine, Technische Universität Dresden, University Hospital Carl Gustav Carus, Fetscherstrasse 74, 01307 Dresden, Germany; kay.engellandt@ukdd.de

* Correspondence: mido.hijazi@ukdd.de; Tel.: +49-1-799-847-820

**Abstract:** Background: Owing to the lack of evidence on the diagnostics, clinical course, treatment, and outcomes of patients with extremely rare spinal intradural abscess (SIA) and spinal epidural abscess (SEA), we retrospectively analyzed and compared a cohort of patients to determine the phenotyping of both entities. Methods: Over a period of 20 years, we retrospectively analyzed the electronic medical records of 78 patients with SIA and SEA. Results: The patients with SIA showed worse motor scores (MS scores) on admission (SIA: $20 \pm 26$ vs. SEA: $75 \pm 34$, $p < 0.001$), more often with an ataxic gait (SIA: 100% vs. SEA: 31.8%, $p < 0.001$), and more frequent bladder or bowel dysfunction (SIA: 91.7% vs. SEA: 27.3%, $p < 0.001$) compared to the SEA patients. Intraoperative specimens showed a higher diagnostic sensitivity in the SEA patients than the SIA patients (SIA: 66.7% vs. SEA: 95.2%, $p = 0.024$), but various pathogens such as *Staphylococcus aureus* (SIA 33.3% vs. SEA: 69.4%) and *Streptococci* and *Enterococci* (SIA 33.3% vs. SEA: 8.1%, $p = 0.038$) were detected in both entities. The patients with SIA developed sepsis more often (SIA: 75.0% vs. SEA: 18.2%, $p < 0.001$), septic embolism (SIA: 33.3% vs. SEA: 8.3%, $p = 0.043$), signs of meningism (SIA: 100% vs. 18.5%, $p < 0.001$), ventriculitis or cerebral abscesses (SIA: 41.7% vs. SEA: 3.0%, $p < 0.001$), and pneumonia (SIA: 58.3% vs. SEA: 13.6%, $p = 0.002$). The mean MS score improved in both patient groups after surgery (SIA: 20 to 35 vs. SEA: 75 to 90); however, the SIA patients showed a poorer MS score at discharge (SIA: $35 \pm 44$ vs. SEA: $90 \pm 20$, $p < 0.001$). C-reactive protein (CrP) (SIA: 159 to 49 vs. SEA: 189 to 27) and leukocyte count (SIA: 15 to 9 vs. SEA: 14 to 7) were reduced at discharge. The SIA patients had higher rates of disease-related mortality (SIA: 33.3% vs. SEA: 1.5%, $p = 0.002$), had more pleural empyema (SIA: 58.3% vs. SEA: 13.6%, $p = 0.002$), required more than one surgery (SIA: 33.3% vs. SEA 13.6%, $p = 0.009$), were treated longer with intravenous antibiotics ($7 \pm 4$ w vs. $3 \pm 2$ w, $p < 0.001$) and antibiotics overall ($12 \pm 10$ w vs. $7 \pm 3$ w, $p = 0.022$), and spent more time in the hospital (SIA: $58 \pm 36$ vs. SEA: $26 \pm 20$, $p < 0.001$) and in the intensive care unit (SIA: $14 \pm 18$ vs. SEA: $4 \pm 8$, $p = 0.002$). Conclusions: Our study highlighted distinct clinical phenotypes and outcomes between both entities, with SIA patients displaying a markedly less favorable disease course in terms of complications and outcomes.

**Keywords:** spinal intradural abscess; spinal epidural abscess; epidural empyema; *Staphylococcus aureus*; spinal infection

**Citation:** Hijazi, M.M.; Siepmann, T.; El-Battrawy, I.; Aweimer, A.; Engellandt, K.; Podlesek, D.; Schackert, G.; Juratli, T.A.; Eyüpoglu, I.Y.; Filis, A. Diagnostics, Management, and Outcomes in Patients with Pyogenic Spinal Intra- or Epidural Abscess. *J. Clin. Med.* **2023**, *12*, 7691. https://doi.org/10.3390/jcm12247691

Academic Editor: Kalliopi Alpantaki

Received: 23 November 2023
Revised: 10 December 2023
Accepted: 13 December 2023
Published: 14 December 2023

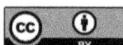

**Copyright:** © 2023 by the authors. Licensee MDPI, Basel, Switzerland. This article is an open access article distributed under the terms and conditions of the Creative Commons Attribution (CC BY) license (https://creativecommons.org/licenses/by/4.0/).

## 1. Introduction

Spinal intradural abscess (SIA) is an extremely rare form of primary spinal infection (PSI) [1]. Together with isolated spinal epidural abscess (SEA) and the most common form, spondylodiscitis (SD), they form PSI [2,3]. While the incidence of PSI was previously reported to be 0.2–3 cases per 100,000 people per year [4–6], the current age-standardized incidence rate in Germany is estimated to be 30 per 250,000 people a year based on data from the Federal Statistical Office (2015) [7].

SIAs are located in the subdural space or in the spinal cord. In contrast to spinal epidural abscesses, intradural abscesses can occur anywhere along the spinal cord or in the spinal cord and are associated with a higher mortality rate. In the first instance, SIA and isolated SEA are due to the hematogenous spread of an infection, but they can also be caused iatrogenically, e.g., by epidural injections [3,8].

In the case of neurological deficits in SIA or SEA patients, the standard recommended treatment is surgical drainage followed by adequate antimicrobial therapy for 4–6 weeks [2,9–12].

The prognosis of an isolated SEA may be better than that of SD with or without an epidural abscess [13]. If SIA is not treated immediately, the prognosis is poor [14,15]. The incidence, clinical course, morbidity, mortality, and optimal standardized treatment of patients with SIA are still unclear, and most evidence is based on case reports and lacks systematic analysis [2,10].

Given the lack of conclusive evidence on the diagnosis, clinical course, treatment, and outcome of patients with SIA and SEA, we retrospectively analyzed a large cohort of 78 patients and compared both populations to determine the phenotyping of the two entities and propose a treatment algorithm for both diseases.

## 2. Materials and Methods

### 2.1. Study Design and Patient Data

#### 2.1.1. Study Design

We retrospectively analyzed the data of 228 patients with PSI. We included all consecutive patients with PSI who underwent surgery at our hospital between 2002 and 2022. Patients were excluded based on one of the following criteria:

- Early or late postoperative local spinal infection
- Only conservative treatment
- Spondylodiscitis

We investigated 78 consecutive patients with SIA and SEA who underwent surgery at our neurosurgical university spine center in Dresden, Germany, between 2002 and 2022 (Figure 1).

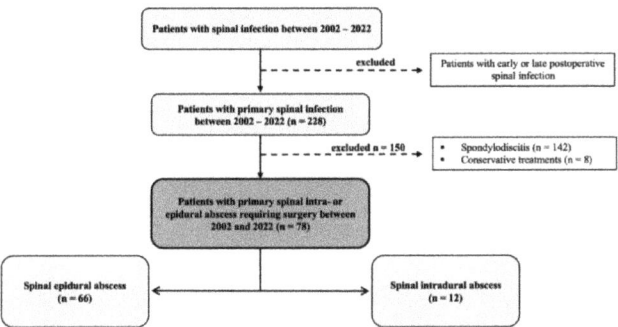

**Figure 1.** Study design. This figure shows our study design in 228 patients with primary spinal infection. One-hundred and fifty patients were excluded due to spondylodiscitis and only receiving conservative treatment.

2.1.2. Institutional Review Board and Electronic Patient Data Software

This study was reviewed and approved by the local ethics committee of the Medical Faculty of the TU Dresden and University Hospital Carl Gustav, Dresden (Ref: BO-EK-17012022). Data on the patients were identified using the ORBIS system (ORBIS, Dedalus, Bonn, Germany), and imaging files were identified using the IMPAX system (IMPAX, Impax Asset Management Group plc, London, UK).

2.1.3. Patient Data

The electronic medical records were pseudonymized and first divided into two groups—SIA or SEA—according to the type of infection. The data collected included sex, age, type of PSI, causative pathogen, detection via (blood cultures, intraoperative specimens, and computer tomography (CT)-guided biopsies), time passed to pathogen detection, type of antibiotic strategy, presence of psoas or pleural abscesses, spinal location of infection, time passed to surgery, incidental dural tears, primary source of infection, surgical and antibiotic treatment, type of surgical procedure, comorbidities (diabetes mellitus, immunodeficiency, obesity, malignancy, hepatic cirrhosis, dialysis, stent or vascular prosthesis, artificial heart valve replacement, osteoporosis, rheumatoid arthritis or elevated rheumatoid factors, gout or elevated uric acid, chronic venous insufficiency, peripheral artery disease, and atrial fibrillation), relapse, sepsis, septic embolism, sign of meningism, reoperation, disease-related mortality, hospitalization, intensive care unit (ICU) stay, ventriculitis or cerebral abscess, deep wound infection, pneumonia, urinary tract infection, presentation of ataxic gait, bladder or bowel dysfunction, number of decompressed levels, number of required surgeries, American Society of Anaesthesiologists (ASA) classification, preoperative and postoperative C-reactive protein (CrP) level and leukocyte count, and motor score based on the American Spinal Injury Association grading system (MS score).

2.2. Clinical Management

We diagnosed SIA and SEA on the basis of the patient's medical history, clinical examination, fever, laboratory values such as leukocyte count, CrP and procalcitonin, typical radiological changes in magnetic resonance imaging (MRI) and CT, as well as pathogen detection in blood cultures, intraoperative specimens, or CT-guided biopsies of paravertebral psoas abscesses. The determination of whether a patient had an SIA or an SEA was based on the intraoperative findings in accordance with the MRI.

Depending on the clinical condition, at least two blood cultures were taken before antibiotic therapy was started for microbiological diagnosis, although some of the patients were initially treated with antibiotics in a peripheral hospital due to their severe clinical condition.

All the patients underwent transthoracic echocardiography (TTE) to rule out infective endocarditis (IE), while the patients with possible or definite IE according to the modified Duke criteria or with proven Gram-positive bacteria received transesophageal echocardiography (TEE).

The SEA and SIA cases were discussed in our neurosurgery–neuroradiology conference or multidisciplinary spine board and treated in collaboration with infectiologists, neuroradiologists, trauma surgeons, and orthopedic surgeons to determine the best treatment strategy for the patients.

2.3. Surgical and Antibiotic Treatment

Surgical treatment of SEA was indicated in the case of source control, epidural abscess with space-occupying effects, or neurological deficits. All the patients with SIA had severe motor deficits and elevated infection parameters and showed obvious intradural findings on their post-contrast MRI. The type of surgical intervention was determined in the multidisciplinary spine board or in the neurosurgical–neuroradiological conference.

The patients with SEA underwent abscess evacuation with epidural suction–irrigation drainage (ESID) or anterior cervical discectomy and fusion (ACDF) for abscesses ventral to the cervical spinal cord with ESID. The patients with SIA were treated via a laminectomy or hemilaminectomy, midline durotomy, and abscess evacuation if the abscess was subdural and extramedullary. In the case of an intramedullary abscess, a limited midline myelotomy with evacuation of the abscess was performed. However, to avoid postoperative cerebrospinal fluid (CSF) leakage, we decided not to use ESID in SIA. Therefore, surgical decision making depended on clinical experience and various defined radiological features.

All the patients received targeted antibiotic treatment (TAT) or empirical antibiotic treatment (EAT) depending on their clinical condition upon admission and according to the recommendations of the local infectious diseases department. It is important to mention that most of the patients with EAT came to us from peripheral hospitals and needed immediate surgery; therefore, the number of EAT patients was high. EAT was switched to TAT as soon as the causative pathogens were isolated.

In the case of a culture-negative spinal infection (blood culture, image-guided biopsy, and open surgery), we initiated EAT. EAT was based on the suspected pathogen, suspected source of infection, clinical condition, epidemiologic risk, and local historical in vitro susceptibility data. In most cases, our therapy consisted of a combination of vancomycin with ceftriaxone or vancomycin with piperacillin/tazobactam.

The first-line therapy in our department for methicillin-sensitive *Staphylococcus aureus* (MSSA) was flucloxacillin (1.5–2 g intravenously (IV) every (e) 4–6 h), β-hemolytic *Streptococci* or penicillin-susceptible *Enterococci* penicillin G (20–24 million units IV e 24 h), *Enterobacteriaceae* or *Pseudomonas aeruginosa* Cefepime (2 g IV e 8–12 h), methicillin-resistant *Staphylococcus aureus* (MRSA), or coagulase-negative *Staphylococci* (CoNS) or penicillin-resistant *Enterococci* Vancomycin (IV 15–20 mg/kg e 12 h with a loading dose and monitoring of serum levels). In the patients with foreign body infections or osteosynthesis material, a combination such as flucloxacillin or vancomycin with rifampicin was used [7,16].

Depending on the clinical condition, infection parameters, and MRI findings, the SIA patients were switched from IV to oral antibiotics after 4 weeks for a further 6–8 weeks. The twelve SIA patients in our study were treated longer on average (7 weeks) with IV antibiotics due to their severe infection after consultation with our infectiologist. The SEA patients were switched from IV antibiotics to oral antibiotics after 2–3 weeks on average for a further 4 weeks.

All the patients who met our recommendation were followed up clinically and radiologically at 3, 6, and 12 months after discharge from the hospital, if possible.

*2.4. Illustrative Case with Spinal Intradural Abscess*

A 49-year-old male patient presented with a three-day history of an increasing ataxic gait, high-grade tetraparesis (MS score 55), urinary and faecal incontinence, meningism sign, and positive Babinski sign. Infectious parameters, including leukocyte count and CrP, were elevated, and MRI scans of the whole spine and cranium with contrast showed an isolated dorsal SIA between the C5 and C7 levels. Intramedullary involvement could not be ruled out. Emergency surgery was performed in the form of a dorsal laminectomy at the C6 level, durotomy, and abscess evacuation, as well as irrigation with gentamycin. Intramedullary involvement was excluded intraoperatively via ultrasound. The postoperative MRI with contrast showed a regression of the SIA, but with residual edema of the spinal cord. *Streptococcus anginosus* was detected, which was treated with antibiotics for a total of 12 weeks (4 weeks intravenously). A source of infection could not be determined through further examinations. Endocarditis and septic embolisms were ruled out. On discharge, the infection parameters were within the normal range, and the tetraparesis had regressed (MS score 85). At the first outpatient follow-up after completion of antibiotic therapy (12 weeks), the patient had no neurological abnormalities, and no recurrence was detected on the postcontrast MRI (Figure 2).

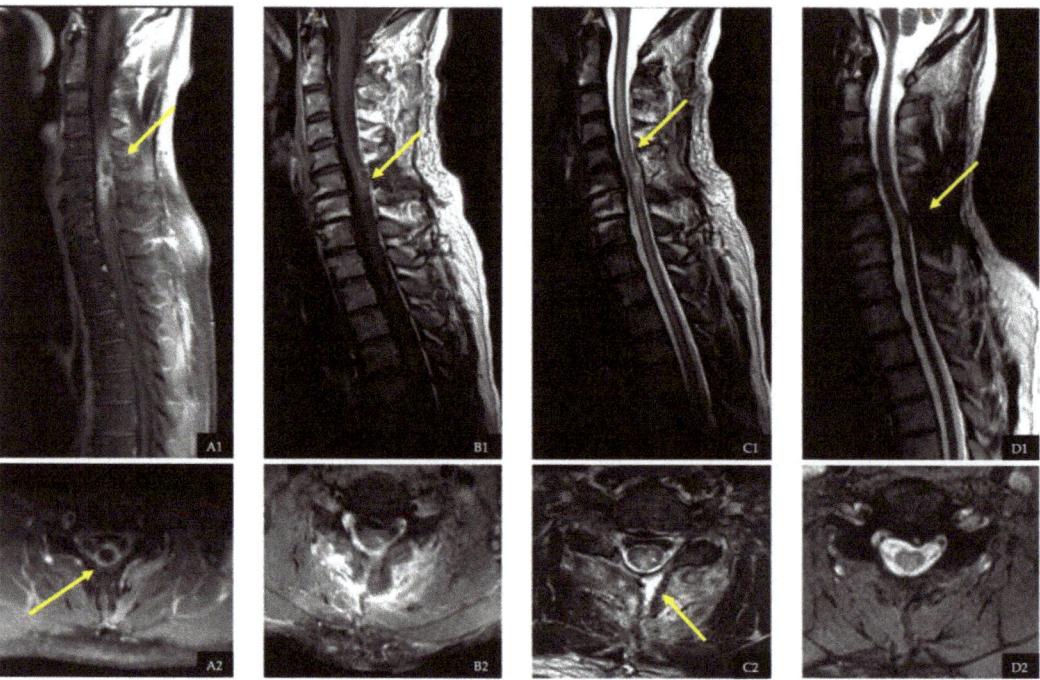

**Figure 2.** Clinical management of spinal intradural abscess. (**A1,A2**): Preoperative sagittal and axial contrast-enhanced T1-weighted MR images of the cervical spine showing a spinal intradural abscess (SIA) on the dorsal part of the spinal cord at the level of C5 to C7. The yellow arrows indicate the SIA. (**B1,B2**): Immediate postoperative sagittal and axial T1-weighted contrast-enhanced MR images of the cervical spine showing postoperative contrast enhancement at the level of C6 (yellow arrow). (**C1,C2**): Immediate postoperative sagittal and axial T2-weighted MR images showing the postoperative intramedullary hyperintense signal (sign of myelopathy, yellow arrow in C1). The yellow arrow in C2 points out the approach. (**D1,D2**): Sagittal and axial T2-weighted MR images after 12 weeks at the time of discontinuation of antibiotics, showing no signs of infection.

### 2.5. Illustrative Case with Spinal Epidural Abscess

A 68-year-old male patient presented to a peripheral hospital with one week of increasing neck pain, signs of meningism, and fever. The infection parameters, including leukocyte count and CrP, were elevated, and *Streptococcus dysgalactiae* was detected in his blood cultures. The patient was then treated with intravenous antibiotics. A postcontrast MRI of the entire spine and cranium revealed a space-occupying isolated SEA at the level of C2 to C7 ventral to the spinal cord. We performed urgent surgery in form of an ACDF at level C5/6, abscess evacuation, and irrigation with Gentamycin through an epidural irrigation catheter up to level C2. The intraoperative specimen also contained *Streptococcus dysgalactiae*. Intravenous antibiotics were administered for 2 weeks and then continued orally for 4 weeks. A source of infection could not be determined through further examinations. Endocarditis and septic embolisms were ruled out. On discharge, the infection parameters were within the normal range and there were no neurological abnormalities. No recurrence was detected during the MRI examination with contrast (Figure 3).

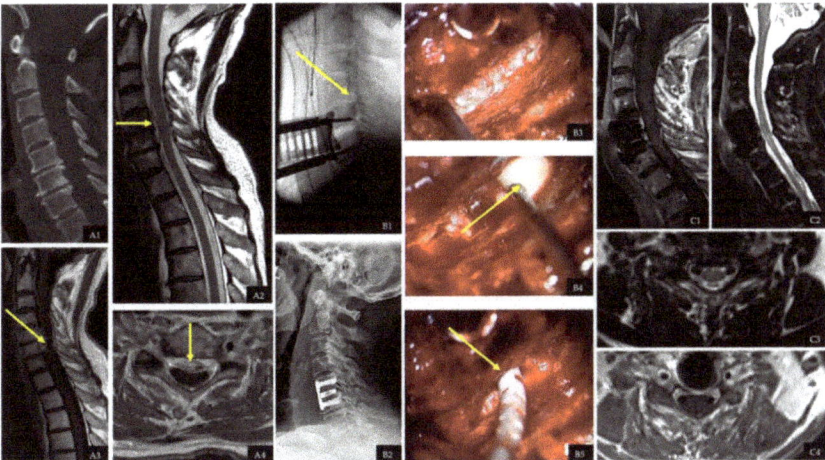

**Figure 3.** Clinical management of spinal epidural abscess. (**A1**): Preoperative sagittal reformatted CT image showing no sign of spondylodiscitis. (**A2**): Preoperative sagittal T2-weighted MR image of the cervical spine showing an isolated spinal epidural abscess (SEA) on the ventral part of the spinal canal at the level of C2 to C7 (yellow arrow). (**A3,A4**): Preoperative sagittal and axial contrast-enhanced T1-weighted MR images presenting the SEA (yellow arrows). (**C3,C4**): Preoperative sagittal and axial contrast-enhanced T1-weighted MR images of the cervical spine showing an SEA (yellow arrows). (**B1**): Intraoperative sagittal X-ray showing the insertion of epidural drainage from the C5/C6 level to C2 (yellow arrow). (**B2**): Postoperative sagittal X-ray image showing the anterior cervical discectomy and fusion (ACDF). (**B3**): Intraoperative image presenting the situation after discectomy of C5/C6 without signs of infection. (**B4**): Intraoperative image showing the pus outflow from the posterior longitudinal ligament after opening it (yellow arrow). (**B5**): Intraoperative image revealing the insertion of the catheter up to the level of C2 (yellow arrow). (**C1–C4**) Sagittal and axial T2-weighted and contrast-enhanced T1-weighted MR images at the time of discontinuation of antibiotics showing no signs of infection.

*2.6. Statistical Analysis*

Statistical analysis of the data was performed using the SPSS software package (SPSS Statistics 29, IBM, Armonk, NY, USA). Descriptive statistics were used, and the categorical variables were tested using Fisher exact tests or chi-square tests. The numerical variables were analyzed using Mann–Whitney U tests. All the statistical tests were two-sided, and a $p$ value ($p < 0.05$) was considered statistically significant.

## 3. Results

*3.1. Baseline Characteristics*

Over a 20-year period, 66 patients were diagnosed with SEA and 12 patients were diagnosed with SIA. The groups did not differ in terms of age, gender, preoperative infection parameters, and spinal localization of the infection.

On admission, a new motor deficit was observed in both groups, with the mean MS score being lower in SIA than in SEA (SIA: 20 ± 26 vs. SEA: 75 ± 34, $p < 0.001$). The patients with SIA had a more ataxic gait (SIA: 12, 100% vs. SEA: 21, 31.8%, $p < 0.001$) and bladder or bowel dysfunction (SIA: 11, 91.7% vs. SEA: 18, 27.3%, $p < 0.001$) compared to the SEA patients.

The most common comorbidities showed only a difference in the distribution of rheumatic diseases (SIA: 0, 0.0% vs. SEA: 9/25, 36.0%, $p = 0.018$) and gout (SIA: 0, 0.0% vs. SEA: 9/21, 42.9%, $p = 0.012$) between the two groups.

The American Society of Anesthesiologists (ASA) class was significantly higher in the SIA patients, such as ASA class IV (SIA: 4, 33.3% vs. SEA: 4, 6.1%, $p = 0.028$), and the distribution of the source of infection, such as skin infection (SIA: 1/6, 16.7% vs. SEA: 14/44, 31.8%, *p* = 0.015) (Table 1).

**Table 1.** Baseline factors between spinal intra- or epidural abscess.

| Variables | SEA (n = 66) | SIA (n = 12) | *p* Value |
|---|---|---|---|
| **Demographics** | | | |
| Age, mean ± SD | 63 ± 13 | 59 ± 21 | 0.739 |
| Male, n (%) | 35 (53.0) | 6 (50.0) | 1.000 |
| **Preoperative symptoms** | | | |
| Preoperative MS score, mean ± SD | 75 ± 34 | 20 ± 26 | **<0.001** |
| Ataxic gait, n (%) | 21 (31.8) | 12 (100) | **<0.001** |
| Bladder or bowel dysfunction, n (%) | 18 (27.3) | 11 (91.7) | **<0.001** |
| **Preoperative infection parameters** | | | |
| CrP level, mg/L, mean ± SD | 189 ± 111 | 159 ± 91 | 0.406 |
| Leukocyte count/L, mean ± SD | 14 + 6 | 15 ± 4 | 0.445 |
| **ASA class, n (%)** | | | |
| I | 3 (4.5) | 0 (0.0) | |
| II | 24 (36.4) | 2 (16.7) | **0.028** |
| III | 35 (53.0) | 6 (50.0) | |
| IV | 4 (6.1) | 4 (33.3) | |
| **Medical history, n (%)** | | | |
| Obesity (BMI > 30 kg/m$^2$) | 29 (43.9) | 3 (25.0) | 0.340 |
| Diabetes mellitus | 18 (27.3) | 3 (25.0) | 1.000 |
| Osteoporosis | 19/58 (32.8) | 1/11 (9.1) | 0.157 |
| Hepatic cirrhosis | 7 (10.6) | 3 (25.0) | 0.178 |
| Dialysis | 1 (1.5) | 2 (16.7) | 0.060 |
| History of malignancy | 12 (18.2) | 4 (33.3) | 0.254 |
| Atrial fibrillation | 8 (12.1) | 1 (8.3) | 1.000 |
| Rheumatic disease or elevated RF | 9/25 (36.0) | 0 (0.0) | **0.018** |
| Immunodeficiency | 7 (10.6) | 2 (16.7) | 0.622 |
| Gout or elevated uric acid | 9/21 (42.9) | 0 (0.0) | **0.012** |
| PAD/CVI | 6 (9.1) | 0 (0.0) | 0.582 |
| History of stent or vascular prosthesis | 2 (3.0) | 0 (0.0) | 1.000 |
| AHVR | 2 (3.0) | 0 (0.0) | 1.000 |
| **Localization, n (%)** | | | |
| Cervical | 7 (10.6) | 1 (8.3) | |
| Cervicothoracic | 5 (7.6) | 2 (16.7) | |
| Thoracic | 13 (19.7) | 5 (41.7) | 0.246 |
| Thoracolumbar | 6 (9.1) | 2 (16.7) | |
| Lumbar | 25 (37.9) | 1 (8.3) | |
| Distributed in the whole spine | 10 (15.2) | 1 (8.3) | |
| **Source of infection, n (%)** | | | |
| Skin infection | 14/44 (31.8) | 1/6 (16.7) | |
| Foreign body-associated infection | 2/44 (4.5) | 0 (0.0) | |
| Following epidural intervention | 15/44 (34.1) | 2/6 (33.3) | |
| Respiratory tract infection | 3/44 (6.8) | 0 (0.0) | |
| Urinary tract infection | 6/44 (13.6) | 0 (0.0) | **0.015** |
| Gastrointestinal tract infection | 0 (0.0) | 2/6 (16.7) | |
| Retropharyngeal infection | 1/44 (2.3) | 0 (0.0) | |
| Odontogenic | 3/44 (6.8) | 1/6 (16.7) | |
| Unknown | 12/66 (18.2) | 6/12 (50.0) | |

SIA: spinal intradural abscess; SEA: spinal epidural abscess; MS: motor score of the American Spinal Injury Association grading system; SD: standard deviation; CrP: C-reactive protein; ASA: American Society of Anesthesiologists; BMI: body mass index, RF: rheumatoid factors; PAD: peripheral arterial disease; CVI: chronic venous insufficiency; AHVR: artificial heart valve replacement. Values in bold are significant results ($p < 0.05$), as indicated in the methods.

## 3.2. Pathogens and Diagnostic Sensetivity

The distribution of pathogens between the two groups was significantly different, such as for MSSA (SIA: 3/9, 33.3% vs. SEA: 43, 69.4%, $p = 0.038$) and *Streptococci* and *Enterococci* (SIA: 3/9, 33.3% vs. SEA: 5, 8.1%, $p = 0.038$).

In SEA, pathogens could always be detected, while no pathogens could be detected in 25.0% of the SIA patients (n = 3). No polymicrobial infections were identified in the SEA patients, while this was the case in 33.3% of the SIA patients (n = 3, $p = 0.003$).

The diagnostic sensitivity of the intraoperative specimens was higher in both groups than that of the blood culture and CT-guided biopsy. The success rate via intraoperative specimens was significantly higher in SEA than in SIA (SIA: 6/9, 66.7% vs. SEA: 59, 95.2%, $p = 0.024$) (Table 2).

**Table 2.** Pathogens and diagnostic sensitivity of spinal intra- or epidural abscess.

| Variables | SEA (n = 66) | SIA (n = 12) | $p$ Value |
|---|---|---|---|
| **Gram stain, n (%)** | | | |
| Gram-positive bacteria | 57 (91.9) | 9/9 (100) | 1.000 |
| Gram-negative bacteria | 8 (8.1) | 0 (0.0) | |
| **Pathogen, n (%)** | | | |
| MSSA | 43 (69.4) | 3/9 (33.3) | |
| *Streptococcus* and *Enterococcus* spp. | 5 (8.1) | 3/9 (33.3) | |
| Enterobacterales | 4 (6.5) | 0 (0.0) | |
| Coagulase-negative *Staphylococci* | 5 (8.1) | 0 (0.0) | **0.038** |
| MRSA | 1 (1.6) | 1/9 (11.1) | |
| Anaerobic bacteria | 3 (4.8) | 2/9 (22.2) | |
| Pseudomonas aeruginosa | 1 (1.6) | 0 (0.0) | |
| **Polymicrobial** | 0 (0.0) | 3/9 (33.3) | **0.003** |
| **Diagnostic sensitivity, n (%)** | | | |
| Blood culture | 29 (46.8) | 5/9 (55.6) | 0.729 |
| Intraoperative specimen | 59 (95.2) | 6/9 (66.7) | **0.024** |
| CT-guided biopsy of psoas abscess | 11/19 (57.9) | 0/2 (0.0) | 0.214 |

SIA: spinal intradural abscess; SEA: spinal epidural abscess; MMSA: methicillin-sensitive *Staphylococcus aureus*; MRSA: methicillin-resistant *Staphylococcus aureus*; CT: computer tomography. Values in bold are significant results ($p < 0.05$), as indicated in the methods.

## 3.3. Antibiotic Management and Surgical Characteristics

The patients with SIA were treated longer with intravenous antibiotics (SIA: 7 ± 4 w vs. SEA: 3 ± 2 w, $p < 0.001$), and they also received prolonged antibiotics overall (SIA: 12 ± 10 w vs. SEA: 7 ± 3 w, $p = 0.022$) compared to the SEA patients. The mean postoperative MS score was lower in the SIA patients than in the SEA patients (SIA: 35 ± 44 vs. SEA: 90 ± 20, $p < 0.001$).

Pleural empyema was observed more frequently in the SIA patients than in the SEA patients (SIA: 7, 58.3% vs. n SEA: 9, 13.6%, $p = 0.002$). The patients with SIA were more likely to require more than one surgery compared to the SEA patients (SIA: 4, 33.3% vs. SEA 9, 13.6%, $p = 0.009$) (Table 3).

## 3.4. Disease Course and Complications

The patients with SIA developed more sepsis (SIA: 9, 75.0% vs. SEA: 12, 18.2%, $p < 0.001$), septic embolism (SIA: 4, 33.3% vs. SEA: 4/48, 8.3%, $p = 0.043$), signs of meningism (SIA: 12, 100% vs. 12/65, 18.5%, $p < 0.001$), ventriculitis or cerebral abscess (SIA: 5, 41.7% vs. SEA: 2, 3.0%, $p < 0.001$), pneumonia (SIA: 7, 58.3% vs. SEA: 9, 13.6%, $p = 0.002$), and disease-related mortality (SIA: 4, 33.3% vs. SEA: 1, 1.5%, $p = 0.002$).

Furthermore, the patients with SIA spent more time in the hospital (SIA: 58 ± 36 vs. SEA: 26 ± 20, $p < 0.001$) and in the intensive care unit (SIA: 14 ± 18 vs. SEA: 4 ± 8, $p = 0.002$) (Table 4).

**Table 3.** Antibiotic management and surgical features of spinal intra- or epidural abscess.

| Variables | SEA (n = 66) | SIA (n = 12) | p Value |
|---|---|---|---|
| **Type of antibiotic strategy, n (%)** | | | |
| EAT | 51 (77.3) | 10 (83.3) | 1.000 |
| TAT | 15 (22.7) | 2 (16.7) | |
| **Antibiotic treatment, mean ± SD** | | | |
| Time passed to TAT, D | 4 ± 3 | 6 ± 3 | 0.366 |
| Duration of intravenous antibiotics, W | 3 ± 2 | 7 ± 4 | **<0.001** |
| Total duration of antibiotics, W | 7 ± 3 | 12 ± 10 | **0.022** |
| CrP level, mg/L | 27 ± 31 | 49 ± 61 | 0.359 |
| Leukocyte count/L | 7 ± 3 | 9 ± 4 | 0.119 |
| **Surgical characteristics** | | | |
| Incidental dural tears, n (%) | 7 (10.6) | -- | -- |
| Time passed to surgery, mean ± SD, D | 2 ± 3 | 2 ± 2 | 0.864 |
| Postoperative MS score, mean ± SD | 90 ± 20 | 35 ± 44 | **<0.001** |
| Paravertebral psoas abscess n (%) | 33 (50.0) | 2 (16.7) | 0.056 |
| Pleural empyema, n (%) | 9 (13.6) | 7 (58.3) | **0.002** |
| **Number of decompressed levels** | | | |
| I | 32 (48.5) | 6 (50.0) | |
| II | 21 (31.8) | 4 (33.3) | |
| III | 6 (9.1) | 2 (16.7) | 0.763 |
| IV | 5 (7.6) | 0 (0.0) | |
| V | 2 (3.0) | 0 (0.0) | |
| **Number of required surgeries, n (%)** | | | |
| I | 57 (86.4) | 8 (66.7) | |
| II | 8 (12.1) | 1 (8.3) | **0.009** |
| III or more | 1 (1.5) | 3 (25.0) | |

SIA: spinal intradural abscess; SEA: spinal epidural abscess; TAT: targeted antibiotic treatment, EAT: empirical antibiotic treatment; SD: standard deviation; D: days; W: weeks; CrP: C-reactive protein; MS: motor score of the American Spinal Injury Association grading system. Values in bold are significant results ($p < 0.05$), as indicated in the methods.

**Table 4.** Complications and hospitalization rates between spinal intra- or epidural abscess patients.

| Variables | SEA (n = 66) | SIA (n = 12) | p Value |
|---|---|---|---|
| **Complications, n (%)** | | | |
| Sepsis | 12 (18.2) | 9 (75.0) | **<0.001** |
| Septic embolism | 4/48 (8.3) | 4 (33.3) | **0.043** |
| Sign of meningism | 12/65 (18.5) | 12 (100) | **<0.001** |
| Infective endocarditis | 1/52 (1.9) | 0 (0.0) | 1.000 |
| Ventriculitis or cerebral abscess | 2 (3.0) | 5 (41.7) | **<0.001** |
| Deep wound infection | 9 (13.6) | 2 (16.7) | 0.675 |
| Pneumonia | 9 (13.6) | 7 (58.3) | **0.002** |
| Urinary tract infection | 10 (15.2) | 4 (33.3) | 0.212 |
| Re-Surgery | 9 (13.6) | 3 (25.0) | 0.383 |
| Relapse | 4/46 (8.7) | 2/8 (25.0) | 0.213 |
| Disease-related mortality | 1 (1.5) | 4 (33.3) | **0.002** |
| **Hospitalization, mean ± SD, D** | | | |
| Hospital stay | 26 ± 20 | 58 ± 36 | **<0.001** |
| ICU stay | 4 ± 8 | 14 ± 18 | **0.002** |

SIA: spinal intradural abscess; SEA: spinal epidural abscess; SD: standard deviation; D: days; ICU: intensive care unit. Values in bold are significant results ($p < 0.05$), as indicated in the methods.

*3.5. Course of the Disease within a Group*

The mean motor deficits based on the MS score improved in both groups (SIA: from 20 to 35 vs. SEA: from 75 to 90) following surgery. In addition, infection parameters such as CrP (SIA: from 159 to 49 vs. SEA: from 189 to 27) and leukocyte count (SIA: from 15 to 9 vs. SEA: from 14 to 7) were reduced at discharge (Figures 4 and 5).

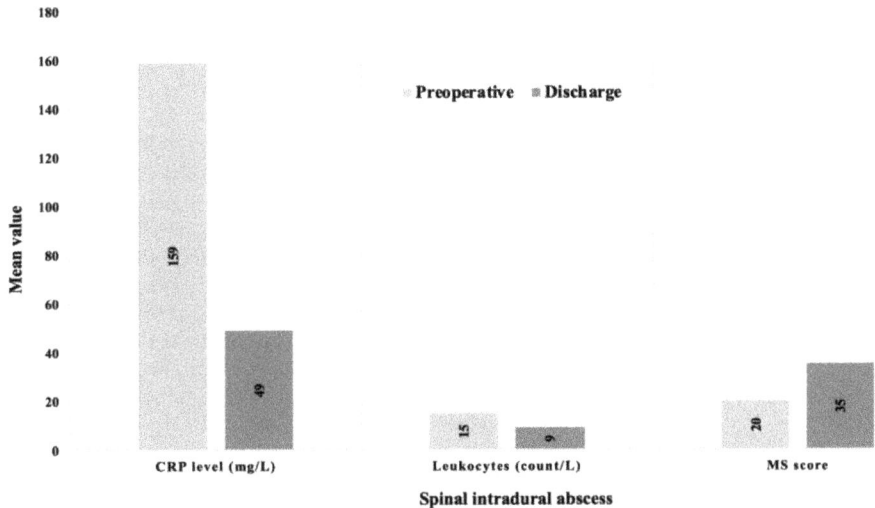

**Figure 4.** Clinical course of spinal intradural abscess. This figure shows the course of CrP (C-reactive protein), leukocyte count, and the MS score for motor deficits (motor score of the American Spinal Injury Association Grading System) in spinal intradural abscess patients.

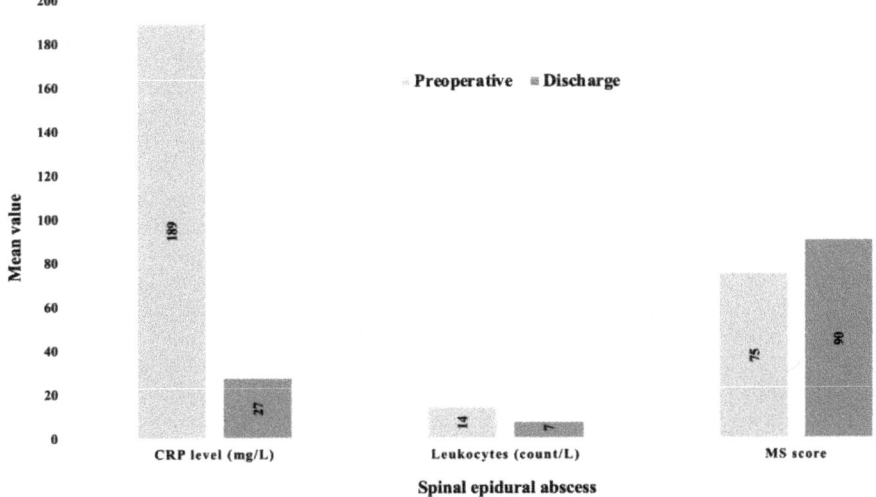

**Figure 5.** Clinical course of spinal epidural abscesses. This figure shows the course of CrP (C-reactive protein), leukocyte count, and the MS score for motor deficits (motor score of the American Spinal Injury Association Grading System) in spinal epidural abscess patients.

## 4. Discussion

The main message of this study and our 20-year experience with SIA and SEA patients is that SIA is a very severe and rare entity with a distinctly less-favorable disease course in terms of complications and outcomes, requiring a long, intensive conservative and surgical treatment.

The baseline demographics of the patients in our study did not differ between the two groups in terms of age, gender, preoperative infection parameters, and spinal localization of the infection. To the best of our knowledge, there are no comparisons in the literature between the two groups, as SIA being a rare disease [2,13,17,18]. A systematic review by Arko et al. showed an average age of 57.2 years in 1099 patients with SEA, which was similar to our SEA patients, with an average age of 59 years [19]. Likewise, a study by Lenga et al. found an average age of 69.6 years in patients with SIA, which is also comparable to our average age of SIA patients of 63 years [2]. Presumably, SEA and SIA are more common in men than in women, which we could not be reproduced in our study [3,19]. In our study, the patients with SEA mostly presented with infections of the lumbar spine, which has also been described in the literature [19]. On the contrary, infection in the thoracic spine was more frequent in the SIA patients in our cohort.

The symptoms on admission, such as new motor deficits based on the MS score, an ataxic gait, and bladder or bowel dysfunction, were worse in the SIA patients compared with the SEA patients in our study, although both groups showed significant improvement at discharge after medical and surgical treatment [2,18,20,21]. This study demonstrates the severity of SIA and the importance of surgical and medical treatment for SIA patients.

Remarkably, the SEA patients had more rheumatic diseases and gout as a concomitant disease. The extent to which these two diseases have an influence on the development of SEA needs to be investigated in a prospective study. Intravenous drug abuse is suggested to be an associated risk factor, and diabetes is the most commonly associated medical comorbidity in SEA patients [19]. In our study, we found that obesity (BMI > 30 kg/m$^2$), diabetes mellitus, osteoporosis, rheumatic diseases, and gout were frequent in the SEA patients, whereas malignancy, liver cirrhosis, diabetes, and obesity were common in the SIA patients. The poorer ASA class in the SIA patients compared to the SEA patients also reflected the severity of the diseases and sequelae.

The primary source of infection in our cohort was different for both entities, with the most common reason being due to epidural intervention followed by skin infection. These two causes have also been identified in the literature as the most common primary sources of infection [3,13,17,18,20,22]. The finding of the primary source of infection is essential in the management of both diseases. We were only able to detect the primary nidus in 50% of the patients with SIA, whereas we identified the primary infectious source in 82% of the SEA patients.

In order to successfully treat a bacterial infection, pathogen isolation is absolutely crucial. In our SEA patients, as known in the literature, MSSA was the most common pathogen, followed by *Streptococci* and *Enterococci* and coagulase-negative *Staphylococci* [13,19]. The patients with SIA in our cohort showed a diverse distribution of pathogens, such that 33% of the patients had polymicrobial infections, 33% had MSSA, and 33% had *Streptococci* and *Enterococci*. Lenga et al. pointed out that MSSA is the most common pathogen in SIA [2].

Open surgery specimens showed the best diagnostic sensitivity for both entities, with SIA patients having a poorer sensitivity. Nevertheless, the collection of blood cultures plays a greater role in pathogen isolation due to its natural non-invasiveness [23].

In our cohort, most of the patients with both entities were treated with the EAT strategy, and it took on average 4–6 days to switch to TAT. Overall, the antibiotic treatment was effective, and both groups showed a decrease in the infection parameters (CrP and leukocyte count) at discharge. The duration of intravenous antibiotic therapy and the total duration of antibiotic therapy were significantly longer in SIA, which is consistent with our algorithm.

Pleural abscesses were more common in our SIA patients than in our SEA patients, whereas the rate of paravertebral psoas abscesses was equal in both groups, indicating the frequent thoracic localization and systematic infection of the SIA patients. On average, the patients were admitted within 2 days of admission. This slight delay is probably due to the extensive diagnostics that these patients needed. An incidental durotomy occurred intraoperatively in approximately 10% of the SEA patients in our cohort. However, the rates of incisional durotomies in lumbar spine surgeries is reported in the literature to be between 1 and 17% [24]. Most of the patients with SEA and SIA were treated equally with one or two levels of spinal decompression and abscess evacuation, with the SIA patients more often requiring more than one surgery on average.

In contrast to our expectations, the occurrence of IE in both entities seemed to be a rarity, whereas PSI patients, such as those with spondylodiscitis with MSSA as a pathogen, showed a higher occurrence of IE in the literature [13,25–27]. All the SIA patients underwent TTE followed by TEE without finding vegetations confirming IE, although some of these patients had septic emboli, brain abscesses, and ventriculitis with proven bacteremia. The largest study of patients with SIA provided no insights into endocarditis as a possible complication or cause in its results [2]. This finding should be investigated in a larger prospective multicenter study. SEA often results from local infection following spinal infiltration or epidural analgesia via a catheter; therefore, IE is less likely.

Both groups showed a recurrence rate of 8–25%, with no significant difference. There were no significant differences in the rates of deep wound infections, between 14–17%, in both groups. Urinary tract infections occurred more frequently in the SIA patients without being significant. The patients with SIA in our cohort developed more sepsis, septic embolism, signs of meningism, ventriculitis or cerebral abscess, and pneumonia. These complications demonstrate the severity of SIA and the difficulties of its management, which requires multidisciplinary assessments.

Disease-related mortality in SEA patients is reported in the literature to be between 1.3% and 31%; however, in our cohort, it was 1.5% [13,28]. Indeed, SIA is associated with high morbidity and mortality rates of up to 45%, which is also similar to our disease-related mortality rate of 33% in our SIA patients [29–31]. Furthermore, we observed in our cohort that the patients with SIA spent more time in the hospital and in the intensive care unit compared to the SEA patients.

*Limitations and Strengths of This Study*

Our study is limited by its retrospective design and a possible bias in the selection of the more severe cases due to the high degree of specialization at our university center. In addition, some of the patients were primarily pre-treated in another hospital and transferred to us secondarily following a clinical deterioration. Furthermore, the generalizability of our observations is limited by the monocentric design of our study. The number of SIA patients treated was limited, with only 12 patients. Nevertheless, our data are based on detailed state-of-the-art clinical, imaging, and microbiological diagnostics with high internal validities. To validate and confirm our results, a large multicenter study with a larger number of SIA patients is needed.

## 5. Conclusions

Our 20-year experience and cohort analysis of the diagnostics and clinical management of SIA and SEA shows that both entities display different clinical phenotypes and outcomes. The patients with SIA had poorer symptoms on admission, higher ASA classes, different primary sources of infection, distinct causative pathogens, and more frequent pleural empyema.

The patients with SIA were more likely to develop sepsis, septic embolism, signs of meningism, ventriculitis or brain abscesses, and pneumonia. Intraoperative sampling has the best diagnostic sensitivity for both entities.

In addition, disease-related mortality was very high in the SIA patients, and these patients required more frequent surgeries, longer durations of intravenous antibiotic therapy, and longer overall durations of antibiotic therapy, as well as prolonged hospital stays and ICU stays.

**Author Contributions:** M.M.H.: conceptualization, methodology, software, validation, formal analysis, investigation, resources, data curation, writing—original draft preparation, project administration, and funding acquisition. I.Y.E., T.A.J., G.S., D.P., T.S., I.E.-B., A.A., K.E., A.F. and M.M.H.: writing—review and editing, visualization, and supervision. All authors have read and agreed to the published version of the manuscript.

**Funding:** This research received no external funding.

**Institutional Review Board Statement:** This study was conducted in accordance with the Declaration of Helsinki and approved by the Institutional Review Board of the local ethics committee at the University Hospital Dresden (protocol code: BO-EK-17012022, January 2022).

**Informed Consent Statement:** Patient consent was waived due to the retrospective, anonymous nature of this study.

**Data Availability Statement:** The original contributions presented in this study are included in the article. Further inquiries can be directed to the corresponding author.

**Conflicts of Interest:** The authors declare no conflict of interest.

## References

1. Greenlee, J.E. Subdural Empyema. *Curr. Treat. Options Neurol.* **2003**, *5*, 13–22. [CrossRef] [PubMed]
2. Lenga, P.; Fedorko, S.; Gulec, G.; Cand, M.; Kiening, K.; Unterberg, A.W.; Ishak, B. Intradural Extramedullary Pyogenic Abscess: Incidence, Management, and Clinical Outcomes in 45 Patients with a Mean follow up of 2 Years. *Glob. Spine J.* **2023**, *9*, 21925682231151640. [CrossRef] [PubMed]
3. Romano, A.; Blandino, A.; Romano, A.; Palizzi, S.; Moltoni, G.; Acqui, M.; Miscusi, M.; Bozzao, A. Intradural abscess: A challenging diagnosis. Case series and review of the literature. *Radiol. Case Rep.* **2023**, *18*, 4140–4144. [CrossRef]
4. Krogsgaard, M.R.; Wagn, P.; Bengtsson, J. Epidemiology of acute vertebral osteomyelitis in Denmark: 137 cases in Denmark 1978-1982, compared to cases reported to the National Patient Register 1991–1993. *Acta Orthop. Scand.* **1998**, *69*, 513–517. [CrossRef] [PubMed]
5. Grammatico, L.; Baron, S.; Rusch, E.; Lepage, B.; Surer, N.; Desenclos, J.C.; Besnier, J.M. Epidemiology of vertebral osteomyelitis (VO) in France: Analysis of hospital-discharge data 2002–2003. *Epidemiol. Infect.* **2008**, *136*, 653–660. [CrossRef] [PubMed]
6. Sapico, F.L.; Montgomerie, J.Z. Pyogenic vertebral osteomyelitis: Report of nine cases and review of the literature. *Rev. Infect. Dis.* **1979**, *1*, 754–776. [CrossRef] [PubMed]
7. Herren, C.; Jung, N.; Pishnamaz, M.; Breuninger, M.; Siewe, J.; Sobottke, R. Spondylodiscitis: Diagnosis and Treatment Options. *Dtsch. Arztebl. Int.* **2017**, *114*, 875–882. [CrossRef]
8. Kulkarni, A.G.; Chu, G.; Fehlings, M.G. Pyogenic intradural abscess: A case report. *Spine* **2007**, *32*, E354–E357. [CrossRef]
9. Thome, C.; Krauss, J.K.; Zevgaridis, D.; Schmiedek, P. Pyogenic abscess of the filum terminale. Case report. *J. Neurosurg.* **2001**, *95*, 100–104. [CrossRef]
10. Lener, S.; Hartmann, S.; Barbagallo, G.M.V.; Certo, F.; Thome, C.; Tschugg, A. Management of spinal infection: A review of the literature. *Acta Neurochir.* **2018**, *160*, 487–496. [CrossRef]
11. Duarte, R.M.; Vaccaro, A.R. Spinal infection: State of the art and management algorithm. *Eur. Spine J.* **2013**, *22*, 2787–2799. [CrossRef] [PubMed]
12. Agarwal, N.; Shah, J.; Hansberry, D.R.; Mammis, A.; Sharer, L.R.; Goldstein, I.M. Presentation of cauda equina syndrome due to an intradural extramedullary abscess: A case report. *Spine J.* **2014**, *14*, e1–e6. [CrossRef]
13. Hijazi, M.M.; Siepmann, T.; El-Battrawy, I.; Glatte, P.; Eyupoglu, I.; Schackert, G.; Juratli, T.A.; Podlesek, D. Clinical phenotyping of spondylodiscitis and isolated spinal epidural empyema: A 20-year experience and cohort study. *Front. Surg.* **2023**, *10*, 1200432. [CrossRef] [PubMed]
14. Velnar, T.; Bunc, G. Abscess of cauda equina presenting as lumboischialgic pain: A case report. *Folia Neuropathol.* **2012**, *50*, 287–292. [CrossRef] [PubMed]
15. Nadkarni, T.; Shah, A.; Kansal, R.; Goel, A. An intradural-extramedullary gas-forming spinal abscess in a patient with diabetes mellitus. *J. Clin. Neurosci.* **2010**, *17*, 263–265. [CrossRef]
16. Berbari, E.F.; Kanj, S.S.; Kowalski, T.J.; Darouiche, R.O.; Widmer, A.F.; Schmitt, S.K.; Hendershot, E.F.; Holtom, P.D.; Huddleston, P.M., 3rd; Petermann, G.W.; et al. 2015 Infectious Diseases Society of America (IDSA) Clinical Practice Guidelines for the Diagnosis and Treatment of Native Vertebral Osteomyelitis in Adults. *Clin. Infect. Dis.* **2015**, *61*, e26–e46. [CrossRef]
17. Sharfman, Z.T.; Gelfand, Y.; Shah, P.; Holtzman, A.J.; Mendelis, J.R.; Kinon, M.D.; Krystal, J.D.; Brook, A.; Yassari, R.; Kramer, D.C. Spinal Epidural Abscess: A Review of Presentation, Management, and Medicolegal Implications. *Asian Spine J.* **2020**, *14*, 742–759. [CrossRef]
18. Rosc-Bereza, K.; Arkuszewski, M.; Ciach-Wysocka, E.; Boczarska-Jedynak, M. Spinal epidural abscess: Common symptoms of an emergency condition. A case report. *Neuroradiol. J.* **2013**, *26*, 464–468. [CrossRef]
19. Arko, L.t.; Quach, E.; Nguyen, V.; Chang, D.; Sukul, V.; Kim, B.S. Medical and surgical management of spinal epidural abscess: A systematic review. *Neurosurg. Focus.* **2014**, *37*, E4. [CrossRef]
20. Darouiche, R.O. Spinal epidural abscess. *N. Engl. J. Med.* **2006**, *355*, 2012–2020. [CrossRef]
21. Turner, A.; Zhao, L.; Gauthier, P.; Chen, S.; Roffey, D.M.; Wai, E.K. Management of cervical spine epidural abscess: A systematic review. *Ther. Adv. Infect. Dis.* **2019**, *6*, 2049936119863940. [CrossRef]
22. Reihsaus, E.; Waldbaur, H.; Seeling, W. Spinal epidural abscess: A meta-analysis of 915 patients. *Neurosurg. Rev.* **2000**, *23*, 175–204, discussion 205. [CrossRef]

23. Hijazi, M.M.; Siepmann, T.; Disch, A.C.; Platz, U.; Juratli, T.A.; Eyupoglu, I.Y.; Podlesek, D. Diagnostic Sensitivity of Blood Culture, Intraoperative Specimen, and Computed Tomography-Guided Biopsy in Patients with Spondylodiscitis and Isolated Spinal Epidural Empyema Requiring Surgical Treatment. *J. Clin. Med.* **2023**, *12*, 3693. [CrossRef]
24. Kalevski, S.K.; Peev, N.A.; Haritonov, D.G. Incidental Dural Tears in lumbar decompressive surgery: Incidence, causes, treatment, results. *Asian J. Neurosurg.* **2010**, *5*, 54–59.
25. Cone, L.A.; Hirschberg, J.; Lopez, C.; Kanna, P.K.; Goldstein, E.J.; Kazi, A.; Gade-Andavolu, R.; Younes, B. Infective endocarditis associated with spondylodiscitis and frequent secondary epidural abscess. *Surg. Neurol.* **2008**, *69*, 121–125. [CrossRef] [PubMed]
26. Carbone, A.; Lieu, A.; Mouhat, B.; Santelli, F.; Philip, M.; Bohbot, Y.; Tessonnier, L.; Peugnet, F.; D'Andrea, A.; Cammilleri, S.; et al. Spondylodiscitis complicating infective endocarditis. *Heart* **2020**, *106*, 1914–1918. [CrossRef] [PubMed]
27. Behmanesh, B.; Gessler, F.; Schnoes, K.; Dubinski, D.; Won, S.Y.; Konczalla, J.; Seifert, V.; Weise, L.; Setzer, M. Infective endocarditis in patients with pyogenic spondylodiscitis: Implications for diagnosis and therapy. *Neurosurg. Focus.* **2019**, *46*, E2. [CrossRef] [PubMed]
28. Kang, T.; Park, S.Y.; Lee, S.H.; Park, J.H.; Suh, S.W. Spinal epidural abscess successfully treated with biportal endoscopic spinal surgery. *Medicine* **2019**, *98*, e18231. [CrossRef]
29. Bartels, R.H.; de Jong, T.R.; Grotenhuis, J.A. Spinal subdural abscess. Case report. *J. Neurosurg.* **1992**, *76*, 307–311. [CrossRef]
30. Kim, M.; Simon, J.; Mirza, K.; Swong, K.; Johans, S.; Riedy, L.; Anderson, D. Spinal Intradural Escherichia coli Abscess Masquerading as a Neoplasm in a Pediatric Patient with History of Neonatal *E. coli* Meningitis: A Case Report and Literature Review. *World Neurosurg.* **2019**, *126*, 619–623. [CrossRef] [PubMed]
31. Lange, M.; Tiecks, F.; Schielke, E.; Yousry, T.; Haberl, R.; Oeckler, R. Diagnosis and results of different treatment regimens in patients with spinal abscesses. *Acta Neurochir.* **1993**, *125*, 105–114. [CrossRef] [PubMed]

**Disclaimer/Publisher's Note:** The statements, opinions and data contained in all publications are solely those of the individual author(s) and contributor(s) and not of MDPI and/or the editor(s). MDPI and/or the editor(s) disclaim responsibility for any injury to people or property resulting from any ideas, methods, instructions or products referred to in the content.

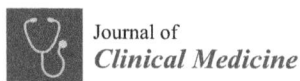 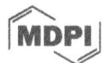

Article

# In-Hospital Mortality from Spondylodiscitis: Insights from a Single-Center Retrospective Study

Ann-Kathrin Joerger *, Carolin Albrecht, Nicole Lange, Bernhard Meyer and Maria Wostrack

Department of Neurosurgery, Klinikum Rechts der Isar, Technical University Munich, 81675 Munich, Germany; maria.wostrack@tum.de (M.W.)
* Correspondence: annkathrin.joerger@tum.de; Tel.: +49-89-4140-2151; Fax: +49-89-4140-4889

**Abstract:** (1) Background: There is a marked proportion of spondylodiscitis patients who die during the early stage of the disease despite the applied therapy. This study investigates this early mortality and explores the associated risk factors. (2) Methods: We conducted a retrospective analysis of spondylodiscitis patients treated at our Level I spine center between 1 January 2018 and 31 December 2022. (3) Results: Among 430 patients, 32 (7.4%) died during their hospital stay, with a median time of 28.5 days (range: 2.0–84.0 days). Six of these patients (18.75%) did not undergo surgery due to dire clinical conditions or death prior to scheduled surgery. Identified causes of in-hospital death included multiorgan failure ($n = 15$), acute bone marrow failure (2), cardiac failure (4), liver failure (2), acute respiratory failure (2), acute renal failure (1), and concomitant oncological disease (1). In a simple logistic regression analysis, advanced age ($p = 0.0006$), diabetes mellitus ($p = 0.0002$), previous steroid medication ($p = 0.0279$), Charlson Comorbidity Index ($p < 0.0001$), and GFR level at admission ($p = 0.0008$) were significant risk factors for in-hospital death. In a multiple logistic regression analysis, advanced age ($p = 0.0038$), diabetes mellitus ($p = 0.0002$), and previous steroid medication ($p = 0.0281$) remained significant. (4) Conclusions: Despite immediate treatment, a subset of spondylodiscitis patients experience early mortality. Particular attention should be given to elderly patients and those with diabetes or a history of steroid medication, as they face an elevated risk of a rapidly progressing and fatal disease.

**Keywords:** in-hospital death spondylodiscitis; vertebral osteomyelitis; spondylodiscitis; spinal infection

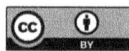

## 1. Introduction

Spondylodiscitis—the infection of the intervertebral disc and the adjacent vertebral bodies—is an infectious disease associated with high morbidity and mortality [1]. It primarily affects patients aged 70 years or older [1]. Men are 1.5 times more likely to be affected than women [1]. The incidence of spondylodiscitis is on the rise in Europe as well as in the United States, leading to a high socioeconomic burden [1–3]. Notably, in Germany, the incidence rose from 10.4 per 100,000 inhabitants in 2010 to 14.4 per 100,000 in 2020 [1]. In the United States, the incidence increased from 2.9 per 100,000 in 1998 to 5.4 per 100,000 in 2013 [2]. This trend can be attributed to the shifting demographic landscape, encompassing an aging population [4], and to an increase in multimorbid and immunocompromised patients [5,6]. Additionally, better diagnostic techniques and broader access to these diagnostic modalities have also contributed to the enhanced detection of spondylodiscitis cases [7]. Spondylodiscitis may arise through different mechanisms, including hematogenous spread from a distant focus of infection, dissemination from nearby tissue, or direct inoculation [8]. When spondylodiscitis is caused by hematogenous spread, it predominantly affects the lumbar spine (58%), followed by the thoracic (30%) and cervical spine (11%) [9]. In cases of hematogenous spread, the infection can extend beyond the bony structures and affect the surrounding tissue. In contrast, spondylodiscitis originating from dissemination from contiguous tissues is rare and is typically associated with adjacent infections such as esophageal fistula [10]. The mode of direct external inoculation is primarily iatrogenic, often arising from infiltrations or prior surgeries [11]. Although diagnostic and therapeutic guidelines have been established to optimize the management of patients with spondylodiscitis [12,13], delay of diagnosis due to the lack of specific symptoms is still a relevant problem [8]. Additionally, therapy for spondylodiscitis is not standardized and differs locally. The duration and method of antibiotic treatment, as well as the effectiveness of conservative versus surgical treatment, are still matters of debate. While numerous studies report favorable outcomes with low relapse and therapy failure rates [14], there is still a marked proportion of patients who die during the early stage of the disease despite adequate therapy [15]. Older age, diabetes, hemodialysis, endocarditis, malignant diseases, and liver cirrhosis have been identified as risk factors for the death of patients with spondylodiscitis [16]. However, the literature data on these severe cases are sparse. Understanding the present epidemiology and clinical characteristics of these severe cases is of utmost importance to ensure effective treatment. This study's aim was to describe the clinical data of patients with spondylodiscitis-related early mortality and to identify the associated risk factors.

## 2. Materials and Methods

### 2.1. Population

We conducted a retrospective study comprising consecutive patients treated for spondylodiscitis of the cervical, thoracic, or lumbosacral spine at a high-volume Level I surgical spine center between 1 January 2018 and 31 December 2022. Patients aged 18 years or older were included. Spondylodiscitis cases were retrieved from the hospital's database by screening for the International Classification of Diseases, Tenth Revision (ICD-10) code for spondylodiscitis. Patients' records, imaging data, laboratory and microbiological results, and surgical reports were analyzed. The following variables were extracted: age, sex, body mass index (BMI), American Association of Anesthesiologists (ASA) risk classification score, substance abuse, previous steroid medication, comorbidities, (previous or current) malignant disease, hepatopathy, diabetes mellitus, Charlson Comorbidity Index (CCI), C-reactive protein (CRP) level, neurologic status at admission and discharge, infective focus, bacteria cultivated, surgical strategy, and complications. The primary outcome measured was in-hospital mortality. Patients were divided into those with early mortality, i.e., who died during the same hospital stay, and those who survived the hospital stay. Patients who died after discharge from the hospital were excluded.

### 2.2. Diagnostics and Treatment

The diagnosis of spondylodiscitis was established based on the typical clinical presentation of the patients, along with the characteristic radiological features, and confirmed by positive pathogen detection in blood cultures or through CT-guided tissue biopsy. Culture-negative, mycobacterial, or fungal cases were also included in our analysis. The date of the hospitalization was assigned as the date of the diagnosis.

Magnetic resonance imaging (MRI) scans of the whole spine were performed in all patients. Computer tomography (CT) and/or positron emission tomography (PET) were performed if the MRI results were not conclusive enough or in patients who were not able to undergo MRI.

Septic condition at admission was defined by fulfilling at least two Systemic Inflammatory Response Syndrome (SIRS) criteria: body temperature over 38 or under 36 degrees Celsius; heart rate greater than 90 beats/minute; respiratory rate greater than 20 breaths/minute or partial pressure of $CO_2$ less than 32 mmHg; and leucocyte count >12,000/mm$^3$ or <4000/mm$^3$, or >10% bands.

In almost all cases, surgical therapy was performed except for severely affected patients with very high perioperative risks or patients who died prior to surgery. Surgery typically involved dorsal fixation with pedicle screws and decompression of the infected intervertebral disc space from the dorsal or ventral/lateral approach, followed by fusion using a cage, and local antibiotic application. Empirical antibiotic therapy, usually consisting of a combination of vancomycin and meropenem, was initiated promptly after biopsy collection or, in cases of severely affected patients with elevated inflammation markers, after the collection of blood cultures. Subsequently, antibiotic therapy was tailored to the specific spectrum of identified pathogens. All patients received a minimum of two weeks of intravenous antibiotic therapy, followed by a long-term oral regimen to complete a total of 12 weeks of antibiotic treatment.

### 2.3. Statistics

Simple logistic regression and multiple logistic regression analysis were used to identify risk factors for in-hospital mortality. A paired t-test (for continuous variables), Fisher's exact test (for categorical variables), and chi-square test (for categorical variables) were used to compare the clinical data of patients who died during the same hospital stay and of those who survived. Statistical analysis was performed with GraphPad Prism 10.0.2 (Boston, MA, USA).

## 3. Results

### 3.1. Demographic Background

Over the course of a five-year study period, we enrolled 430 patients with a median age of 72 years (ranging from 30 to 94 years) in our research cohort. Among these participants, 271 (63.0%) were male and 159 (37.0%) were female (Table 1). In total, 32 (7.4%) patients died during the same hospital stay (early mortality group) after a median time of 28.5 days (2.0–84.0 days), while 14 (3.3%) died after being discharged from hospital after a median time of 313 days (54–990 days). These 14 patients were subsequently excluded from further analysis. Consequently, 384 patients (98.3%) successfully survived throughout the study period, with a median follow-up duration of 86 days (ranging from 20 to 1232 days). The median hospital stay for surviving patients was 14 days (2–110 days). This was primarily determined by the duration of intravenous antibiotics.

Notably, the patients in the early mortality group were significantly older than those who survived ($p = 0.0018$) (Table 1). Furthermore, there were significant disparities in the American Association of Anesthesiologists (ASA) risk classification scores between the two groups ($p < 0.0001$). Specifically, patients in the early mortality group were more likely to have a more severe ASA score (IV and V) compared to their counterparts who survived. Additionally, the early mortality group exhibited a notably higher Charlson Comorbidity Index (CCI) compared to those who survived ($p < 0.0001$).

While both groups were comparable regarding body mass index (BMI), alcohol abuse, IV drug abuse, hepatopathy, and history of malignant diseases, the proportion of patients on steroid medication ($p = 0.0242$) and with diabetes mellitus ($p = 0.0004$) was significantly higher in the early mortality group (Table 1).

### 3.2. Characterization of Spondylodiscitis

In most instances, spondylodiscitis was acquired endogenously, indicating that it occurred without any prior spinal surgery on the same spinal level (Table 2). For both groups, the lumbosacral region emerged as the predominant site for spondylodiscitis (Figure 1A,B). However, it is noteworthy that 25.0% of patients who experienced early mortality had multifocal spondylodiscitis, whereas this occurred in only 11.7% of patients who survived ($p = 0.0477$). Among the surviving patients, there was a trend, albeit statistically non-significant, towards less frequent occurrences of epidural empyema and paravertebral abscess compared to patients with early mortality (Table 2).

Table 1. Demographic overview. Shows a comparison of the patients' baseline characteristics. ASA = American Association of Anesthesiologists, BMI = body mass index, CCI = Charlson Comorbidity Index. A paired *t*-test (for continuous variables) and Fisher's exact test/chi-square test (for categorical variables) were used.

|  | All N (%) | Surviving (S) N (%) | In-Hospital Mortality (M) N (%) | *p*-Value (S vs. M) |
|---|---|---|---|---|
| Total | 430 | 384 | 32 | |
| Age (y) | | | | |
| Median | 72.0 | 70.5 | 76.5 | 0.0018 |
| Min. | 30.0 | 30.0 | 62.0 | |
| Max. | 94.0 | 94.0 | 91.0 | |
| Sex | | | | |
| Male | 271 (63.02) | 238 (61.98) | 24 (75.00) | n.s. |
| Female | 159 (36.98) | 146 (38.02) | 8 (25.00) | |
| BMI (kg/m$^2$) | | | | |
| Mean | 26.7 | 26.9 | 26.8 | n.s. |
| STD | 6.4 | 6.1 | 4.7 | |
| ASA | | | | |
| I | 8 (1.86) | 8 (2.08) | 0 (0.00) | |
| II | 117 (27.21) | 111 (28.91) | 4 (12.50) | n.a. |
| III | 259 (60.23) | 232 (60.42) | 16 (50.00) | |
| IV | 41 (9.53) | 32 (8.33) | 8 (25.00) | |
| V | 5 (1.16) | 1 (0.26) | 4 (12.50) | |
| ASA | | | | |
| I–III | 384 (89.30) | 351 (91.40) | 20 (62.50) | <0.0001 |
| IV–V | 46 (10.70) | 33 (8.60) | 12 (37.50) | |
| CCI | | | | |
| Median | 4.0 | 4.0 | 6.5 | <0.0001 |
| Min. | 0.0 | 0.0 | 3.0 | |
| Max. | 12.0 | 12.0 | 12.0 | |
| Alcohol abuse | | | | n.s. |
| Present | 24 (5.58) | 22 (5.73) | 2 (6.25) | |
| Absent | 406 (94.42) | 362 (94.27) | 30 (93.75) | |
| Drugs IV | | | | |
| Present | 18 (4.19) | 18 (4.69) | 0 (0.00) | n.s. |
| Absent | 412 (95.81) | 366 (95.31) | 32 (100.00) | |
| Diabetes mellitus | | | | 0.0004 |
| Present | 125 (29.07) | 103 (26.82) | 19 (59.38) | |
| Absent | 305 (70.93) | 281 (73.18) | 13 (40.62) | |
| Hepatopathy | | | | |
| Present | 46 (10.70) | 39 (10.16) | 4 (12.50) | n.s. |
| Absent | 384 (89.30) | 345 (89.84) | 28 (87.50) | |
| Steroids | | | | |
| Present | 23 (5.35) | 18 (4.69) | 5 (15.62) | 0.0242 |
| Absent | 407 (94.65) | 366 (95.31) | 27 (84.38) | |
| Malignant disease | | | | n.s. |
| Present | 56 (13.02) | 46 (11.98) | 5 (15.62) | |
| Absent | 374 (86.98) | 338 (88.02) | 27 (84.38) | |

n.s. = non significant; n.a. = not applicable.

**Table 2.** Details of spondylodiscitis. Compares the details of spondylodiscitis between the different groups. Secondarily acquired was defined as prior spinal surgery on the same spinal level. CRP = C-reactive protein. A paired *t*-test (for continuous variables) and Fisher's exact test/chi-square test (for categorical variables) were used.

|  | All N (%) | Surviving (S) N (%) | In-Hospital Mortality (M) N (%) | *p*-Value (S vs. M) |
|---|---|---|---|---|
| Total | 430 | 384 | 32 |  |
| **Etiology** |  |  |  | 0.0058 |
| Endogenously | 318 (73.95) | 278 (72.40) | 30 (93.75) |  |
| Secondarily | 112 (26.05) | 106 (27.60) | 2 (6.25) |  |
| **Localization** |  |  |  | n.a. |
| Cervical | 47 (10.93) | 43 (11.20) | 3 (9.38) |  |
| Thoracic | 68 (15.81) | 61 (15.89) | 5 (15.63) |  |
| Lumbosacral | 260 (60.47) | 235 (61.20) | 16 (50.00) |  |
| Multifocal | 55 (12.79) | 45 (11.72) | 8 (25.00) |  |
| Unifocal | 375 (87.21) | 339 (88.28) | 24 (75.00) | 0.0477 |
| Multifocal | 55 (12.79) | 45 (11.72) | 8 (25.00) |  |
| **Epidural empyema** |  |  |  | n.s. |
| Present | 200 (46.51) | 177 (46.09) | 16 (50.00) |  |
| Absent | 230 (53.49) | 207 (53.91) | 16 (50.00) |  |
| **Paravertebral abscess** |  |  |  | n.s. |
| Present | 161 (37.44) | 141 (36.72) | 16 (50.00) |  |
| Absent | 269 (62.56) | 243 (63.82) | 16 (50.00) |  |
| **CRP (mg/dL)** |  |  |  | 0.0437 |
| Median | 8.1 | 7.5 | 12.2 |  |
| Min. | 0.1 | 0.1 | 1.6 |  |
| Max. | 50.4 | 50.4 | 41.2 |  |
| **Treated surgically** |  |  |  | 0.0003 |
| Yes | 415 (96.51) | 376 (97.92) | 26 (81.25) |  |
| No | 15 (3.49) | 8 (2.08) | 6 (18.75) |  |

n.s. = non significant; n.a. = not applicable.

C-reactive protein (CRP) level at admission was significantly higher for patients who died during the same hospital stay.

Interestingly, only five (15.6%) patients experiencing early mortality were admitted in a clinically compromised state necessitating intensive care therapy. The vast majority (84.4%) initially presented in a stable general condition but experienced rapid deterioration during their hospitalization. Of the surviving patients, 20.8% had sepsis at admission and 10.2% suffered from sepsis-induced hepatopathy. Of patients with in-hospital mortality, 50.0% had sepsis when admitted to hospital and 12.5% suffered from hepatopathy. While almost all surviving patients were treated surgically, 18.8% of patients in the early mortality group did not receive surgical treatment due to their swift deterioration and death before scheduled surgery.

Table 3 provides an overview of patients' neurological status at admission. Patients with early mortality were more likely to exhibit significant motor deficits (as indicated by a Medical Research Council Scale for Muscle Strength score of 3 or less) ($p = 0.0064$) or bowel/bladder dysfunction ($p = 0.0054$) compared to those who survived.

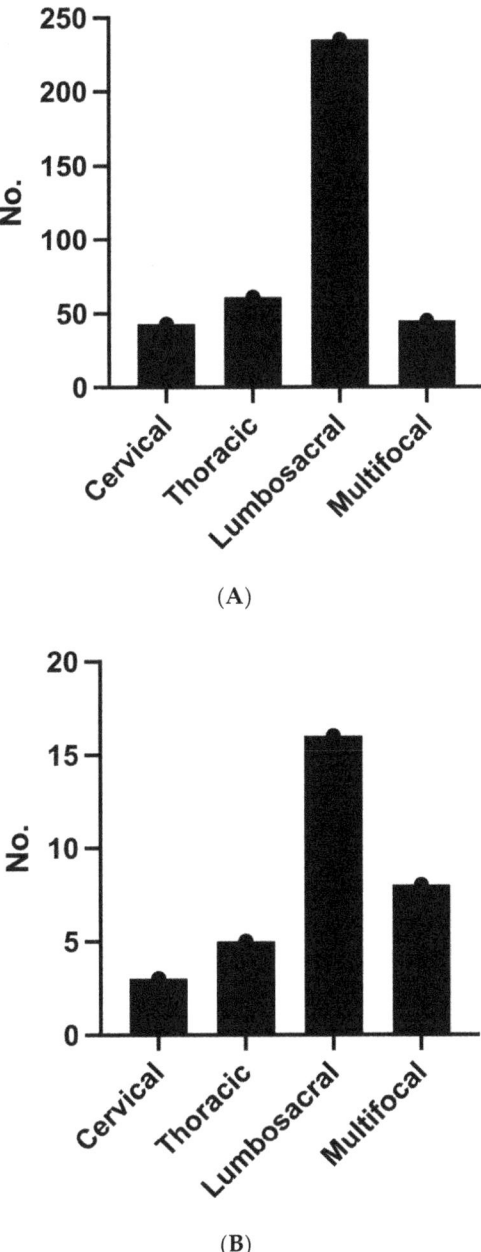

**Figure 1.** (**A**): Localization of spondylodiscitis in the survivor group. Cervical: $n = 43$; thoracic: $n = 61$; lumbosacral: $n = 235$; multifocal: $n = 45$. (**B**): Localization of spondylodiscitis in early mortality group. Cervical: $n = 3$; thoracic: $n = 5$; lumbosacral: $n = 16$; multifocal: $n = 8$.

### 3.3. Focus of Spondylodiscitis and Microbiology

Among patients in the early mortality group, the most prevalent sources of infection were joint empyema (21.9%), urosepsis (18.8%), and leg ulcers (15.6%), respectively (Table 4). In contrast, for surviving patients, the primary source of infection was prior spinal surgery

(29.4%) (Table 5). Notably, 4 out of 32 patients (12.5%) in the early mortality group were afflicted with endocarditis (Table 4), in comparison to 19 out of 384 surviving patients (4.9%), although this difference was not statistically significant. Patients with endocarditis in the early mortality group exhibited a significantly worse ASA score than those without endocarditis in the same group ($p = 0.0138$).

**Table 3.** Neurological examination. Shows the neurological status at admission to the hospital indicated by muscle strength grades according to the Medical Research Council (MRC) scale, with 0 representing the worst and 5 the best muscle strength grade. Fisher's exact test was used.

|  | Surviving (S) N (%) | In-Hospital Mortality (M) N (%) | $p$-Value (S vs. M) |
|---|---|---|---|
| Total | 384 | 32 |  |
| MRC |  |  |  |
| 5 | 250 (65.10) | 15 (46.88) |  |
| 4 | 60 (15.63) | 2 (6.25) |  |
| 3 | 22 (5.73) | 2 (6.25) | n.a. |
| 2 | 16 (4.17) | 6 (18.75) |  |
| 1 | 12 (3.13) | 1 (3.13) |  |
| 0 | 20 (5.21) | 3 (9.38) |  |
| n.a. | 4 (1.04) | 3 (9.38) |  |
| MRC |  |  |  |
| 5–4 | 310 (80.73) | 17 (53.12) |  |
| 3–0 | 70 (18.23) | 12 (37.50) | 0.0064 |
| n.a. | 4 (1.04) | 3 (9.38) |  |
| Bladder/bowel dysfunction |  |  |  |
| Yes | 51 (13.28) | 9 (28.13) | 0.0054 |
| No | 331 (86.20) | 16 (50.00) |  |
| n.a. | 2 (0.52) | 7 (21.88) |  |

n.a. = not applicable.

**Table 4.** Infective focus of the early mortality group. Depicts the infective focus of patients in the early mortality group. In six cases, more than one focus was found.

| Infective Focus | N (%) 32 |
|---|---|
| Joint empyema | 7 (21.9) |
| Urogenital tract | 6 (18.8) |
| Leg ulcers | 5 (15.6) |
| Endocarditis | 4 (12.5) |
| Prior spinal surgery | 2 (6.3) |
| Pulmonal | 2 (6.3) |
| Catheter-associated | 2 (6.3) |
| Teeth | 1 (3.1) |
| Ears–Nose–Throat | 1 (3.1) |
| Not found | 7 (21.9) |

Table 5. Infective focus of the survivor group. Shows the infective focus of patients in the survivor group. In 36 cases, more than one focus was found.

| Infective Focus | N (%) 384 |
|---|---|
| Prior spinal surgery | 113 (29.4) |
| Joint empyema | 38 (9.9) |
| Urogenital tract | 37 (9.6) |
| Teeth | 36 (9.4) |
| Leg ulcers | 29 (7.6) |
| Endocarditis | 19 (4.9) |
| Prior spinal infiltration | 16 (4.2) |
| Pulmonal | 11 (2.9) |
| Catheter-associated | 10 (2.6) |
| Ears–Nose–Throat | 10 (2.6) |
| Peritonitis | 3 (0.8) |
| Hepatic abscess | 1 (0.3) |
| Cholangitis | 1 (0.3) |
| Infected aortic prosthesis | 1 (0.3) |
| Not found | 95 (24.7) |

Bacterial cultures of infected disc tissue were successfully obtained in 78.9% of surviving patients and 81.3% of patients with early mortality, respectively. In both groups, the most frequently isolated pathogen was *Staphylococcus aureus*, followed by *Staphylococcus epidermidis* and *Cutibacterium acnes* (Figure 2A,B). *Mycobacterium tuberculosis* was found in three cases (0.8%) among surviving patients and in none of the patients with early mortality. A fungal infection with *Candida albicans* was detected in three cases (0.8%) among the surviving patients, whereas in patients with early mortality, it was observed in one case (3.1%).

*3.4. In-Hospital Mortality: Causes and Risk Factors*

The overall in-hospital mortality rate was 7.4%, comprising 32 out of 430 patients. The documented causes of in-hospital mortality were multiorgan failure ($n = 15$), acute bone marrow failure ($n = 2$), cardiac failure ($n = 4$), cirrhosis-related liver failure ($n = 2$), acute respiratory failure ($n = 2$), acute renal failure ($n = 1$), and the presence of concomitant oncological disease ($n = 1$). In five cases, a single specific cause of death could not be identified.

In a simple logistic regression analysis, advanced age ($p = 0.0006$), diabetes mellitus ($p = 0.0002$), previous steroid medication ($p = 0.0279$), Charlson Comorbidity Index (CCI) ($p < 0.0001$), and glomerular filtration rate (GFR) level at admission ($p = 0.0008$) were significant risk factors for in-hospital death (Supplementary Table S1). However, variables such as BMI, CRP level at admission, history of malignant disease, alcohol abuse, hepatopathy, endocarditis, paraspinal abscess, and intraspinal empyema did not reach statistical significance. A multiple logistic regression analysis identified advanced age ($p = 0.0038$), diabetes mellitus ($p = 0.0002$), and previous steroid medication ($p = 0.0281$) as significant risk factors for in-hospital death (Supplementary Table S2).

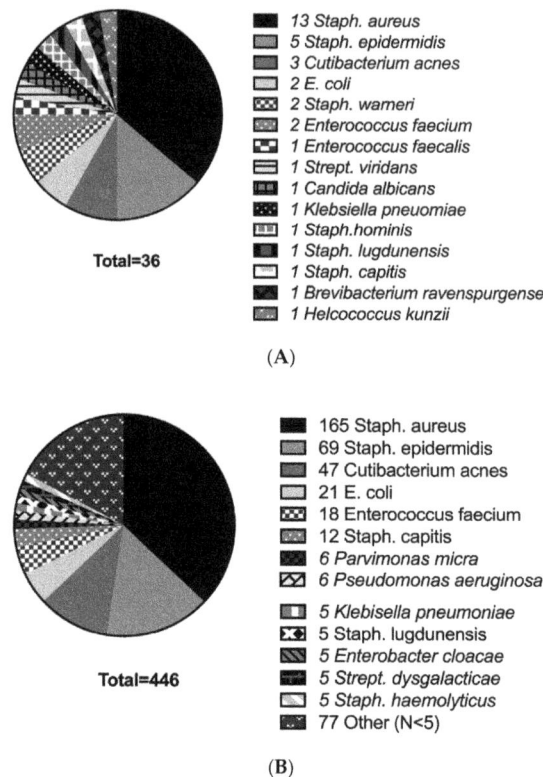

**Figure 2.** (**A**). Microbiological results of the early mortality group. (**A**) shows the results of microbiological cultivation (blood cultures and tissue) in the early mortality group. E. = *Eschericha*; *Staph.* = *Staphylococcus*; *Strept.* = *Streptococcus*. (**B**). Microbiological results of the survivor group. (**B**) shows the results of microbiological cultivation (blood cultures and tissue) in the survivor group. For the sake of clarity, bacteria that were detected fewer than 5 times were grouped under the category "Other". E. = *Eschericha*; *Staph.* = *Staphylococcus*; *Strept.* = *Streptococcus*.

## 4. Discussion

This study aimed to investigate the rate of in-hospital mortality in patients with spondylodiscitis and explore its associated risk factors.

Over the five-year study period, the in-hospital mortality rate was 7.4% (32 out of 430). This rate is consistent with findings from a large-scale Japanese study (6%) [16] and a smaller study conducted in the United Kingdom (7%) [17]. However, recent German studies reported even higher in-hospital mortality rates ranging from 10 to 14% [15,18–20]. This persistently high mortality underscores that spondylodiscitis remains a potentially life-threatening disease, despite advancements in diagnostic and treatment approaches. It should be recognized and treated not merely as a localized infection of bones and intervertebral discs but also as a systemic disease. As a result, the primary treatment objectives must focus on managing the infection by addressing the underlying systemic condition and eliminating the source of infection. Antibiotic therapy should be tailored to the results of microbiological cultivation. In our study, the majority of patients were treated surgically. Conservative treatment options can effectively manage many cases; however, they may not always be sufficient. In general, surgical intervention should be considered when conservative treatment proves ineffective and when symptoms or imaging results indicate disease progression [8]. Immediate surgical intervention is essential when patients present with neurologic impairments, septic disease progression, or progressive deformity [21]. We and many other centers are opting for early surgery including cases without neurologic impairments or deformity as complications arising from immobilization and ongoing infection can be particularly severe in today's older and comorbid population. Moreover, during the early stages of the infection, minimally invasive procedures reducing surgical trauma, intraoperative blood loss, and postoperative complications [22] may still be viable, while extensive strategies are required at later stages with significant bony destruction and deformity.

Our data revealed that patients with early mortality often presented with a more extensive infection, characterized by a higher prevalence of paravertebral manifestations, neurological deficits, and septic condition. Interestingly, only a small percentage of patients with early mortality were admitted in an unstable general condition necessitating intensive care therapy. This suggests that clinical deterioration may occur later in the disease course in a certain subset of patients, emphasizing the importance of identifying risk factors for rapid deterioration at an early stage of the disease.

For patients with early mortality, the most prevalent sources of infection were joint empyema (21.9%), urosepsis (18.8%), and leg ulcers (15.6%), while for surviving patients, the primary source of infection was a prior spinal surgery (29.4%). These data are in line with results from Lener et al. [23]: they reported that deceased patients were more frequently affected by primary acquired spondylodiscitis compared to surviving patients. In a large-scale nationwide study of 10,695 spondylodiscitis patients, Kim et al. [24] documented the most frequent concurrent infections as urinary tract infections (11.3%), intra-abdominal infections (9.4%), pneumonia (8.5%), and septic arthritis (4.6%). Moreover, they found that patients with concurrent infection had a four-fold higher mortality than those without. Kim et al. registered concurrent infections, whereas we identified the infective focus of spondylodiscitis. This explains why typical hospital-acquired infections were numerically predominant in the study by Kim et al. On the other hand, in some infections, such as endocarditis or joint empyema, retrospectively, it will never be possible to distinguish whether they are the infective focus of spondylodiscitis or concurrent infections. However, for clinical practice, this distinction is not relevant, as the treatment does not differ. In both cases, the infection must be addressed.

Known risk factors for the development of spondylodiscitis in general include advanced age, obesity, diabetes mellitus, substance abuse, immunodeficiency, and long-term steroid medication [8]. The present study identified advanced age, diabetes mellitus, previous steroid medication, higher CCI, and lower glomerular filtration rate (GFR) level at admission as significant risk factors for in-hospital death from spondylodiscitis. A recent German study reported increasing age, elevated creatinine and CRP levels, and the presence of rheumatoid arthritis as significant risk factors for in-hospital mortality from spondylodiscitis [15], whereas in the present study, CRP level at admission did not reach statistical significance. Additionally, unlike a study from Ohio that identified epidural empyema, neurologic deficits, in-hospital acquisition, and time to diagnosis as risk factors for an adverse outcome [25], our study did not find epidural empyema to be a significant factor. Contrary to findings from a Japanese study [16], in the present study, a history of malignant disease, hepatopathy, and endocarditis were not associated with an elevated risk for in-hospital death from spondylodiscitis.

Interestingly, the bacterial spectrum did not differ between patients with early mortality and surviving patients. For both groups, the most frequently detected bacterium was *Staphylococcus aureus*, which is the most common pathogen for spondylodiscitis in Europe [26–28]. Other studies have reported increased mortality, complication rates, and treatment failure rates for spondylodiscitis patients with *Staphylococcus aureus* bacteremia [15,20,28,29].

Our study has several limitations. First, being retrospective, it relies on historical data, which may not be as comprehensive as those provided by prospective trials, particularly regarding comorbidities, prior medication, and prior clinical course before admission to hospital. Second, group sizes differed significantly, a fact that is inherent to the nature of the matter and cannot be overcome. Third, the follow-up period for surviving patients was not standardized. However, the primary outcome was in-hospital death compared to patients who survived this period, not long-term outcomes. Additionally, some potentially predictive factors were not considered in our analysis, either due to their perceived lack of relevance or unavailability in a retrospective setting.

However, it is important to note that one of the study's strengths lies in its substantial sample size, encompassing consecutive patients treated at a single specialized center known for its high treatment standards, over an extended five-year period.

## 5. Conclusions

The present study demonstrates that even if admitted in a moderate clinical condition and if maximum medical treatment is applied immediately, a certain proportion of patients with spondylodiscitis die during their hospital stay. Special attention should be paid to elderly patients and to patients with diabetes or steroid medication who harbor an elevated risk for a fulminant disease with fatal consequences.

**Supplementary Materials:** The following supporting information can be downloaded at: https://www.mdpi.com/article/10.3390/jcm12237228/s1, Table S1: Results of simple logistic regression analysis. Table S2: Results of multiple logistic regression analysis.

**Author Contributions:** Conceptualization: B.M., M.W. and A.-K.J.; formal analysis: A.-K.J. and N.L.; investigation: A.-K.J., N.L. and C.A.; data curation: A.-K.J. and C.A.; writing—original draft preparation: A.-K.J. and M.W.; writing— review and editing: A.-K.J., C.A., N.L., B.M. and M.W.; visualization: A.-K.J.; supervision, B.M. and M.W.; project administration, A.-K.J. and M.W. All authors have read and agreed to the published version of the manuscript.

**Funding:** This research received no external funding.

**Institutional Review Board Statement:** The study was approved by the ethics committee of our university (reference number 2023-324-S-SR) and conducted in accordance with the Declaration of Helsinki. The need for informed consent was waived by the ethical committee as it was a retrospective study.

**Informed Consent Statement:** The need for informed consent was waived by the ethical committee as this was a retrospective study.

**Data Availability Statement:** The data presented in this study are available on request from the corresponding author.

**Conflicts of Interest:** B.M. received honoraria, consulting fees, and research grants from Medtronic (Meerbusch, Germany), Icotec AG (Altstätten, Switzerland), and Relievant Medsystems Inc. (Sunnyvale, CA, USA), honoraria and research grants from Ulrich Medical (Ulm, Germany), honoraria and consulting fees from Spineart Deutschland GmbH (Frankfurt, Germany) and DePuy Synthes (West Chester, PA, USA), and royalties from Spineart Deutschland GmbH (Frankfurt, Germany). B.M. is a consultant for Brainlab AG (Munich, Germany). M.W. is a consultant for Medacta International (Castel San Pietro, Switzerland) and Ulrich Medical (Ulm, Germany). A.-K.J., N.L., and C.A. do not have any financial stake. All authors declare that they have no conflict of interest concerning this research.

## References

1. Lang, S.; Walter, N.; Schindler, M.; Baertl, S.; Szymski, D.; Loibl, M.; Alt, V.; Rupp, M. The Epidemiology of Spondylodiscitis in Germany: A Descriptive Report of Incidence Rates, Pathogens, In-Hospital Mortality, and Hospital Stays between 2010 and 2020. *J. Clin. Med.* **2023**, *12*, 3373. [CrossRef] [PubMed]
2. Issa, K.; Diebo, B.G.; Faloon, M.; Naziri, Q.; Pourtaheri, S.; Paulino, C.B.; Emami, A. The Epidemiology of Vertebral Osteomyelitis in the United States from 1998 to 2013. *Clin. Spine Surg.* **2018**, *31*, E102–E108. [CrossRef] [PubMed]
3. Conan, Y.; Laurent, E.; Belin, Y.; Lacasse, M.; Amelot, A.; Mulleman, D.; Rosset, P.; Bernard, L.; Grammatico-Guillon, L. Large increase of vertebral osteomyelitis in France: A 2010–2019 cross-sectional study. *Epidemiol. Infect.* **2021**, *149*, e227. [CrossRef] [PubMed]
4. Kehrer, M.; Pedersen, C.; Jensen, T.G.; Lassen, A.T. Increasing incidence of pyogenic spondylodiscitis: A 14-year population-based study. *J. Infect.* **2014**, *68*, 313–320. [CrossRef] [PubMed]

5. Puth, M.T.; Weckbecker, K.; Schmid, M.; Munster, E. Prevalence of multimorbidity in Germany: Impact of age and educational level in a cross-sectional study on 19,294 adults. *BMC Public Health* **2017**, *17*, 826. [CrossRef]
6. Herren, C.; von der Hoeh, N.H.; Zwingenberger, S.; Sauer, D.; Jung, N.; Pieroh, P.; Drange, S.; Pumberger, M.; Scheyerer, M.J.; Spine Section of the German Society for Orthopaedics and Trauma. Spondylodiscitis in Geriatric Patients: What Are the Issues? *Global Spine J.* **2023**, *13*, 73S–84S. [CrossRef] [PubMed]
7. Kouijzer, I.J.E.; Scheper, H.; de Rooy, J.W.J.; Bloem, J.L.; Janssen, M.J.R.; van den Hoven, L.; Hosman, A.J.F.; Visser, L.G.; Oyen, W.J.G.; Bleeker-Rovers, C.P.; et al. The diagnostic value of (18)F-FDG-PET/CT and MRI in suspected vertebral osteomyelitis—A prospective study. *Eur. J. Nucl. Med. Mol. Imaging* **2018**, *45*, 798–805. [CrossRef] [PubMed]
8. Lener, S.; Hartmann, S.; Barbagallo, G.M.V.; Certo, F.; Thome, C.; Tschugg, A. Management of spinal infection: A review of the literature. *Acta Neurochir.* **2018**, *160*, 487–496. [CrossRef]
9. Mylona, E.; Samarkos, M.; Kakalou, E.; Fanourgiakis, P.; Skoutelis, A. Pyogenic vertebral osteomyelitis: A systematic review of clinical characteristics. *Semin. Arthritis Rheum.* **2009**, *39*, 10–17. [CrossRef]
10. Janssen, I.; Shiban, E.; Rienmuller, A.; Ryang, Y.M.; Chaker, A.M.; Meyer, B. Treatment considerations for cervical and cervicothoracic spondylodiscitis associated with esophageal fistula due to cancer history or accidental injury: A 9-patient case series. *Acta Neurochir.* **2019**, *161*, 1877–1886. [CrossRef]
11. Silber, J.S.; Anderson, D.G.; Vaccaro, A.R.; Anderson, P.A.; McCormick, P. Management of postprocedural discitis. *Spine J.* **2002**, *2*, 279–287. [CrossRef] [PubMed]
12. Herren, C.; von der Höh, N.; im Namen der Leitlinienkommission der Deutschen, W. Zusammenfassung der S2K-Leitlinie "Diagnostik und Therapie der Spondylodiszitis" (Stand 08/2020). *Die Wirbelsäule* **2021**, *5*, 18–20. [CrossRef]
13. Berbari, E.F.; Kanj, S.S.; Kowalski, T.J.; Darouiche, R.O.; Widmer, A.F.; Schmitt, S.K.; Hendershot, E.F.; Holtom, P.D.; Huddleston, P.M., 3rd; Petermann, G.W.; et al. 2015 Infectious Diseases Society of America (IDSA) Clinical Practice Guidelines for the Diagnosis and Treatment of Native Vertebral Osteomyelitis in Adults. *Clin. Infect. Dis.* **2015**, *61*, e26–e46. [CrossRef] [PubMed]
14. Rutges, J.P.; Kempen, D.H.; van Dijk, M.; Oner, F.C. Outcome of conservative and surgical treatment of pyogenic spondylodiscitis: A systematic literature review. *Eur. Spine J.* **2016**, *25*, 983–999. [CrossRef] [PubMed]
15. Heuer, A.; Strahl, A.; Viezens, L.; Koepke, L.G.; Stangenberg, M.; Dreimann, M. The Hamburg Spondylodiscitis Assessment Score (HSAS) for Immediate Evaluation of Mortality Risk on Hospital Admission. *J. Clin. Med.* **2022**, *11*, 660. [CrossRef] [PubMed]
16. Akiyama, T.; Chikuda, H.; Yasunaga, H.; Horiguchi, H.; Fushimi, K.; Saita, K. Incidence and risk factors for mortality of vertebral osteomyelitis: A retrospective analysis using the Japanese diagnosis procedure combination database. *BMJ Open* **2013**, *3*, e002412. [CrossRef] [PubMed]
17. Widdrington, J.D.; Emmerson, I.; Cullinan, M.; Narayanan, M.; Klejnow, E.; Watson, A.; Ong, E.L.C.; Schmid, M.L.; Price, D.A.; Schwab, U.; et al. Pyogenic Spondylodiscitis: Risk Factors for Adverse Clinical Outcome in Routine Clinical Practice. *Med. Sci.* **2018**, *6*, 96. [CrossRef] [PubMed]
18. Lang, S.; Fromming, A.; Walter, N.; Freigang, V.; Neumann, C.; Loibl, M.; Ehrenschwender, M.; Alt, V.; Rupp, M. Is There a Difference in Clinical Features, Microbiological Epidemiology and Effective Empiric Antimicrobial Therapy Comparing Healthcare-Associated and Community-Acquired Vertebral Osteomyelitis? *Antibiotics* **2021**, *10*, 1410. [CrossRef]
19. Lenz, M.; Harland, A.; Egenolf, P.; Horbach, M.; von Hodenberg, C.; Brinkkoetter, P.T.; Benzing, T.; Eysel, P.; Scheyerer, M.J. Correlation between kidney function and mortality in pyogenic spondylodiscitis: The glomerular filtration rate (GFR) as new predictive parameter? *Eur. Spine J.* **2023**, *32*, 1455–1462. [CrossRef]
20. Loibl, M.; Stoyanov, L.; Doenitz, C.; Brawanski, A.; Wiggermann, P.; Krutsch, W.; Nerlich, M.; Oszwald, M.; Neumann, C.; Salzberger, B.; et al. Outcome-related co-factors in 105 cases of vertebral osteomyelitis in a tertiary care hospital. *Infection* **2014**, *42*, 503–510. [CrossRef]
21. Ryang, Y.M.; Akbar, M. Pyogenic spondylodiscitis: Symptoms, diagnostics and therapeutic strategies. *Orthopade* **2020**, *49*, 691–701. [CrossRef] [PubMed]
22. Janssen, I.K.; Jorger, A.K.; Barz, M.; Sarkar, C.; Wostrack, M.; Meyer, B. Minimally invasive posterior pedicle screw fixation versus open instrumentation in patients with thoracolumbar spondylodiscitis. *Acta Neurochir.* **2021**, *163*, 1553–1560. [CrossRef] [PubMed]
23. Lener, S.; Wipplinger, C.; Stocsits, A.; Hartmann, S.; Hofer, A.; Thome, C. Early surgery may lower mortality in patients suffering from severe spinal infection. *Acta Neurochir.* **2020**, *162*, 2887–2894. [CrossRef]
24. Kim, J.; Oh, S.H.; Kim, S.W.; Kim, T.H. The epidemiology of concurrent infection in patients with pyogenic spine infection and its association with early mortality: A nationwide cohort study based on 10,695 patients. *J. Infect. Public Health* **2023**, *16*, 981–988. [CrossRef] [PubMed]
25. McHenry, M.C.; Easley, K.A.; Locker, G.A. Vertebral osteomyelitis: Long-term outcome for 253 patients from 7 Cleveland-area hospitals. *Clin. Infect. Dis.* **2002**, *34*, 1342–1350. [CrossRef] [PubMed]
26. Lackermair, S.; Egermann, H.; Muller, A. Distribution of Underlying Causative Organisms, Patient Age, and Survival in Spontaneous spondylodiscitis with Special Focus on Elderly Patients. *J. Neurol. Surg. A Cent. Eur. Neurosurg.* **2023**, *84*, 8–13. [CrossRef] [PubMed]
27. Herren, C.; Jung, N.; Pishnamaz, M.; Breuninger, M.; Siewe, J.; Sobottke, R. Spondylodiscitis: Diagnosis and Treatment Options. *Dtsch. Arztebl. Int.* **2017**, *114*, 875–882. [CrossRef]

28. Bernard, L.; Dinh, A.; Ghout, I.; Simo, D.; Zeller, V.; Issartel, B.; Le Moing, V.; Belmatoug, N.; Lesprit, P.; Bru, J.P.; et al. Antibiotic treatment for 6 weeks versus 12 weeks in patients with pyogenic vertebral osteomyelitis: An open-label, non-inferiority, randomised, controlled trial. *Lancet* **2015**, *385*, 875–882. [CrossRef]
29. Stangenberg, M.; Mende, K.C.; Mohme, M.; Kratzig, T.; Viezens, L.; Both, A.; Rohde, H.; Dreimann, M. Influence of microbiological diagnosis on the clinical course of spondylodiscitis. *Infection* **2021**, *49*, 1017–1027. [CrossRef]

**Disclaimer/Publisher's Note:** The statements, opinions and data contained in all publications are solely those of the individual author(s) and contributor(s) and not of MDPI and/or the editor(s). MDPI and/or the editor(s) disclaim responsibility for any injury to people or property resulting from any ideas, methods, instructions or products referred to in the content.

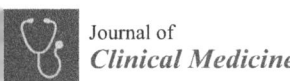 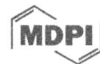

*Article*

# The Efficacy of Daily Local Antibiotic Lavage via an Epidural Suction–Irrigation Drainage Technique in Spondylodiscitis and Isolated Spinal Epidural Empyema: A 20-Year Experience of a Single Spine Center

Mido Max Hijazi [1,*], Timo Siepmann [2], Ibrahim El-Battrawy [3], Percy Schröttner [4], Dino Podlesek [1], Kay Engellandt [5], Gabriele Schackert [1], Tareq A. Juratli [1], Ilker Y. Eyüpoglu [1] and Andreas Filis [1]

1. Technische Universität Dresden, Faculty of Medicine, and University Hospital Carl Gustav Carus, Department of Neurosurgery, Division of Spine Surgery, Fetscherstrasse 74, 01307 Dresden, Germany; dino.podlesek@ukdd.de (D.P.); gabriele.schackert@ukdd.de (G.S.); tareq.juratli@ukdd.de (T.A.J.); ilker.eyuepoglu@ukdd.de (I.Y.E.); afilis@neuromaster.gr (A.F.)
2. Technische Universität Dresden, Faculty of Medicine, and University Hospital Carl Gustav Carus, Department of Neurology, Fetscherstrasse 74, 01307 Dresden, Germany; timo.siepmann@ukdd.de
3. Bergmannsheil University Hospitals Bergmannsheil, Ruhr University Bochum, Department of Cardiology, Bürkle de la Camp-Platz 1, 44789 Bochum, Germany; ibrahim.elbattrawy2006@gmail.com
4. Technische Universität Dresden, Faculty of Medicine, and University Hospital Carl Gustav Carus, Institute for Microbiology and Virology, Fetscherstrasse 74, 01307 Dresden, Germany; percy.schroettner@ukdd.de
5. Technische Universität Dresden, Faculty of Medicine, and University Hospital Carl Gustav Carus, Institute of Diagnostic and Interventional Neuroradiology, Fetscherstrasse 74, 01307 Dresden, Germany; kay.engellandt@ukdd.de
* Correspondence: mido.hijazi@ukdd.de; Tel.: +49-1-799-847-820

**Citation:** Hijazi, M.M.; Siepmann, T.; El-Battrawy, I.; Schröttner, P.; Podlesek, D.; Engellandt, K.; Schackert, G.; Juratli, T.A.; Eyüpoglu, I.Y.; Filis, A. The Efficacy of Daily Local Antibiotic Lavage via an Epidural Suction–Irrigation Drainage Technique in Spondylodiscitis and Isolated Spinal Epidural Empyema: A 20-Year Experience of a Single Spine Center. *J. Clin. Med.* **2023**, *12*, 5078. https://doi.org/10.3390/jcm12155078

Academic Editor: Kalliopi Alpantaki

Received: 8 July 2023
Revised: 29 July 2023
Accepted: 31 July 2023
Published: 2 August 2023

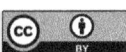

**Copyright:** © 2023 by the authors. Licensee MDPI, Basel, Switzerland. This article is an open access article distributed under the terms and conditions of the Creative Commons Attribution (CC BY) license (https://creativecommons.org/licenses/by/4.0/).

**Abstract:** Background: Various treatment modalities are available for local antibiotic therapy in spondylodiscitis (SD) and isolated spinal epidural empyema (ISEE), but there is no evidence-based recommendation. Postoperative epidural suction–irrigation drainage (ESID) is thought to reduce bacterial load, which may prevent the development of relapse, wound healing, hematogenous spread, and systemic complications. We evaluated the efficacy of postoperative ESID over 20 years on disease progression and outcome in SD and ISEE. Methods: Detailed demographic, clinical, imaging, laboratory, and microbiological characteristics were examined in our cohorts of 208 SD and ISEE patients treated with and without ESID at a university spine center in Germany between 2002 and 2022. Between-group comparisons were performed to identify meaningful differences for the procedure. Results: We included data from 208 patients (142 SD, 68.3% vs. 66 ISEE, 31.7%) of whom 146 were ESID patients (87 SD, 59.6% vs. 59 ISEE, 40.4%) and 62 were NON-ESID patients (55 SD, 88.7% vs. 7 ISEE, 11.3%). ESID patients with SD showed more frequent SSI (ESID: 22, 25.3% vs. NON-ESID: 3, 5.5%, $p = 0.003$), reoperations due to empyema persistence or instability (ESID: 37, 42.5% vs. NON-ESID: 12, 21.8%, $p = 0.012$), and a higher relapse rate (ESID: 21, 37.5% vs. NON-ESID: 6, 16.7%, $p = 0.037$) than NON-ESID patients with SD. The success rate in NON-ESID patients with SD was higher than in ESID patients with SD (ESID: 26, 29.9% vs. NON-ESID: 36, 65.6%, $p < 0.001$). Multivariate binary logistic regression analysis showed that ESID therapy ($p < 0.001$; OR: 0.201; 95% CI: 0.089–0.451) was a significant independent risk factor for treatment failure in patients with SD. Conclusions: Our retrospective cohort study with more than 20 years of experience in ESID technique shows a negative effect in patients with SD in terms of surgical site infections and relapse rate.

**Keywords:** spondylodiscitis; isolated spinal epidural empyema; epidural suction–irrigation drainage; surgical site infection; complications; relapse

## 1. Introduction

Successful treatment of primary spinal infections (PSI), including spondylodiscitis (SD) and isolated spinal epidural empyema (ISEE), is a clinical challenge and can be addressed with a variety of surgical techniques [1]. Once the pathogen is identified, the focus is on systematic therapy, whereby the use of local antibiotic irrigation during and after surgery is an important adjunctive treatment [2]. The primary purpose of local antibiotic irrigation is to reduce the bacterial load, which may prevent the development of recurrence, wound healing, hematogenous spread, and systemic complications by shortening the duration of antibiotic therapy [2].

Several techniques for local antibiotic irrigation have been reported, but none of them has yet gained acceptance. Some authors reported on a small number of patients with continuous or onetime epidural irrigation and drainage as an effective method to reduce the residual infection and the risk of nosocomial complication [3–5]. Other authors proposed CT-guided percutaneous needle drainage with irrigation showing its efficacy in ISEE [6]. The endoscopic application in this setting has increased recently, with many authors reporting posterolateral endoscopic debridement followed by percutaneous drainage for irrigation [7,8].

One disadvantage of local antibiotic therapy using collagen carriers or antibiotic irrigation is increased seroma formation [9,10]. Löhr et al. reported an increased risk of epidural fluid stasis following the use of postoperative suction–irrigation drainage with no beneficial effects on outcome [11]. It is not known whether local antibiotic irrigation after surgical debridement promotes fusion [2].

Postoperative epidural suction–irrigation drainage (ESID) has been reported to have potential advantages and disadvantages; however, previous studies did not examine the short- and long-term outcome of ESID on SD and ISEE. The purpose of this study was to determine the efficacy of postoperative ESID on disease course and outcome on SD and ISEE, and to identify the benefits and drawbacks of this technique.

## 2. Materials and Methods

### 2.1. Study Design and Patient Data

#### 2.1.1. Study Design

Retrospective data from 208 patients with SD and ISEE managed with ESID or NON-ESID were analyzed. Consecutive patients with PSI who underwent surgery at our neurosurgical university spine center in Dresden, Germany, between 2002 and 2022 were included. Patients with early or late postoperative secondary spinal infections, patients with intradural infections (subdural abscess or spinal cord abscess) on admission, or patients with only conservative treatment were excluded from this study.

#### 2.1.2. Institutional Review Board and Electronic Patient Data Software

The study was approved by the local ethics committee of the Medical Faculty of the TU Dresden and University Hospital Carl Gustav, Dresden (Ref: BO-EK-17012022). Data on patients were identified via the ORBIS system (ORBIS, Dedalus, Bonn, Germany) and imaging files via the IMPAX system (IMPAX, Impax Asset Management Group plc, London, UK).

#### 2.1.3. Patient Data

Electronic medical records were pseudonymized and first divided into two groups—ISEE or SD—according to the type of infection. In addition, we examined the SD and ISEE groups to determine whether patients were treated with ESID or not (NON-ESID). Thereby, we formed 4 groups.

Baseline data were analyzed, along with age, gender, type of antibiotic therapy strategy (empirical or targeted), presence of paravertebral psoas abscess or pleural abscess, localization of infection in the spine, type of bacterial group, primary infectious source, time to surgery, time to pathogen detection, incidental dural tears, intraoperative local antibiotic irrigation, and type of surgery such as only abscess evacuation, one- or two-stage surgery.

In a next step, risk factors such as immunosuppression, diabetes mellitus, obesity, malignancy, liver cirrhosis, dialysis, stent or vascular prosthesis, artificial valve replacement, osteoporosis, rheumatoid arthritis or increased rheumatoid factors, gout or increased uric acid, chronic venous insufficiency, peripheral artery disease, and atrial fibrillation were analyzed.

Subsequently, disease-related complications such as sepsis, septic embolism, meningism, endocarditis with vegetations, surgical site infections (SSI), reoperations due to SSI, reoperations due to persistent empyema or increased spinal instability, relapse rate, mortality, length of hospital and intensive care unit (ICU) stay, duration of intravenous antibiotic administration, and total duration of antibiotic administration were analyzed.

We determined the success rate in the PSI and SD groups with and without ESID, whereas treatment failure was present in cases of persistent empyema, instability, SSI with or without reoperation, relapse rate, or death. Last, we determined the independent risk factors in multivariate binary logistic regression analysis for treatment failure. Sex, age over 65 years, methicillin-sensitive *Staphylococcus aureus* (MSSA), time to pathogen detection, empirical antibiotic treatment (EAT), time to surgery, diabetes mellitus, hepatic cirrhosis, malignancy, paravertebral psoas abscess, pleural abscess, incidental dural tears, and ESID were evaluated in multivariate binary logistic regression analysis.

*2.2. Clinical Management and Microbiological Assessment*

2.2.1. Assessment of Clinical, Microbiological, and Radiological Diagnostics

We determined the diagnosis of SD or ISEE based on the medical history; clinical examination; fever; laboratory values such as leukocyte count, C-reactive protein (CrP), and Procalcitonin; typical radiological changes on magnetic resonance imaging (MRI) and computed tomography (CT); and pathogen detection in blood cultures, intraoperative specimens, or CT-guided biopsies of paravertebral psoas abscess. A transoesophageal echocardiogram (TEE) was obtained in patients with suspected infective endocarditis according to the modified DUKE criteria.

Depending on the clinical condition, at least two blood cultures were taken before antibiotic therapy was started for microbiological diagnosis, although some patients were initially treated with antibiotics due to their severe clinical condition. Tissue samples collected during open surgery and samples obtained by CT-guided biopsies were used for microbiological analysis.

In our multidisciplinary spine board or neurosurgical–neuroradiology conference, the diagnosis of ISEE or SD was performed depending on clinical, laboratory, and radiological findings. From 2002 to 2015, cases were discussed in our neurosurgical–neuroradiology conference and treated in collaboration with infectiologists when possible. Since 2015, we have established a multidisciplinary spine board that includes neuroradiologists, neurosurgeons, trauma surgeons, orthopedic surgeons, and infectiologists when appropriate in order to determine the best treatment strategy for patients.

2.2.2. Antibiotic and Surgical Management

Surgical Treatment

First-line treatment was usually conservative with intravenous antibiotics, although surgical treatment was indicated in cases of source control, epidural abscess, neurologic deficits, or spinal instability. The type of surgical intervention was determined in the multidisciplinary spine board or neurosurgical–neuroradiology conference. All of our patients in this study required surgery and were treated with various surgical procedures.

Patients with ISEE underwent abscess evacuation with ESID or anterior cervical discectomy and fusion (ACDF) for abscesses ventral to the cervical spinal cord with ESID. Patients with SD were treated with either abscess evacuation alone or one- or two-stage instrumentation due to spinal instability, deformity, and pain-related immobility. Therefore, surgical decision-making depends on clinical experience and various defined radiological features. To assess bony integrity, preoperative CT scans were obtained from all patients who received spinal instrumentation.

Choice between ESID and NON-ESID Techniques in ISEE and SD

Of the 66 ISEE patients, only 7 did not receive ESID. In reviewing the medical records, no clear reason was identified explaining why the surgeons opted for NON-ESID. In 2 cases, the ESID was removed immediately postoperatively when the patient was repositioned. Incidental dural tears or reactive tissue without evidence of pus as the cause have not been reported in the remaining cases. The placement of an ESID in SD patients was based on surgeon experience and intraoperative findings, although patients treated with single-stage surgical abscess evacuation and simultaneous fixation were treated up to 81% without an ESID.

Epidural Suction–Irrigation Drainage

During abscess evacuation in patients with SD and ISEE, we placed one or two ESIDs in the spinal canal, when possible, with one ESID inserted cranially and one caudally. Beginning on the first postoperative day, the ESIDs were irrigated twice daily with gentamycin (5 mg in 5 mL), and samples were collected daily from the irrigation drainages for microbiological examination before irrigation. In case the identified pathogen was resistant to gentamycin, ESIDs were irrigated with vancomycin whenever possible. During irrigation, the suction drainage was closed and reopened after half an hour. If there were three bacteria-free microbiological results from the ESIDs on three consecutive days, the ESIDs were removed, and in most cases, the drainages were removed between postoperative days 8 and 14.

Antibiotic Treatment

Either targeted antibiotic treatment (TAT) or EAT was administered to all patients, depending on the clinical condition at admission and according to the recommendations from the local infectious disease department. However, it is important to mention that the majority of patients with EAT presented to us from secondary hospitals and required immediate surgery, therefore the number of EAT patients was high. The EAT was switched to TAT after detection of the causative pathogens.

In case of SD, intravenous antibiotic therapy was administered for about 4–6 weeks and then switched to oral antibiotics for total duration of 10 and 12 weeks. On the other hand, ISEE patients received intravenous antibiotic treatment for about 2 weeks and then switched to oral administration for a total duration of 4 to 6 weeks. Follow-up clinical and radiological examinations were conducted in all patients who complied with our recommendation at 3, 6, and 12 months after hospital discharge, if possible.

*2.3. Illustrative Cases*

We selected two different cases to describe our strategy for managing patients with ISEE and SD using ESID.

2.3.1. First Case with Isolated Spinal Epidural Empyema

Our first case was a 71-year-old female patient with distal weakness on lower extremities and urosepsis. MRI of the whole spine revealed ISEE at the level of L2 to S1. *Escherichia coli* was detected twice in blood cultures from two different peripheral regions and once in urine. Immediate microsurgical decompression with abscess evacuation and insertion of ESIDs was performed. Epidural irrigation was performed twice daily with gentamycin (5 mg in 5 mL), and samples from the irrigation drainage were collected daily before administration of local antibiotics. Once three times no bacteria were detected in the samples from the irrigation drainages, the ESIDs were removed, in this case it was the tenth postoperative day. *E. coli* was also isolated in intraoperative specimens and in the ESID samples, subsequently treated with ampicillin IV 4 g thrice daily for four weeks, and then switched to oral co-trimoxazole 160 mg/800 mg twice daily for an additional six weeks. The patient was discharged home after approximately four weeks on oral antibiotics. Follow-up showed no recurrence, so the antibiotics could be stopped after a total of ten weeks (Figure 1).

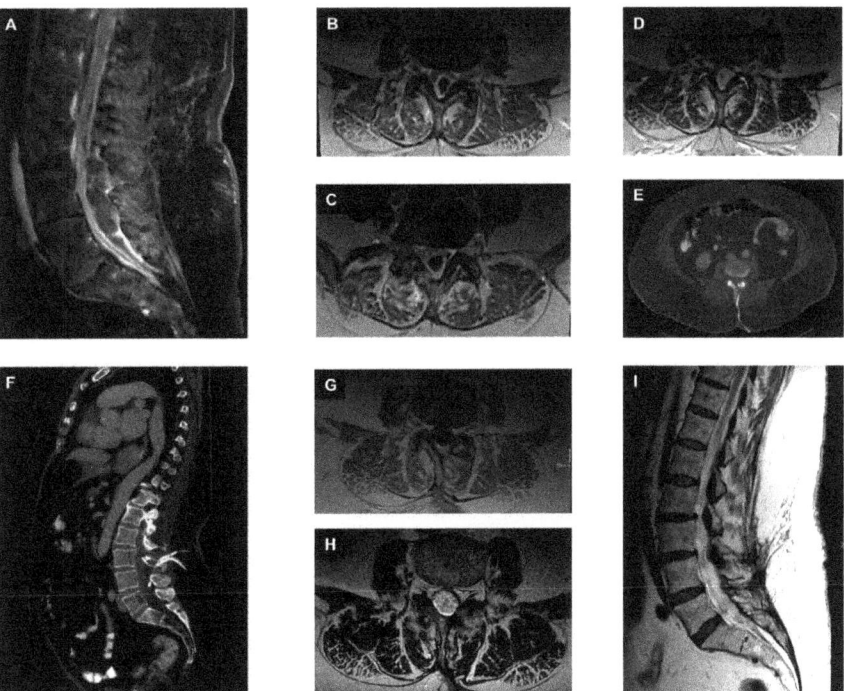

**Figure 1.** Management of ISEE with epidural suction–irrigation drainages. (**A**): A preoperative sagittal fat-saturated contrast-enhanced T1-weighted MR image of the lumbar spine shows isolated spinal epidural empyema in the dorsal part of the spinal canal at the level of L3 to S1. (**B–D**): Different preoperative axial T1-weighted contrast-enhanced MR images of the lumbar spine at the level of L3, L4, and L5. (**E,F**) Postoperative axial and sagittal reformatted CT images showing the previously placed suction–irrigation drainages cranially and caudally in the spinal canal at the level of L3/L4. (**G**): Axial T1-weighted contrast-enhanced MR image at 10 weeks at the time of antibiotic discontinuation. (**H**): Axial T2-weighted MR image at 10 weeks at the time of antibiotic discontinuation. (**I**): Sagittal T2-weighted MR image at 10 weeks at the time of antibiotic discontinuation.

2.3.2. Second Case with Spondylodiscitis and Epidural Empyema

A 72-year-old male patient from a secondary hospital presented with MSSA bacteraemia detected twice in blood cultures, with increasing infection parameters, severe back pain, and immobility due to pain with lower extremities weakness that was difficult to evaluate. Therapy with intravenous flucloxacillin 2 g four times daily was started externally. Whole-spine MRI was performed showing SD at the level of L2/L3 with spinal epidural empyema at the level of L2 to L5. In addition, a calcified disc herniation at the level of L2/L3 was seen on CT with abnormal narrowing of the spinal canal. We immediately performed a microsurgical decompression at the level L2/L3 with abscess evacuation and insertion of two ESIDs. The patient was postoperatively transferred to our ICU and subsequently transferred to normal ward in stable cardiopulmonary condition. MSSA was detected twice from the ESIDs. The ESIDs were irrigated twice a day with local antibiotics. After three sterile results, the ESIDs were removed on the ninth postoperative day. After two weeks, the patient, who was in favorable general condition, had no neurologic deficits, and was able to mobilize on the ward, was transferred to a secondary hospital near to his home for continuation of antibiotic therapy. Intravenous therapy with flucloxacillin was continued for a total of six weeks and then switched to oral antibiotics for an additional five weeks. Presentation to our outpatient clinic for stopping the antibiotics with a recent MRI and CT showed increasing bone destruction at the level of L2/L3 with instability, but no epidural empyema was noted. We discontinued the antibiotics for two days. After a two-day antibiotic-free period, we performed an extreme lateral interbody fusion (XLIF) on the right side at the level L2/L3 with specimen collection followed by dorsal instrumentation in terms of a single-stage 360-degree instrumentation in a two-position. Intraoperative findings showed an abscess-free situs after SD with reactive tissue. The pathogen could not be detected in the blood cultures and in the intraoperative specimens. The patient received two weeks additional intravenous antibiotic treatment with flucloxacillin, and rifampicin followed by four weeks more of oral levofloxacin and rifampicin. After completion of antibiotics, the patient presented to our outpatient clinic with a recent MRI and CT of the lumbar spine. This showed favorable results with no evidence of relapse. The patient stated well-being and showed absence of any weakness on the lower extremities and the infection parameters were normal (Figure 2).

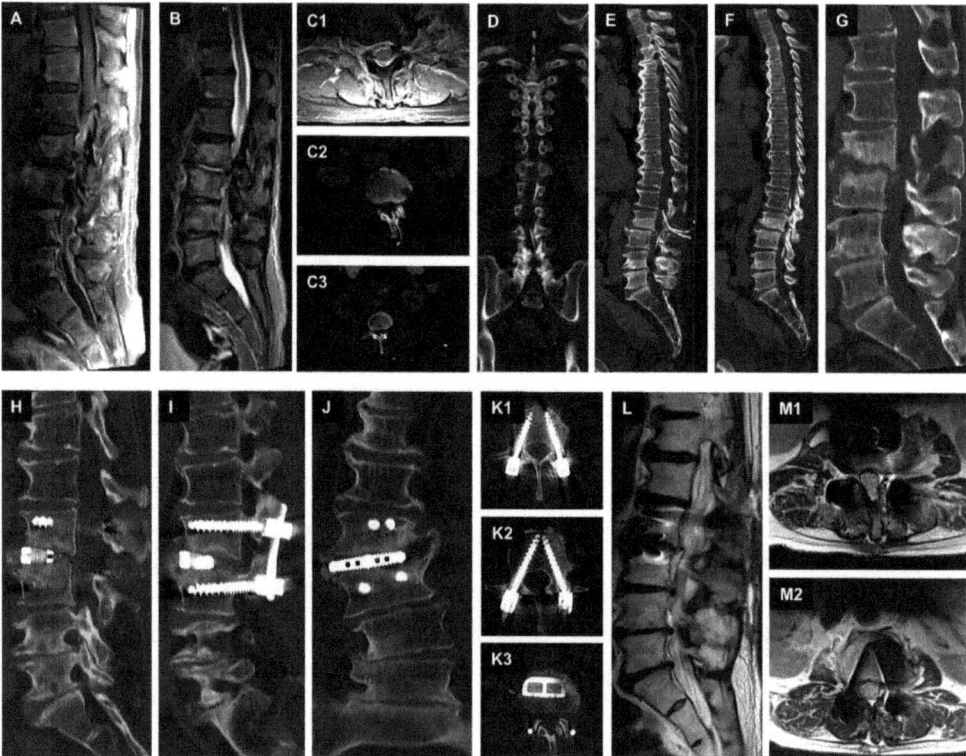

**Figure 2.** Management of SD with epidural suction–irrigation drainages. (**A**): A preoperative sagittal T1-weighted fat-saturated contrast-enhanced MR image of the lumbar spine shows spondylodiscitis at the L2/L3 level with epidural spinal empyema at the level of L2 to L5. (**B**): A preoperative sagittal

T2-weighted MR image of the lumbar spine. (**C1**): Preoperative axial T1-weighted fat-saturated contrast-enhanced MR image of the level L2/L3. (**C2–F**): Postoperative axial, coronal, and sagittal reformatted CT images showing the placed epidural suction-irrigation drainages cranially and caudally in the spinal canal at the level of L3/L4. (**G**): Sagittal reformatted CT image showing bone destruction at the level of L2/L3 at 11 weeks at the time of proposed antibiotic discontinuation. (**H–K3**): Postoperative sagittal, coronal, and axial reformatted CT images showing the result of the single-stage 360-degree instrumentation in a two position. (**L–M2**): Sagittal and axial T2-weighted MR images displaying the result after stopping the antibiotics.

*2.4. Statistical Analysis*

Statistical analysis of the data was performed using the SPSS software package (SPSS Statistics 29, IBM, Armonk, NY, USA). Descriptive statistics were used, and categorical variables were tested by Fisher exact tests or chi-square tests. Numerical variables were analyzed with Mann–Whitney U tests. All statistical tests were two-sided, and a $p$ value $p < 0.05$ was considered statistically significant. The dependent variable was treatment failure in SD patients, and a backward multivariate binary logistic regression analysis was performed. In this way, the regression equation was established and the relative risk value for treatment failure (odds ratio) and 95% confidence interval (CI) were determined.

## 3. Results

*3.1. General Baseline Characteristics*

Our study included 208 patients (men: 136, 65.4% vs. women: 72, 34.6%, $p < 0.001$) with PSI, of whom 142 patients presented with SD (68.3%) and 66 patients with ISEE (31.7%). In our collectives, 146 patients (70.2%) received intraoperative ESID and 62 patients (29.8%) were not treated with ESID. A total of 61.3% of SD patients were treated with ESID (87 patients), while the remaining 55 SD patients (38.7%) were treated with NON-ESID. The ISEE group was 89.4% managed with ESID (59 patients) and only 7 patients with NON-ESID. ISEE-NON-ESID group was small (7 patients), therefore only the SD patients were analyzed in detail.

*3.2. ESID Group vs. NON-ESID Group*

3.2.1. Baseline Factors

The ESID and NON-ESID group did not differ in age distribution over 65 years (ESID: 74, 50.7% vs. NON-ESID: 39, 62.9%, $p = 0.0128$) and gender (ESID: 55 females, 37.7% vs. NON-ESID: 17 females 27.4%, $p = 0.202$) (Table 1). ESID group was more frequently treated with EAT strategy than NON-ESID (ESID: 105, 71.9% vs. 35, 56.5%, $p = 0.036$). Paravertebral psoas abscesses (ESID: 92, 63.0% vs. NON-ESID: 36, 58.1%, $p = 0.535$) and pleural abscesses (ESID: 28, 19.2% vs. NON-ESID: 14, 22.2%, $p = 0.576$) were found equally frequently in both groups. The distribution of detected infections in the cervical spine (CS), thoracic spine (TS), lumbar spine (LS), and in more than one part of the spine was equally common in both groups. MSSA was detected more frequently in ESID than in NON-ESID (ESID: 82/135, 60.7% vs. NON-ESID: 18/52, 34.6%, $p = 0.002$). Other bacterial groups (Streptococci/Enterococci, Enterobacterales, and coagulase-negative Staphylococci (CoNS)) did not show different distribution in both groups. Likewise, there were no differences in the distribution of the primary source of infection in the two groups ($p = 0.143$). The time from suspicion of SD or ISEE on imaging to performing surgery was significantly shorter in the ESID group (ESID: 2 [1–4] d vs. NON-ESID: 4 [1–13] d, $p < 0.001$). The time from suspicion of SD or ISEE to isolation of the pathogen was equally frequent in both groups (ESID: 4 [3–7] d vs. 5 [3–10] d, $p = 0.198$). Incidental dural tear during surgery was distributed equally in both groups (ESID: 16, 11% vs. NON-ESID: 10, 16.1%, $p = 0.360$). In the ESID group, intraoperative local antibiotic irrigation with gentamycin, vancomycin, or both was performed more frequently (ESID: 129, 88.4% vs. NON-ESID: 44, 71.0%, $p = 0.004$). Patients with ESID underwent more frequently abscess evacuation only (ESID: 82, 56.2% vs. NON-ESID: 11, 17.7%, $p < 0.001$) and more often two-stage surgery (ESID: 32, 21% vs.

5, 8.1%, $p = 0.017$). One-stage surgery was performed more frequently in patients with NON-ESIDS (ESID: 32, 21.9% vs. 46, 74.2%, $p < 0.001$).

**Table 1.** Baseline factors between ESID and NON-ESID.

| Baseline Factors | ESID (n = 146, 70.2%) | NON-ESID (n = 62, 29.8%) | p-Value |
|---|---|---|---|
| Age > 65 years | 74/146 (50.7%) | 39/62 (62.9%) | 0.128 [1] |
| Gender | F: 55 vs. M: 91 | F: 17 vs. M: 45 | 0.202 [1] |
| EAT | 105/146 (71.9%) | 35/62 (56.5%) | 0.036 [1] |
| TAT | 41/146 (28.1%) | 27/62 (43.5%) | |
| Paravertebral psoas abscesses | 92/146 (63.0%) | 36/62 (58.1%) | 0.535 [1] |
| Pleural abscesses | 28/146 (19.2%) | 14/62 (22.6%) | 0.576 [1] |
| CS | 43/146 (29.5%) | 18/62 (29.0%) | 1.000 [1] |
| TS | 58/146 (39.7%) | 24/62 (38.7%) | 1.000 [1] |
| LS | 101/146 (69.2%) | 36/62 (58.1%) | 0.150 [1] |
| More than one part of spine | 43/146 (29.5%) | 14/62 (22.6%) | 0.396 [1] |
| MSSA (n = 187) | 82/135 (60.7%) | 18/52 (34.6%) | **0.002** [1] |
| SE (n = 187) | 19/135 (14.1%) | 12/52 (23.1%) | 0.187 [1] |
| Enterobacterales (n = 187) | 12/135 (8.9%) | 8/52 (15.4%) | 0.198 [1] |
| CoNS (n = 187) | 12/135 (8.9%) | 8/52 (15.4%) | 0.198 [1] |
| Primary infectious sources (n = 145) | -- | -- | 0.143 [2] |
| Time to surgery | 2 [1–4] d * | 4 [1–13] d * | **<0.001** [2] |
| Time to pathogen detection | 4 [3–7] d * | 5 [3–10] d * | 0.198 [2] |
| Incidental dural tears | 16/146 (11.0%) | 10/62 (16.1%) | 0.360 [1] |
| Intraoperative antibiotic Irrigation | 129/146 (88.4%) | 44/62 (71.0%) | **0.004** [1] |
| Only abscess evacuation | 82/146 (56.2%) | 11/62 (17.7%) | **<0.001** [1] |
| One-stage surgery | 32/146 (21.9%) | 46/62 (74.2%) | **<0.001** [1] |
| Two-stage surgery | 32/146 (21.9%) | 5/62 (8.1%) | **0.017** [1] |

ESID: epidural suction–irrigation drainage group; NON-ESID: group without epidural suction–irrigation drainage; EAT: empirical antibiotic treatment; TAT: targeted antibiotic treatment; CS: cervical spine, TS: thoracic spine; LS: lumbar spine; MSSA: methicillin-sensitive *Staphylococcus* aureus; SE: *Streptococcus* spp. and *Enterococcus* spp.; CoNS: coagulase-negative *Staphylococci*; *: median [interquartile range]; (1): Fisher exact test; (2): Mann–Whitney U test. One-stage surgery: simultaneous abscess evacuation and fixation; Two-stage surgery: initial abscess evacuation and then fixation. Bold values are significant results ($p < 0.05$) as indicated in the methods.

3.2.2. Risk Factors

Risk factors such as immunosuppression (ESID: 22, 15.1% vs. 13, 21.0%, $p = 0.315$), diabetes mellitus (ESID: 52, 36.6% vs. 25, 40.3%, $p = 0.534$), obesity (ESID: 48, 32.9% vs. 18, 29.0%, $p = 0.628$), malignancy (ESID: 25, 17.1% vs. 13, 21.0%, $p = 0.558$), hepatic cirrhosis (ESID: 32, 21.9% vs. 13, 21.0%, $p = 1.000$), dialysis (ESID: 5, 3.4% vs. 3, 4.8%, $p = 0.698$), presence of a stent or vascular prosthesis (ESID: 13, 8.9% vs. 4, 6.5%, $p = 0.783$), osteoporosis (ESID: 51/129, 39.5% vs. 31/60, 51.7%, $p = 0.156$), rheumatoid arthritis or increased rheumatoid factors (ESID: 29/67, 43.3% vs. 8/24, 33.3%, $p = 0.472$), gout or increased uric acid (ESID: 28/63, 44.4% vs. 17/29, 58.6%, $p = 0.263$), chronic venous insufficiency (ESID: 5, 3.4% vs. 2, 3.2%, $p = 1.000$), peripheral artery disease (ESID: 7, 4.8% vs. 6, 9.7%, $p = 0.214$), and atrial fibrillation (ESID: 31, 21.2% vs. 20, 32.3%, $p = 0.113$) were equally distributed in both groups (Table 2).

**Table 2.** Risk factors between ESID and NON-ESID.

| Risk Factors | ESID (n = 146, 70.2%) | NON-ESID (n = 62, 29.8%) | $p$-Value |
|---|---|---|---|
| Immunosuppression | 22/146 (15.1%) | 13/62 (21.0%) | 0.315 [1] |
| Diabetes mellitus | 52/146 (36.6%) | 25/62 (40.3%) | 0.534 [1] |
| Obesity (BMI > 30 kg/m$^2$) | 48/146 (32.9%) | 18/62 (29.0%) | 0.628 [1] |
| Malignancy | 25/146 (17.1%) | 13/62 (21.0%) | 0.558 [1] |
| Hepatic cirrhosis | 32/146 (21.9%) | 13/62 (21.0%) | 1.000 [1] |
| Dialysis | 5/146 (3.4%) | 3/62 (4.8%) | 0.698 [1] |
| Stent or vascular prosthesis | 13/146 (8.9%) | 4/62 (6.5%) | 0.783 [1] |
| Artificial heart valve replacement | 5/146 (3.4%) | 7/62 (11.3%) | **0.045** [1] |
| Osteoporosis (n = 189) | 51/129 (39.5%) | 31/60 (51.7%) | 0.156 [1] |
| RA or increased RF (n = 91) | 29/67 (43.3%) | 8/24 (33.3%) | 0.472 [1] |
| Gout or increased uric acid (n = 92) | 28/63 (44.4%) | 17/29 (58.6%) | 0.263 [1] |
| Chronic venous insufficiency | 5/146 (3.4%) | 2/62 (3.2%) | 1.000 [1] |
| Peripheral artery disease | 7/146 (4.8%) | 6/62 (9.7%) | 0.214 [1] |
| Atrial fibrillation | 31/146 (21.2%) | 20/62 (32.3%) | 0.113 [1] |

ESID: epidural suction–irrigation drainage group; NON-ESID: group without epidural suction–irrigation drainage; BMI: body mass index; RA: rheumatoid arthritis; RF: rheumatoid factors; [1]: Fisher exact test. Bold values are significant results ($p < 0.05$) as indicated in the methods.

### 3.2.3. Disease-Related Complications

SSI (ESID: 29, 19.9% vs. NON-ESID: 4, 6.5%, $p = 0.021$) and reoperations due to SSI (ESID: 24, 16.4% vs. NON-ESID: 3, 4.8%, $p = 0.024$) were significantly more common in the ESID group than in the NON-ESID group (Table 3). We found no differences in both groups in terms of complications such as sepsis (ESID: 69, 47.3% vs. NON-ESID: 37, 59.7%, $p = 0.129$), septic embolism (ESID: 34/108, 31.5% vs. NON-ESID: 22/57, 38.6%, $p = 0.390$), meningism (ESID: 22/141, 15.6% vs. NON-ESID: 15/61, 24.6%, $p = 0.165$), endocarditis with vegetation (ESID: 17/121, 14.0% vs. NON-ESID: 7/56, 12.5%, $p = 1.000$), reoperations due to persistence or instability of empyema (ESID: 41, 28.1% vs. NON-ESID: 12, 19.4%, $p = 0.225$), recurrence rate (ESID: 25/98, 25.5% vs. NON-ESID: 6/40, 15.0%, $p = 0.261$), mortality (ESID: 6, 4.1% vs. NON-ESID: 6, 9.7%, $p = 0.189$), hospital stay (ESID: 31 [22–48] d vs. NON-ESID: 35 [24–490] d, $p = 0.512$), ICU stay (ESID: 1 [0–8] d vs. 2 [0–13] d, $p = 0.423$), intravenous antibiotic duration (ESID: 4 [3–6] w vs. NON-ESID: 4 [3–6] w, $p = 0.426$), and total antibiotic duration (ESID: 8 [6–12] w vs. NON-ESID: 10 [6–12] w, $p = 0.301$).

**Table 3.** Disease-related complications between ESID and NON-ESID.

| Variable | ESID (n = 146, 70.2%) | NON-ESID (n = 62, 29.8%) | $p$-Value |
|---|---|---|---|
| Sepsis | 69/146 (47.3%) | 37/62 (59.7%) | 0.129 [1] |
| Septic embolism (n = 165) | 34/108 (31.5%) | 22/57 (38.6%) | 0.390 [1] |
| Meningism (n = 202) | 22/141 (15.6%) | 15/61 (24.6%) | 0.165 [1] |
| Endocarditis with vegetation (n = 177) | 17/121 (14.0%) | 7/56 (12.5%) | 1.000 [1] |
| SSI | 29/146 (19.9%) | 4/62 (6.5%) | **0.021** [1] |
| Reoperation due SSI | 24/146 (16.4%) | 3/62 (4.8%) | **0.024** [1] |

**Table 3.** *Cont.*

| Variable | ESID (n = 146, 70.2%) | NON-ESID (n = 62, 29.8%) | *p*-Value |
|---|---|---|---|
| Reoperation (empyema or instability) | 41/146 (28.1%) | 12/62 (19.4%) | 0.225 (1) |
| Relapse rate (n = 138) | 25/98 (25.5%) | 6/40 (15.0%) | 0.261 (1) |
| Mortality | 6/146 (4.1%) | 6/62 (9.7%) | 0.189 (1) |
| Hospital stay | 31 [22–48] d * | 35 [24–49] d * | 0.512 (2) |
| ICU stay | 1 [0–8] d * | 2 [0–13] d * | 0.423 (2) |
| Intravenous antibiotic duration | 4 [3–6] w * | 4 [3–6] w * | 0.426 (2) |
| Total antibiotic duration | 8 [6–12] w * | 10 [6–12] w * | 0.301 (2) |

ESID: epidural suction–irrigation drainage group; NON-ESID: group without epidural suction–irrigation drainage; SSI: surgical site infection; ICU: intensive care unit; *: median [interquartile range]; (1): Fisher exact test; (2): Mann–Whitney U test. Bold values are significant results ($p < 0.05$) as indicated in the methods.

### 3.3. ESID Group vs. NON-ESID Group in Spondylodiscitis

#### 3.3.1. Baseline Factors

Age over 65 years, gender, EAT/TAT, paravertebral psoas abscesses, pleural abscesses, and distribution in the spine (CS, TS, LS, and more than part of the spine) were equally distributed in the ESID and NON-ESID groups (Table 4). MSSA were detected more frequently in patients with ESID than in patients without ESID (ESID: 44/80, 55.0% vs. NON-ESID: 13/45, 28.9%, $p = 0.005$); however, Streptococci/Enterococci, Enterobacterales, and CoNS showed no differences between the two groups. The primary sources of infection were equally distributed in both groups ($p = 0.0676$). The time to surgery was significantly longer in the NON-ESID group than in the ESID group (ESID: 2 [1–6] d vs. NON-ESID: 5 [2–14] d, $p = 0.004$), although the time to pathogen detection was the same in both groups (ESID: 5 [3–8] d vs. NON-ESID: 6 [3–11] d, $p = 0.470$). There were no differences between both groups in incidental dural tears (ESID: 11, 12.6% vs. NON-ESID: 8, 14.5%, $p = 0.803$). Patients with ESID were more likely to be irrigated intraoperatively with a local antibiotic (ESID: 80, 92.0% vs. NON-ESID: 40, 72.7%, $p = 0.004$). ESID patients underwent more often abscess evacuation only (ESID: 25, 28.7% vs. NON-ESID: 5, 9.1%, $p < 0.006$) and more often two-stage surgery (ESID: 32, 36.8% vs. 5, 9.1%, $p < 0.001$). One-stage surgery was performed more frequently in patients with NON-ESIDS (ESID: 30, 34.5% vs. 45, 81.8%, $p < 0.001$).

**Table 4.** Baseline factors between ESID and NON-ESID in SD.

| Baseline Factors | SD (n = 142, 68.3%) | | |
|---|---|---|---|
| | ESID (n = 87, 61.3%) | NON-ESID (n = 55, 38.7%) | *p*-Value |
| Age > 65 years | 53/87 (60.9%) | 35/55 (63.6%) | 0.859 (1) |
| Gender | F: 29 vs. M: 58 | F: 12 vs. M: 43 | 0.184 (1) |
| EAT | 58/87 (66.7%) | 31/55 (56.4%) | 0.285 (1) |
| TAT | 29/87 (33.3%) | 24/55 (43.6%) | |
| Paravertebral psoas abscesses | 62/87 (71.3%) | 33/55 (60.0%) | 0.201 (1) |
| Pleural abscesses | 20/87 (23.0%) | 13/55 (23.6%) | 1.000 (1) |
| CS | 24/87 (27.6%) | 15/55 (27.3%) | 1.000 (1) |
| TS | 30/87 (34.5%) | 19/55 (34.5%) | 1.000 (1) |
| LS | 62/87 (71.3%) | 34/55 (61.8%) | 0.272 (1) |

Table 4. Cont.

| Baseline Factors | SD (n = 142, 68.3%) | | |
|---|---|---|---|
| | ESID (n = 87, 61.3%) | NON-ESID (n = 55, 38.7%) | p-Value |
| More than one part of spine | 25/87 (28.7%) | 11/55 (20.0%) | 0.322 [1] |
| MSSA (n= 187) | 44/80 (55.0%) | 13/45 (28.9%) | **0.005** [1] |
| SE (n = 187) | 14/80 (17.5%) | 12/45 (26.7%) | 0.255 [1] |
| Enterobacterales (n= 187) | 8/80 (10.0%) | 8/45 (17.8%) | 0.267 [1] |
| CoNS (n = 187) | 8/80 (10.0%) | 7/45 (15.6%) | 0.397 [1] |
| Primary infectious sources (n = 145) | -- | -- | 0.676 [2] |
| Time to surgery | 2 [1–6] d * | 5 [2–14] d * | **0.004** [2] |
| Time to pathogen detection | 5 [3–8] d * | 6 [3–11] d * | 0.470 [2] |
| Incidental dural tears | 11/87 (12.6%) | 8/55 (14.5%) | 0.803 [1] |
| Intraoperative antibiotic Irrigation | 80/87 (92.0%) | 40/55 (72.7%) | **0.004** [1] |
| Only abscess evacuation | 25/87 (28.7%) | 5/55 (9.1%) | **0.006** [1] |
| One-stage surgery | 30/87 (34.5%) | 45/55 (81.8%) | **<0.001** [1] |
| Two-stage surgery | 32/87 (36.8%) | 5/55 (9.1%) | **<0.001** [1] |

ESID: epidural suction–irrigation drainage group; NON-ESID: group without epidural suction–irrigation drainage; SD: spondylodiscitis; EAT: empirical antibiotic treatment; TAT: targeted antibiotic treatment; CS: cervical spine; TS: thoracic spine; LS: lumbar spine; MSSA: methicillin-sensitive *Staphylococcus* aureus; SE: *Streptococcus* spp. and *Enterococcus* spp.; CoNS: coagulase-negative *Staphylococci*; *: median [interquartile range]; One-stage surgery: simultaneous abscess evacuation and fixation; Two-stage surgery: initial abscess evacuation and then fixation. (1): Fisher exact test; (2): Mann–Whitney U test. Bold values are significant results ($p < 0.05$) as indicated in the methods.

3.3.2. Risk Factors

Patients with ESID were less frequently to have artificial valve replacement than patients without ESID (ESID: 3, 3.4% vs. 7, 12.7%, $p = 0.046$). No differences were seen between the two groups for other risk factors (Table 5).

Table 5. Risk factors between ESID and NON-ESID in SD.

| Risk Factors | SD (n = 142, 68.3%) | | |
|---|---|---|---|
| | ESID (n = 87, 61.3%) | NON-ESID (n = 55, 38.7%) | p-Value |
| Immunosuppression | 16/87 (18.4%) | 12/55 (21.8%) | 0.668 [1] |
| Diabetes Mellitus | 35/87 (40.2%) | 24/55 (43.6%) | 0.729 [1] |
| Obesity (BMI > 30 kg/m$^2$) | 23/87 (26.4%) | 14/55 (25.5%) | 1.000 [1] |
| Malignancy | 14/87 (16.1%) | 12/55 (21.8%) | 0.505 [1] |
| Hepatic cirrhosis | 25/87 (28.7%) | 13/55 (23.6%) | 0.563 [1] |
| Dialysis | 4/87 (4.6%) | 3/55 (5.5%) | 1.000 [1] |
| Stent or vascular prosthesis | 11/87 (12.6%) | 4/55 (7.3%) | 0.406 [1] |
| Artificial heart valve replacement | 3/87 (3.4%) | 7/55 (12.7%) | **0.046** [1] |
| Osteoporosis (n = 189) | 33/76 (43.4%) | 30/55 (54.5%) | 0.221 [1] |
| RA or increased RF (n = 91) | 20/44 (45.5%) | 8/22 (36.4%) | 0.600 [1] |

**Table 5.** Cont.

| Risk Factors | SD (n = 142, 68.3%) | | |
|---|---|---|---|
| | ESID (n = 87, 61.3%) | NON-ESID (n = 55, 38.7%) | p-Value |
| Gout or increased uric acid (n = 92) | 19/42 (45.2%) | 17/29 (58.6%) | 0.337 [1] |
| Chronic venous insufficiency | 1/87 (1.1%) | 2/55 (3.6%) | 0.560 [1] |
| Peripheral artery disease | 5/87 (5.7%) | 6/55 (10.9%) | 0.337 [1] |
| Atrial fibrillation | 23/87 (26.4%) | 20/55 (36.4%) | 0.261 [1] |

ESID: epidural suction–irrigation drainage group; NON-ESID: group without epidural suction–irrigation drainage; SD: spondylodiscitis; BMI: body mass index; RA: rheumatoid arthritis; RF: rheumatoid factors; (1): Fisher exact test. Bold values are significant results ($p < 0.05$) as indicated in the methods.

### 3.3.3. Disease-Related Complications

SSI (ESID: 22, 25.3% vs. NON-ESID: 3, 5.5%, $p = 0.003$), reoperations due to SSI (ESID: 20, 23.0% vs. NON-ESID: 2, 3.6%, $p = 0.002$), and reoperations due to empyema persistence or instability (ESID: 37, 42.5% vs. NON-ESID: 12, 21.8%, $p = 0.012$) were significantly more frequent in the ESID group than in the NON-ESID group (Table 6). The relapse rate was also higher in patients with ESID than in patients with NON-ESID (ESID: 21, 37.5% vs. NON-ESID: 6, 16.7%, $p = 0.037$). No differences were found between the two groups for other disease-related complications.

**Table 6.** Disease-related complications between ESID and NON-ESID in SD.

| Variable | SD (n = 142, 68.3%) | | |
|---|---|---|---|
| | ESID (n = 87, 61.3%) | NON-ESID (n = 55, 38.7%) | p-Value |
| Sepsis | 59/87 (67.8%) | 35/55 (37.2%) | 0.716 [1] |
| Septic embolism (n = 165) | 31/67 (46.3%) | 21/50 (42.0%) | 0.709 [1] |
| Meningism (n = 202) | 12/83 (14.5%) | 13/54 (24.1%) | 0.178 [1] |
| Endocarditis with vegetation (n = 177) | 16/75 (21.3%) | 7/50 (14.0%) | 0.352 [1] |
| SSI | 22/87 (25.3%) | 3/55 (5.5%) | **0.003** [1] |
| Reoperation due SSI | 20/87 (23.0%) | 2/55 (3.6%) | **0.002** [1] |
| Reoperation (empyema or instability) | 37/87 (42.5%) | 12/55 (21.8%) | **0.012** [1] |
| Relapse rate (n = 138) | 21/56 (37.5%) | 6/36 (16.7%) | **0.037** [1] |
| Mortality | 5/87 (5.7%) | 6/55 (10.9%) | 0.337 [1] |
| Hospital stay | 40 [31–56] d * | 35 [26–51] d * | 0.139 [2] |
| ICU stay | 3 [0–13] d * | 2 [0–12] d * | 0.893 [2] |
| Intravenous antibiotic duration | 5 [4–6] w * | 4 [3–7] w * | 0.189 [2] |
| Total antibiotic duration | 10 [8–12] w * | 10 [7–12] w * | 0.789 [2] |

ESID: epidural suction–irrigation drainage group; NON-ESID: group without epidural suction–irrigation drainage; SD: spondylodiscitis; SSI: surgical site infection; ICU: intensive care unit; *: median [interquartile range]; (1): Fisher exact test; (2): Mann–Whitney U test. Bold values are significant results ($p < 0.05$) as indicated in the methods.

### 3.4. Success Rate

Success rate was defined as a single (one- or two-stage surgical strategy) uncomplicated ESID or NON-ESID treatment. Treatment failure was present in persistent empyema, instability, or SSI with or without reoperation, and relapse or fatality. Overall, the success rate was lower in PSI patients with ESID than NON-ESID patients (ESID: 73, 50.0% vs. NON-ESID: 42, 67.7%, $p = 0.022$). SD patients without ESID showed a better success rate than patients with ESID (ESID: 26, 29.9% vs. NON-ESID: 36, 65.6%, $p < 0.001$) (Table 7, Figure 3).

Table 7. Success rate in patients with PSI or SD treated with/without ESID.

| Infection | ESID | NON-ESID | $p$-Value |
|---|---|---|---|
| Primary spinal infection (n = 208) | 73/146 (50.0%) | 42/62 (67.7%) | **0.022** [1] |
| Spondylodiscitis (n = 142) | 26/87 (29.9%) | 36/55 (65.5%) | **<0.001** [1] |

ESID: epidural suction–irrigation drainage group; NON-ESID: group without epidural suction–irrigation drainage; (1): Fisher exact test. Bold values are significant results ($p < 0.05$) as indicated in the methods.

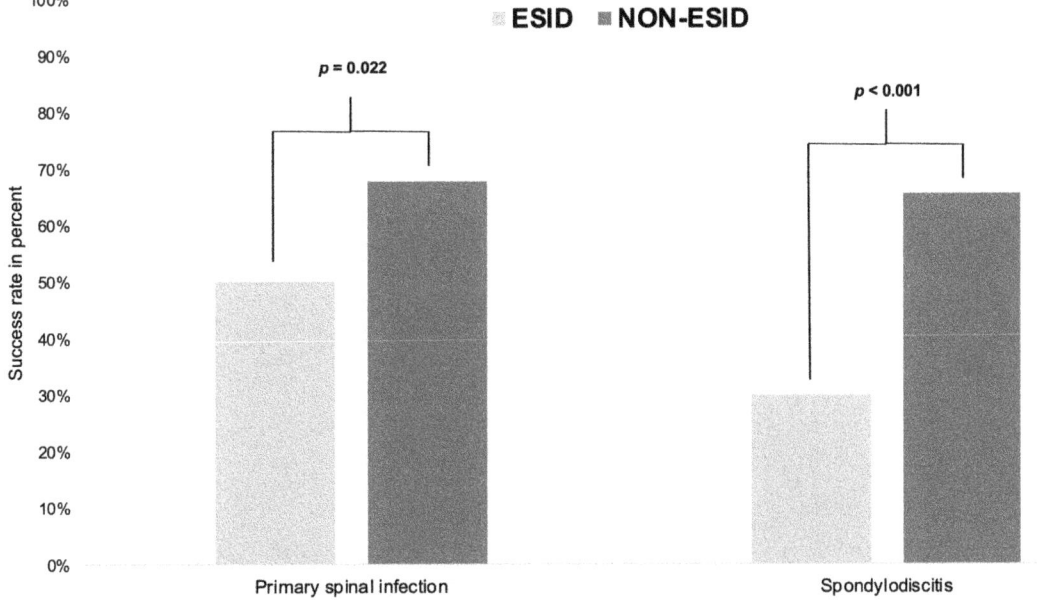

Figure 3. Success rate in patients with primary spinal infection or spondylodiscitis treated with/without ESID. ESID: epidural suction–irrigation drainage group; NON-ESID: group without epidural suction–irrigation drainage; The $p$-values are significant when $p < 0.05$, as indicated in the methods according to the Fisher exact test.

### 3.5. Multivariate Analyses

Multivariate binary logistic regression analyses are summarized in Table 8. Treatment with ESID ($p < 0.001$; OR: 0.201; 95% CI: 0.089–0.451) was identified as a significant independent risk factor for treatment failure in patients with SD in our cohort.

**Table 8.** Multivariate binary logistic regression analysis to identify independent risk factors for treatment failure in patients with SD.

| Variables | Multivariate Logistic Regression | |
|---|---|---|
| | OR (95% CI) | *p*-Value |
| Males | 0.487 (0.200–1.185) | 0.113 |
| Age > 65 years | 0.629 (0.257–1.542) | 0.311 |
| Methicillin-sensitive *Staphylococcus* aureus | 0.928 (0.370–2.329) | 0.874 |
| Time to pathogen detection | 0.938 (0.877–1.002) | 0.058 |
| Empirical antibiotic therapy | 1.707 (0.738–3.948) | 0.211 |
| Time to surgery | 0.992 (0.947–1.040) | 0.748 |
| Diabetes mellitus | 0.612 (0.265–1.415) | 0.251 |
| Hepatic cirrhosis | 0.895 (0.312–2.568) | 0.837 |
| Malignancy | 0.539 (0.174–1.676) | 0.286 |
| Paravertebral psoas abscess | 0.468 (0.208–1.053) | 0.067 |
| Pleural abscess | 0.472 (0.174–1.281) | 0.141 |
| Incidental dural tears | 0.382 (0.111–1.315) | 0.127 |
| Epidural suction-irrigation drainage | 0.201 (0.089–0.451) | **<0.001** |

OR: odds ratio, CI: confidence interval. Bold values are significant results ($p < 0.05$) as indicated in the methods.

Sex ($p = 0.113$; OR: 0.487; 95% CI: 0.200–1.185), age over 65 years ($p = 0.311$; OR: 0.629; 95% CI: 0.257–1.542), MSSA ($p = 0.311$; OR: 0.928; 95% CI: 0.370–2.329), time to pathogen detection ($p = 0.058$; OR: 0.938; 95% CI: 0.877–1.002), EAT ($p = 0.211$; OR: 1.707; 95% CI: 0.738–3.948), time to surgery ($p = 0.748$; OR: 0.992; 95% CI: 0.947–1.040), diabetes mellitus ($p = 0.251$; OR: 0.612; 95% CI: 0.265–1.415), hepatic cirrhosis ($p = 0.837$; OR: 0.895; 95% CI: 0.312–2.568), malignancy ($p = 0.286$; OR: 0.539; 95% CI: 0.174–1.676), paravertebral psoas abscess ($p = 0.067$; OR: 0.468; 95% CI: 0.208–1.053), pleural abscess ($p = 0.141$; OR: 0.472; 95% CI: 0.174–1.281), and incidental dural tears ($p = 0.127$; OR: 0.382; 95% CI: 0.111–1.315) showed no significance in multivariate analysis.

## 4. Discussion

The key message of this study and our 20-year experience with the ESID technique showed that ESID did not confer any benefits in SD patients, possibly even disadvantages in terms of worsening short- and long-term outcomes, such as required reoperations and increased relapse rate. In the ISEE patients, we were unable to perform any meaningful comparisons between ESID and NON-ESID patients due to the small number of ISEE patients. The adverse effects in SD patients were mainly due to SSI and local persistence of infection, probably caused by seroma formation.

*Baseline factors:*

The following baseline factors were equally distributed between both ESID and NON-ESID, even when considering SD patients separately: Age over 65 years, gender, paravertebral psoas abscess or pleural abscess, location in the spine, bacterial groups such as Streptococci and Enterococci, Enterobacterales, CoNS, primary sources of infection, time to pathogen detection, and incidental dural tears.

In total, ESID patients were more often treated with EAT than TAT compared to NON-ESID. In SD patients alone, we found no difference between the ESID and NON-ESID in terms of TAT/EAT. Overall, the number of patients with EAT in our cohort is greater than with TAT because patients were referred to us for immediate surgical treatment and had EAT upfront.

Baseline factors such as MSSA bacterial group, time to surgery, intraoperative antibiotic irrigation, and type of surgery (abscess evacuation only, one- or two-stage surgery) showed a difference between ESID and NON-ESID in PSI and SD patients alone.

In SD patients, MSSA were detected more frequently in the ESID group than in the NON-ESID group, although this may be an incidental finding since MSSA is a typical pathogen of SD [12–14].

In our SD cohort, the time from the suspected clinical radiological diagnosis to surgery was shorter in the ESID group than in the NON-ESID group. Authors reported that early surgery in SD showed better clinical outcomes [15]. Thus, the ESID group in SD has an advantage over NON-ESID, if the assumption were accurate. The time from symptom onset to first surgical treatment was reported differently in the literature, varying from 17 to 69 days [16,17].

More than 70% of the ESID and NON-ESID groups in SD patients were irrigated intraoperatively with local antibiotics, which may have affected the outcomes; however, the ESID group was irrigated intraoperatively more frequently than the NON-ESID group.

The NON-ESID group was treated mainly with single-stage surgery, whereas the three procedures were equally distributed in the ESID group. In a retrospective study of 118 patients, Bydon et al. reported no differences in recurrence and revision rates in patients with abscess evacuation and instrumentation and patients with only abscess evacuation [18]. Dietz et al. demonstrated significant benefits of additive fusion in a population of 2662 patients in terms of recurrence, revision rate, and postoperative complications [19].

*Risk factors:*

Risk factors such as immunosuppression, diabetes mellitus, obesity, malignancy, liver cirrhosis, dialysis, stent or vascular prosthesis, osteoporosis, rheumatoid arthritis or increased rheumatoid factors, gout or increased uric acid, chronic venous insufficiency, peripheral arterial disease, and atrial fibrillation showed no between-group differences. Artificial heart valve replacement was found more frequently in SD patients in the NON-ESID group than in the ESID group.

*Disease-related complications:*

We found a significant increased SSI (19.9%) with required revisions due to SSI (16.4%) in ESID patients with PSI compared to NON-ESID patients with PSI (SSI: 6.5%, revision due to SSI: 4.8%). The ESID technique carries an increased risk of epidural fluid stasis due to irrigation [11], which probably led to SSI.

However, all other disease-related complications such as sepsis, septic embolism, meningism, endocarditis with vegetations, reoperation for persistent empyema or increased spinal instability, relapse rate, mortality, length of hospital and ICU stay, duration of intravenous antibiotic administration, and total duration of antibiotic administration were equally distributed between ESID and NON-ESID patients with PSI in our cohort.

SD cohort showed an increased rate of SSI, relapse, revisions due to SSI, persistent empyema, or instability in ESID patients compared with NON-ESID.

*Success rate:*

ESID showed a worse success rate in PSI and especially in SD patients, and the inefficacy of this technique can only be explained by the accumulation of fluid with the formation of seromas and the resulting increasing bacterial load.

*Multivariate analyses:*

The multivariate regression analysis showed that ESID technique was an independent risk factor for treatment failure in patients with SD, which was suggested in the previous study by Löhr [11].

*Limitations and strengths of this study*

Our study is limited by its retrospective design and a possible selection bias toward more severe cases due to the high degree of specialization at our university center. The number of ISEE patients treated with NON-ESID is very limited, with only seven patients. Nevertheless, our data are derived from detailed clinical, imaging, and microbiological state-of-the-art diagnostic assessment with high internal validity and a meaningful sample size. Finally, the generalizability of our observations is limited by the monocentric design of our study.

## 5. Conclusions

Our retrospective cohort study and more than 20 years of experience with the ESID technique suggest a negative effect in patients with SD in terms of SSI and relapse rate. The evaluation of ISEE patients is limited due to the small number of NON-ESID patients. In SD patients, the unfavorable effects were mainly due to SSI and local persistence of infection, probably caused by seroma formation.

**Author Contributions:** M.M.H.: conceptualization, methodology, software, validation, formal analysis, investigation, resources, data curation, writing—original draft preparation, project administration, and funding acquisition; I.Y.E., T.A.J., G.S., D.P., T.S., I.E.-B., P.S., K.E., A.F. and M.M.H.: writing—review and editing, visualization, and supervision. All authors have read and agreed to the published version of the manuscript.

**Funding:** This research received no external funding.

**Institutional Review Board Statement:** The study was conducted in accordance with the Declaration of Helsinki and approved by the Institutional Review Board of the local ethics committee at the University Hospital Dresden (protocol code: BO-EK-17012022, January 2022).

**Informed Consent Statement:** Patient consent was waived due to the retrospective, anonymous character of this study.

**Data Availability Statement:** The original contributions presented in the study are included in the article; further inquiries can be directed to the corresponding author/s.

**Conflicts of Interest:** The authors declare no conflict of interest.

## References

1. Lener, S.; Hartmann, S.; Barbagallo, G.M.V.; Certo, F.; Thome, C.; Tschugg, A. Management of spinal infection: A review of the literature. *Acta Neurochir.* **2018**, *160*, 487–496. [CrossRef] [PubMed]
2. Fleege, C.; Rauschmann, M.; Arabmotlagh, M.; Rickert, M. Development and current use of local antibiotic carriers in spondylodiscitis: Pilot study on reduction of duration of systemic treatment. *Orthopade* **2020**, *49*, 714–723. [CrossRef] [PubMed]
3. Zhou, B.; Kang, Y.J.; Chen, W.H. Continuous Epidural Irrigation and Drainage Combined with Posterior Debridement and Posterior Lumbar Inter-Body Fusion for the Management of Single-Segment Lumbar Pyogenic Spondylodiscitis. *Surg. Infect.* **2020**, *21*, 262–267. [CrossRef] [PubMed]
4. Tschoeke, S.K.; Kayser, R.; Gulow, J.; Hoeh, N.; Salis-Soglio, G.; Heyde, C. Single-stage epidural catheter lavage with posterior spondylodesis in lumbar pyogenic spondylodiscitis with multilevel epidural abscess formation. *J. Neurol. Surg. A Cent. Eur. Neurosurg.* **2014**, *75*, 447–452. [CrossRef] [PubMed]
5. Mauer, U.M.; Kunz, U. Spinal epidural empyema. Limited surgical treatment combined with continuous irrigation and drainage. *Unfallchirurg* **2007**, *110*, 250–254. [CrossRef] [PubMed]
6. Ran, B.; Chen, X.; Zhong, Q.; Fu, M.; Wei, J. CT-guided minimally invasive treatment for an extensive spinal epidural abscess: A case report and literature review. *Eur. Spine J.* **2018**, *27*, 380–385. [CrossRef]
7. Ito, M.; Abumi, K.; Kotani, Y.; Kadoya, K.; Minami, A. Clinical outcome of posterolateral endoscopic surgery for pyogenic spondylodiscitis: Results of 15 patients with serious comorbid conditions. *Spine* **2007**, *32*, 200–206. [CrossRef]
8. Yang, S.C.; Fu, T.S.; Chen, H.S.; Kao, Y.H.; Yu, S.W.; Tu, Y.K. Minimally invasive endoscopic treatment for lumbar infectious spondylitis: A retrospective study in a tertiary referral center. *BMC Musculoskelet Disord.* **2014**, *15*, 105. [CrossRef] [PubMed]
9. Mehta, S.; Humphrey, J.S.; Schenkman, D.I.; Seaber, A.V.; Vail, T.P. Gentamicin distribution from a collagen carrier. *J. Orthop. Res.* **1996**, *14*, 749–754. [CrossRef]
10. Ascherl, R.; Stemberg, A.; Lechner, F.; Blumel, G. Local treatment of infection with collagen gentamicin. *Aktuelle Probl. Chir. Orthop.* **1990**, *34*, 85–93.
11. Lohr, M.; Reithmeier, T.; Ernestus, R.I.; Ebel, H.; Klug, N. Spinal epidural abscess: Prognostic factors and comparison of different surgical treatment strategies. *Acta Neurochir.* **2005**, *147*, 159–166; discussion 166. [CrossRef] [PubMed]

12. Hijazi, M.M.; Siepmann, T.; El-Battrawy, I.; Glatte, P.; Eyupoglu, I.; Schackert, G.; Juratli, T.A.; Podlesek, D. Clinical phenotyping of spondylodiscitis and isolated spinal epidural empyema: A 20-year experience and cohort study. *Front. Surg.* **2023**, *10*, 1200432. [CrossRef] [PubMed]
13. Ryang, Y.M.; Akbar, M. Pyogenic spondylodiscitis: Symptoms, diagnostics and therapeutic strategies. *Orthopade* **2020**, *49*, 691–701. [CrossRef] [PubMed]
14. Herren, C.; Jung, N.; Pishnamaz, M.; Breuninger, M.; Siewe, J.; Sobottke, R. Spondylodiscitis: Diagnosis and Treatment Options. *Dtsch. Arztebl. Int.* **2017**, *114*, 875–882. [CrossRef] [PubMed]
15. Tsai, T.T.; Yang, S.C.; Niu, C.C.; Lai, P.L.; Lee, M.H.; Chen, L.H.; Chen, W.J. Early surgery with antibiotics treatment had better clinical outcomes than antibiotics treatment alone in patients with pyogenic spondylodiscitis: A retrospective cohort study. *BMC Musculoskelet. Disord.* **2017**, *18*, 175. [CrossRef] [PubMed]
16. Homagk, L.; Homagk, N.; Klauss, J.R.; Roehl, K.; Hofmann, G.O.; Marmelstein, D. Spondylodiscitis severity code: Scoring system for the classification and treatment of non-specific spondylodiscitis. *Eur. Spine J.* **2016**, *25*, 1012–1020. [CrossRef] [PubMed]
17. Pojskic, M.; Carl, B.; Schmockel, V.; Vollger, B.; Nimsky, C.; Sabeta, B. Neurosurgical Management and Outcome Parameters in 237 Patients with Spondylodiscitis. *Brain Sci.* **2021**, *11*, 1019. [CrossRef] [PubMed]
18. Bydon, M.; De la Garza-Ramos, R.; Macki, M.; Naumann, M.; Sciubba, D.M.; Wolinsky, J.P.; Bydon, A.; Gokaslan, Z.L.; Witham, T.F. Spinal instrumentation in patients with primary spinal infections does not lead to greater recurrent infection rates: An analysis of 118 cases. *World Neurosurg.* **2014**, *82*, e807–e814. [CrossRef] [PubMed]
19. Dietz, N.; Sharma, M.; Alhourani, A.; Ugiliweneza, B.; Wang, D.; Nuno, M.; Drazin, D.; Boakye, M. Outcomes of decompression and fusion for treatment of spinal infection. *Neurosurg. Focus* **2019**, *46*, E7. [CrossRef]

**Disclaimer/Publisher's Note:** The statements, opinions and data contained in all publications are solely those of the individual author(s) and contributor(s) and not of MDPI and/or the editor(s). MDPI and/or the editor(s) disclaim responsibility for any injury to people or property resulting from any ideas, methods, instructions or products referred to in the content.

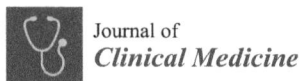
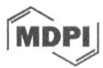

Article

# Risk Factors for the In-Hospital Mortality in Pyogenic Vertebral Osteomyelitis: A Cross-Sectional Study on 9753 Patients

Tomasz Piotr Ziarko [1], Nike Walter [1,2], Melanie Schindler [1], Volker Alt [1], Markus Rupp [1,*] and Siegmund Lang [1,*]

[1] Department for Trauma Surgery, University Hospital Regensburg, 93053 Regensburg, Germany
[2] Department for Psychosomatic Medicine, University Hospital Regensburg, 93053 Regensburg, Germany
* Correspondence: markus.rupp@ukr.de (M.R.); siegmund.lang@ukr.de (S.L.)

**Citation:** Ziarko, T.P.; Walter, N.; Schindler, M.; Alt, V.; Rupp, M.; Lang, S. Risk Factors for the In-Hospital Mortality in Pyogenic Vertebral Osteomyelitis: A Cross-Sectional Study on 9753 Patients. *J. Clin. Med.* **2023**, *12*, 4805. https://doi.org/10.3390/jcm12144805

Academic Editor: Kalliopi Alpantaki

Received: 22 June 2023
Revised: 17 July 2023
Accepted: 19 July 2023
Published: 21 July 2023

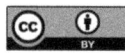

**Copyright:** © 2023 by the authors. Licensee MDPI, Basel, Switzerland. This article is an open access article distributed under the terms and conditions of the Creative Commons Attribution (CC BY) license (https://creativecommons.org/licenses/by/4.0/).

**Abstract:** Background: Pyogenic vertebral osteomyelitis represents a clinical challenge associated with significant morbidity and mortality. The aim of this study was to analyze potential risk factors for the in-hospital mortality of vertebral osteomyelitis (VO) patients. Methods: Based on the International Classification of Diseases, 10th Revision (ICD-10) codes for VO ("M46.2-", "M46.3-", and "M46.4-") data for total case numbers, secondary diagnoses, and numbers of in-hospital deaths were extracted from the Institute for the Hospital Remuneration System (InEK GmbH). Odds ratios (OR) for death were calculated for several secondary diseases and factors of interest. Results: Despite age, certain comorbidities were found to be strongly associated with increased mortality risk: Heart failure (OR = 2.80; 95% CI 2.45 to 3.20; $p < 0.01$), chronic kidney disease (OR = 1.83; 95% CI 1.57 to 2.13; $p < 0.01$), and diabetes with complications (OR = 1.86; 95% CI 1.46 to 2.38; $p < 0.01$). Among the complications, acute liver failure showed the highest risk for in-hospital mortality (OR = 42.41; 95% CI 23.47 to 76.62; $p < 0.01$). Additionally, stage III kidney failure (OR = 9.81; 95% CI 7.96 to 12.08; $p < 0.01$), sepsis (OR = 5.94; 95% CI 5.02 to 7.03; $p < 0.01$), acute respiratory failure (OR = 5.31; 95% CI 4.61 to 6.12; $p < 0.01$), and systemic inflammatory response syndrome (SIRS) (OR = 5.19; 95% CI 3.69 to 5.19; $p < 0.01$) were associated with in-hospital mortality. When analyzing the influence of pathogens, documented infection with *Pseudomonas aeruginosa* had the highest risk for mortality (OR = 2.74; 95% CI 2.07 to 3.63; $p < 0.01$), followed by Streptococci, *Escherichia coli*, and *Staphylococcus aureus* infections. Conclusions: An early assessment of individual patient risk factors may be beneficial in the care and treatment of VO to help reduce the risks of mortality. These findings emphasize the importance of closely monitoring VO patients with chronic organ diseases, early detection and treatment of sepsis, and tailored empirical antibiotic therapy. The identification of specific pathogens and antibiotic susceptibility testing should be prioritized to improve patient outcomes in this high-risk population.

**Keywords:** pyogenic vertebral osteomyelitis; mortality; risk-factors

## 1. Introduction

Musculoskeletal infections present a significant challenge in the fields of orthopedics and trauma surgery [1]. When infections of the spine occur without prior surgery or implanted devices, they are known as pyogenic vertebral osteomyelitis (VO), also referred to as spinal osteomyelitis or spondylodiscitis [2]. Hospitalization is often necessary for patients with VO [3]. Delayed diagnosis is common, particularly in cases involving low-virulence pathogens, and this can lead to high morbidity and mortality rates [4]. It is crucial to highlight the increasing importance of infections caused by coagulase-negative staphylococci (CONS) in this context [5–7]. Epidemiological studies have consistently reported a rise in the incidence of VO, indicating an ongoing challenge for healthcare systems [8–10]. Additionally, the treatment of elderly patients continues to be of great importance to musculoskeletal surgeons [11]. This trend can be attributed to the increasing number of comorbidities in an aging population, as well as advancements in imaging techniques that have improved diagnostics and resulted in a higher number of documented VO cases [12–15]. Furthermore, the standardization of pathogen identification methods has contributed to the detection of VO [16]. Recent publications have provided updated diagnostic and therapeutic approaches to VO treatment [17,18]. However, a significant heterogeneity remains in reports on the epidemiology of VO, with limited analyses of nationwide databases and an incomplete understanding of the risk factors associated with in-hospital mortality [8,10,19].

Therefore, this study aimed to analyze potential risk factors for in-hospital mortality among VO patients.

## 2. Materials and Methods

### 2.1. Data Source

In accordance with section 17b of the German Hospital Financing Act (KHG), a universal and performance-based remuneration system has been established for the provision of general hospital services. This includes a flat-rate compensation approach based on the German Diagnosis Related Groups system (G-DRG system). Each inpatient treatment case is thus remunerated via a corresponding DRG lump sum payment, providing standardized compensation aimed at maintaining uniformity across the healthcare system.

The Institute for the Remuneration System in Hospitals (InEK GmbH) serves as a substantial data source, providing in-depth data on primary and secondary diagnoses, all classified using the International Classification of Diseases, 10th Revision (ICD-10) system. Moreover, it presents data regarding patient demographics such as age and gender, as well as reasons for discharge, including mortality-related circumstances.

The InEK DatenBrowser facilitates a comprehensive analysis of these data, offering a cross-sectional view of healthcare trends and outcomes, and it includes information extending back to the year 2019.

Pre- and post-stationary services are included in the datasets as per § 1 para. 6 FPV. In the remuneration area "PSY", cases with equivalent inpatient psychiatric treatment are also included in the base population.

For cases with partial inpatient care in the remuneration area "DRG", counting is based on the number of transmitted data records, not adhering to the provisions of § 9 FPV where cases with regular or multiple treatments per quarter are counted as one case. This may result in a higher or lower case number compared to the number of delivered data records, and evaluation results for partially inpatient care must be interpreted considering these limitations.

For the purposes of this study, an analysis was conducted specifically for the year 2020. The focus was on the ICD-10 codes for vertebral osteomyelitis (VO)—"M46.2-", "M46.3-", and "M46.4-". The extracted data encompassed total case numbers, secondary diagnoses coding for comorbidities and complications, and instances of in-hospital deaths related to VO. This enabled an insightful exploration of the prevalence and outcomes associated with this specific condition. To ensure relevance, we chose to exclusively report on conditions that accounted for a minimum of 0.5% of the total cases by default.

### 2.2. Statistical Analysis

Statistical analysis was carried out using SPSS software version 28 (SPSS Inc, Chicago, IL, USA). The frequencies of secondary diagnoses, identified through coded data, are represented both as absolute numbers and as proportions of the total cases. To enhance interpretability, these diagnoses were segregated into two distinct categories: comorbidities and complications. Separately, coded data pertaining to pathogens were scrutinized.

In this study, univariate analysis was utilized to individually analyze each variable for its potential as a risk factor associated with in-hospital mortality among patients diagnosed with vertebral osteomyelitis (VO) in the year 2020. The dataset used for this examination included a wide spectrum of patient outcomes, including both cases with and without documented in-hospital deaths.

The statistical strength of the association between exposure to certain factors and the occurrence of the defined outcome—in-hospital mortality, in this case—was quantified using odds ratios (OR). An OR < 1.0 signified a negative association, indicating that the exposure to the variable under consideration was associated with lower odds of in-hospital mortality. Conversely, an OR > 1.0 represented a positive association, implying that the exposure was linked with higher odds of the defined outcome. ORs were calculated for several comorbidities and complications of interest. To complement these ORs, lower and upper 95% Confidence Intervals (CI) were also derived, furnishing an estimate of the range in which the true OR lies with a 95% probability. A $X^2$ (Chi-square) test of independence was conducted to examine the relationship between in-hospital mortality and each variable under consideration. A statistical significance level (alpha) of 0.05 was chosen; hence, a $p$-value less than this threshold would denote a statistically significant association between the factor and in-hospital mortality.

## 2.3. Ethical Considerations

The Informed Consent and Investigational Review Board (IRB) was not required for this cross-sectional study as it used data from an anonymous, de-identified, administrative database.

## 3. Results

The current study describes the secondary diagnoses of a previously published cohort of de-identified patients [20]. Briefly, the cohort of 9753 VO cases in 2020 consisted of mainly elderly patients, with 6.066 (62.6%) patients aged 70 years or older and a male/female ratio of 1.5.

In total, 150.958 secondary diagnoses were documented per 9753 cases in 2020. This results in 16 secondary diagnoses per case on average. The most common comorbidities were arterial hypertension (55.6%), type II diabetes (28.9%), and congestive heart failure (25.9%). Analysis of complications revealed hypokalemia (34.9%) and anemia due to bleeding (20.9%) followed by spinal abscess (intra- and extradural, 16.5%) to be the most documented (Table 1).

**Table 1.** Most common secondary diagnoses for comorbidities and complications in VO cases: Total numbers and share of all cases in 2020.

| | Secondary Diagnosis | ICD-10 Code | [n] | Percentage of All Cases |
|---|---|---|---|---|
| Comorbidity | Arterial Hypertension | I10.- | 5424 | 55.6% |
| | Type II diabetes | E11.- | 2819 | 28.9% |
| | Congestive heart failure | I50.- | 2522 | 25.9% |
| | Atrial fibrillation | I48.- | 2365 | 24.3% |
| | Chronic kidney disease | N18.1-; N19 | 2325 | 23.8% |
| | Coronary arterial disease | I25.0; I25.10-.19 | 1655 | 17.0% |
| | Hypothyreosis | E03.8; -.9 | 1264 | 13.0% |
| | Adipositas | E66.0-.99 | 997 | 10.2% |
| | Malignancy | C01; C10.–C97 | 736 | 7.6% |
| | Malnutrition | E43–E46 | 559 | 5.7% |
| | Implant-associated vertebral osteomyelitis | T81.4 | 431 | 4.4% |
| | Liver cirrhosis | K74.6; .-70-72 | 365 | 3.7% |
| | Dialysis | Z99.2 | 154 | 1.6% |
| | Cachexia | R64 | 107 | 1.1% |

Table 1. Cont.

| | Secondary Diagnosis | ICD-10 Code | [n] | Percentage of All Cases |
|---|---|---|---|---|
| Complications | Hypokalemia | E87.6 | 3408 | 34.9% |
| | Anemia, bleeding | D62 | 2039 | 20.9% |
| | Spinal abscess | G06.1; -.2 | 1612 | 16.5% |
| | Urinal tract infection | N39.0 | 1595 | 16.4% |
| | Pleural infusion | J90; J91 | 1576 | 16.2% |
| | Acute respiratory insufficiency | J96.01; J96.00 | 1441 | 14.8% |
| | Acute kidney failure | N17.0-; N17.81-3, -9-; N17.91-3, -9 | 1185 | 12.2% |
| | Pneumonia | J12.8–J18.9 | 1066 | 10.9% |
| | Infectious myositis | M60.05 | 1010 | 10.4% |
| | SIRS | R65.0-.3 | 980 | 10.1% |
| | Sepsis | A40.1–8; A41.1–9 | 854 | 8.8% |
| | COVID-19 | U07.1, .2 | 332 | 3.4% |
| | Infective Endocarditis | I33.0 | 222 | 2.3% |
| | Acute liver failure | K72.0 | 59 | 0.6% |

*Risk Factors for In-Hospital Mortality*

Risk factors for in-hospital mortality were examined and several significant associations were identified. Patient age was found to have a significant impact on mortality, with higher age categories showing increased risk (65 years and older: OR = 1.28; 95% CI 1.14 to 1.44; 75 years or older: OR = 1.57; 95% CI 1.39 to 1.78; 80 years or older: OR = 1.81; 95% CI 1.58 to 2.08; all $p < 0.01$) (Figure 1).

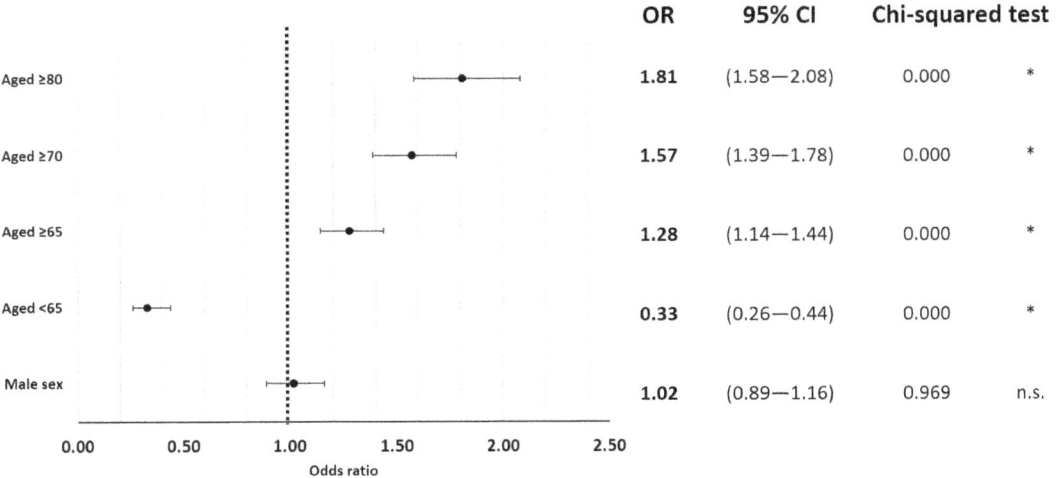

Figure 1. The in-hospital mortality odds ratio for epidemiological factors. * indicates $p < 0.05$.

Specific comorbidities were also significantly correlated with inpatient mortality. Heart failure was identified as a high-risk factor (OR = 2.80; 95% CI 2.45 to 3.20; $p < 0.01$), as well as chronic kidney disease (OR = 1.83; 95% CI 1.57 to 2.13; $p < 0.01$). Diabetes with complications (OR = 1.86; 95% CI 1.46 to 2.38; $p < 0.01$) and liver failure (OR = 42.41; 95% CI 23.47 to 76.62; $p < 0.01$) were also notable risk factors for in-hospital death. Anemia showed a significant increase in mortality risk (OR = 2.14; 95% CI 1.84 to 2.49; $p < 0.01$) (Figure 2).

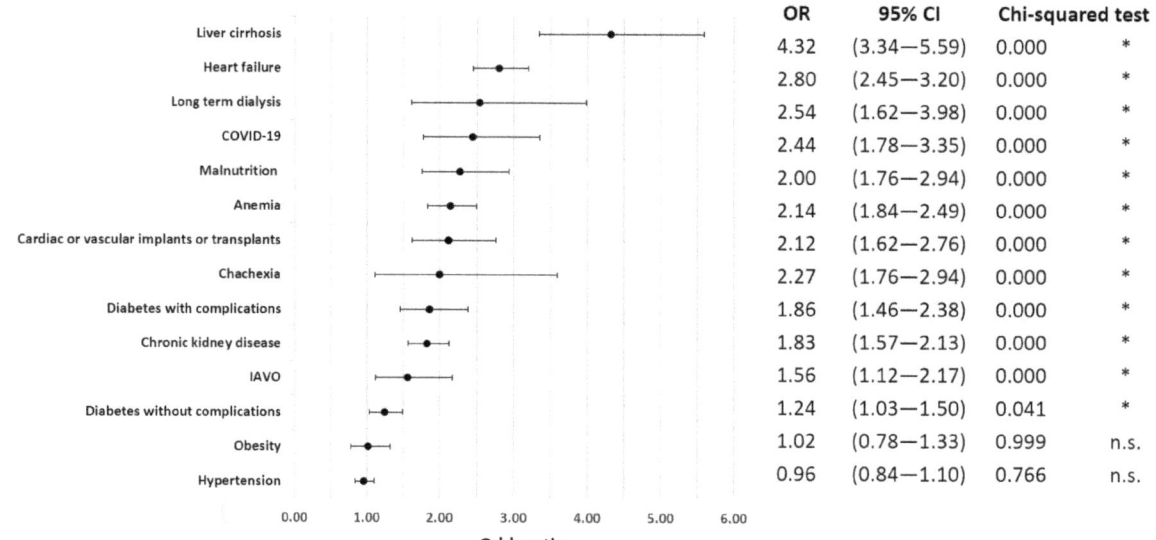

**Figure 2.** In-hospital mortality odds ratio for comorbidities. * indicates $p < 0.05$.

Interestingly, despite their relatively low prevalence (cachexia: 1.10%, malnutrition: 5.73% of all cases), cachexia (OR = 2.00; 95% CI 1.11 to 3.59; $p = 0.123$) and malnutrition (OR = 2.27; 95% CI 1.76 to 2.94; $p < 0.01$) were associated with a significantly increased risk of mortality. In contrast, obesity had a negligible effect on in-hospital mortality (OR = 1.02; 95% CI 0.78 to 1.33; $p = 0.999$).

Among the complications, acute liver failure showed the highest risk for in-hospital mortality (OR = 42.41; 95% CI 23.47 to 76.62; $p < 0.01$). Additionally, stage III kidney failure (OR = 9.81; 95% CI 7.96 to 12.08; $p < 0.01$), sepsis (OR = 5.94; 95% CI 5.02 to 7.03; $p < 0.01$), acute respiratory failure (OR = 5.31; 95% CI 4.61 to 6.12; $p < 0.01$), and systemic inflammatory response syndrome (SIRS) (OR = 5.19; 95% CI 3.69 to 5.19; $p < 0.01$) were associated with in-hospital mortality (Figure 3).

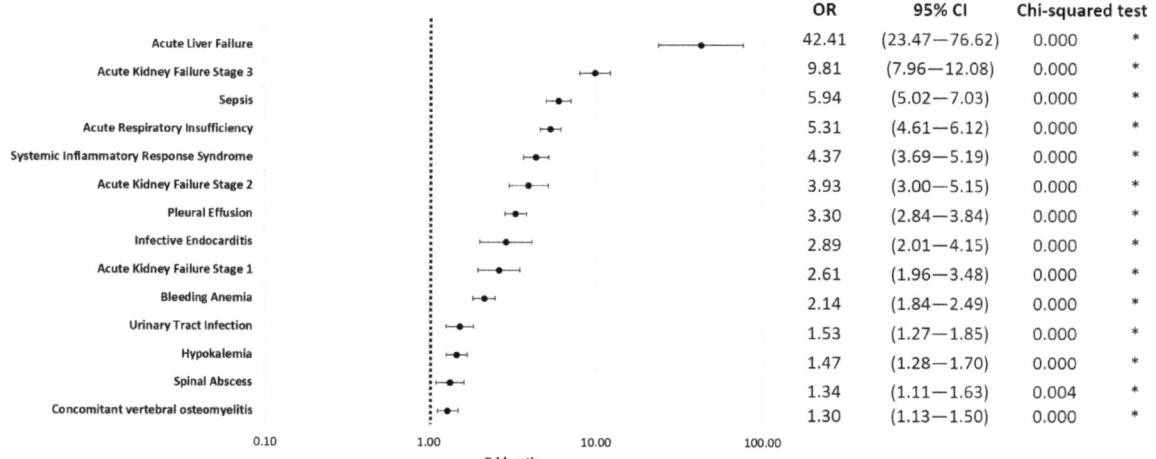

**Figure 3.** In-hospital mortality odds ratio for complications, logarithmically scaled. * indicates $p < 0.05$.

Information about coded pathogens in the current population has been published previously [20]. Briefly, pathogens were documented in 77.8% of the cases, with "other/unspecified staphylococci", *E. coli*, *S. aureus*, and streptococci being most prevalent. When analyzing the influence of pathogens, documented infection with *Pseudomonas aeruginosa* had the highest risk of mortality (OR = 2.74; 95% CI 2.07 to 3.63; $p < 0.01$), followed by Streptococci, *Escherichia coli*, and *Staphylococcus aureus* infections. (Figure 4A). Antimicrobial resistance codes were present in 12.9% of these cases, predominantly among gram-positive pathogens [20]. Overall, the presence of any resistant pathogen increased mortality risk (OR = 1.58; 95% CI 1.27 to 1.96; $p < 0.000$). Among gram-negative pathogens, a significant increase in mortality risk was observed (OR = 1.92; 95% CI 1.32 to 2.78; $p = 0.004$). Similarly, gram-positive pathogens also showed a significant association (OR = 1.78; 95% CI 1.37 to 2.32; $p < 0.000$). *Pseudomonas aeruginosa* with multidrug-resistance excluding carbapenems (3MRGN), although not statistically significant (OR = 2.8; 95% CI 1.16 to 6.73; $p = 0.120$), and glycopeptide antibiotic-resistant *Enterococcus faecium* (*E. faecium*) (OR = 2.33; 95% CI 1.68 to 3.24; $p < 0.000$) were associated with elevated mortality risk. However, *Methicillin-resistant Staphylococcus* aureus (*MRSA*) and *E. coli* 3MRGN did not show a significant impact on mortality ($p > 0.05$ for both, Figure 4B).

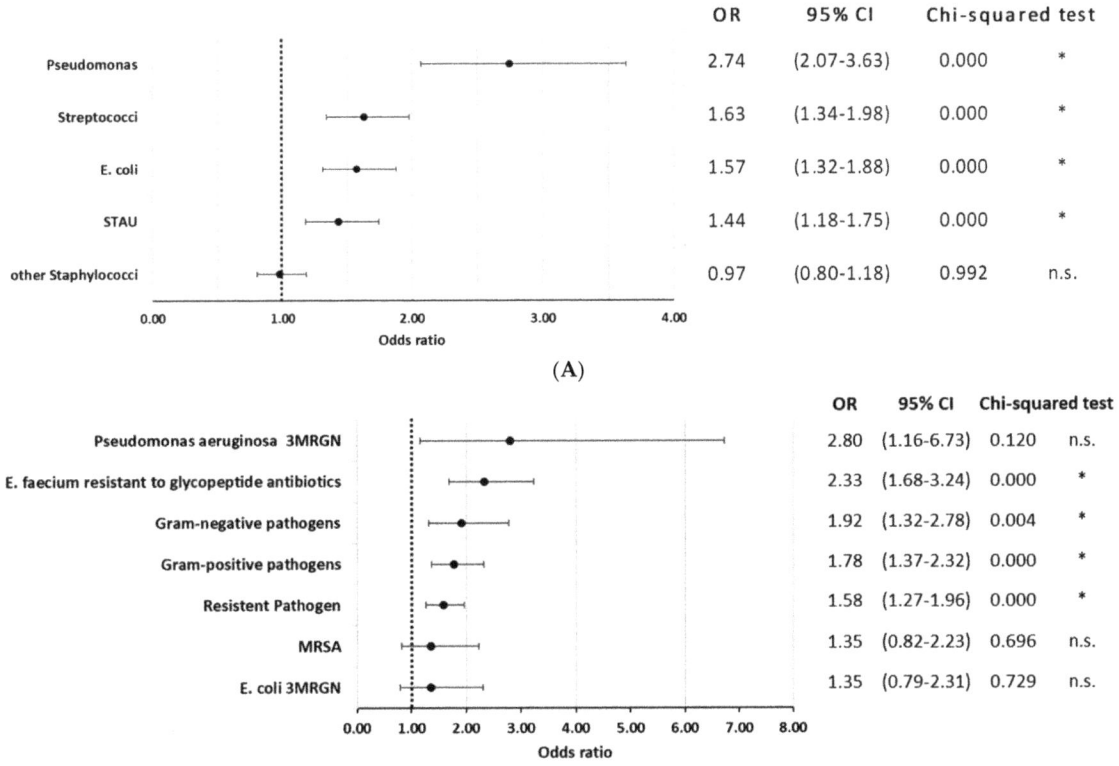

**Figure 4.** (**A**) In-hospital mortality odds ratio for coded pathogen. STAU = *S. aureus*. * indicates $p < 0.05$. (**B**) In-hospital mortality odds ratio for coded pathogen with antimicrobial resistance. * indicates $p < 0.05$.

## 4. Discussion

### 4.1. The Risk Factors for Mortality after VO

Associated risk factors for mortality after VO were examined in this nationwide evaluation analysis. As anticipated and previously reported, the risk of mortality increased with age, with patients aged 80 years or older having an odds ratio (OR) of 1.81 [21,22].

Additionally, secondary diagnoses contributing to frailty were associated with an increased risk. Liver cirrhosis (OR = 4.32), congestive heart failure (OR = 2.80), and the need for kidney dialysis (OR = 2.54) presented as the highest risk factors. Interestingly, obesity did not show an elevated risk in our analysis (OR = 1.02), whereas malnutrition (OR = 2.27) and cachexia (OR = 2.00) were associated with increased risk. In contrast to risk analyses reported by Vettivel et al. [21], the location or multiple levels of vertebral osteomyelitis (VO) were not identified as relevant risk factors in our study.

In a recent retrospective analysis of 155 patients with pyogenic VO, the in-hospital mortality rate was 12.9% [6]. Septic symptoms were observed in 21.9% of the patients. Yagdiran et al. reported 1- and 2-year mortality rates of 20% and 23%, respectively [23]. Vettivel et al. conducted a single-center study on 76 patients with pyogenic VO and reported a mortality rate of 5.2% at 30 days and 22.3% at 1 year. They identified the presence of frailty (OR = 13.62) and chronic renal failure (OR = 13.40) as risk factors for elevated 30-day mortality [21]. These findings closely resemble the current results, which encompassed the entirety of hospitalized patients.

Complications associated with in-hospital mortality include liver failure (OR = 42.41) and stage III acute kidney failure (OR = 9.81). Additionally, infectious complications such as endocarditis, pleural effusion, and systemic inflammatory response syndrome (SIRS) were significant factors. The presence of sepsis resulted in an odds ratio of 5.94 for in-hospital mortality. It is estimated that the global mortality rate for in-hospital-treated sepsis is approximately 25% for sepsis and 35% for severe sepsis at 30 days [24,25]. Sepsis-associated acute kidney injury is a common complication in critically ill patients and is associated with high morbidity and mortality [26,27]. Conversely, acute kidney injury has been identified as a risk factor for sepsis and its adverse outcomes [28]. Similarly, acute and acute-on-chronic liver failure have a negative impact on the prognosis of sepsis and serve as independent predictors of mortality in the intensive care unit [29–31]. There is limited evidence regarding organ failure as a risk factor for mortality in vertebral osteomyelitis (VO). This evaluation, to the best of our knowledge, identifies chronic and acute kidney and liver diseases and failure as significant risk factors for in-hospital mortality.

Apart from Staphylococcus aureus infections (OR = 1.44), the presence of gram-negative pathogens was associated with higher mortality. Specifically, Pseudomonas aeruginosa infection was identified as a relevant risk factor (OR = 2.74). The current results underscore the challenge that antimicrobial resistance poses in VO management. Particularly, *Pseudomonas aeruginosa* 3MRGN (OR = 2.80) and glycopeptide antibiotic-resistant *Enterococcus faecium* (OR = 2.33) showed a substantial contribution to mortality risk, stressing the importance of considering local resistance patterns in empirical antibiotic therapy for VO. These findings emphasize the need for tailored antibacterial strategies and antibiotic stewardship in tackling resistant pathogens in VO, as previously suggested [6]. In a retrospective analysis of 344 cases, Kang et al. found that patients with pyogenic spondylitis caused by gram-negative pathogens had a higher frequency of severe sepsis (24.2% vs. 11.3%), but the mortality rate did not significantly differ compared to infections with gram-positive pathogens (6.0% vs. 5.2%) [32].

Our results suggest that VO patients with chronic organ diseases should be closely monitored, and early detection and treatment of sepsis are crucial [33]. One possible approach could be the implementation of broad empirical antibiotic treatment tailored to local pathogens in this at-risk group, including cases of culture-negative VO. Identifying the specific pathogen and conducting antibiotic susceptibility testing are essential and should be pursued in all cases [34,35].

*4.2. Strengths and Limitations*

One notable strength of this epidemiological evaluation is its utilization of registry data comprising ICD-10 diagnosis codes from all medical institutions in Germany. The availability of these datasets facilitated a univariate analysis of risk factors for in-hospital mortality rates. The findings of this study should be interpreted within the scope of its limitations. In general, registry studies are commonly not accepted by design to allow causative relationships to be made. The limitations of our study include the inherent challenges of coding, which constrains the precise identification of certain pathogens, beyond the given ICD-10 codes. Further, the assessment of one-year or long-term mortality was not feasible. It is important to note that only inpatient data were accessible, and the detailed analysis focused solely on primary diagnoses. Additionally, this analysis does not provide information on treatment modalities such as surgery or antimicrobial therapy, thus precluding their consideration in the risk analysis. A significant limitation of this study is the lack of information regarding the administration of antimicrobials to patients. The ICD-10-based dataset does not capture specific therapeutic interventions, including antimicrobial use. This constraint precludes the assessment of the potential impact of antimicrobial administration on patient outcomes. Therefore, it is important to carefully interpret the data and consider alternative approaches to such prospective studies to gain a deeper understanding of the association between the tested risk factors and in-hospital mortality.

## 5. Conclusions

This analysis identified several comorbidities and complications as potential risk factors for elevated in-hospital mortality in pyogenic VO cases on a national scale. Advanced age, secondary diagnoses contributing to frailty, and specific comorbidities such as liver cirrhosis, congestive heart failure, and the need for kidney dialysis were identified as significant risk factors. Notably, obesity did not show an increased risk, while malnutrition and cachexia were associated with higher mortality rates. The presence of sepsis, gram-negative pathogens, particularly *Pseudomonas aeruginosa* infection, and acute kidney and liver failure were also associated with increased mortality. These findings emphasize the importance of closely monitoring VO patients with chronic organ diseases, early detection and treatment of sepsis, and tailored empirical antibiotic therapy. The identification of specific pathogens and antibiotic susceptibility testing should be prioritized to improve patient outcomes in this high-risk population, mainly geriatric patients.

**Author Contributions:** Conceptualization, S.L., T.P.Z., and M.R.; methodology, T.P.Z., M.S., and N.W.; validation, M.R., V.A. and M.R.; formal analysis, T.P.Z.; investigation, T.P.Z., N.W., M.S., and S.L.; writing—original draft preparation, T.P.Z..; writing—review and editing, N.W., M.S., S.L., M.R., and V.A.; supervision, S.L. and N.W. project administration, M.R. and V.A. All authors have read and agreed to the published version of the manuscript.

**Funding:** This research received no external funding.

**Institutional Review Board Statement:** The study was conducted in accordance with the Declaration of Helsinki. Methods were carried out following local data privacy guidelines and ethical regulations. As only anonymized data from a national, open-access databank were evaluated, no approval of the local ethic committee was necessary: the Informed Consent and Investigational Review Board (IRB) was not required for this study as it used data from an anonymous, de-identified, administrative database.

**Informed Consent Statement:** Patient consent was waived as only anonymized data from a national, open-access databank were used. No studies on humans or animals were conducted by the authors for this paper.

**Data Availability Statement:** All data presented in this study are available on request from the corresponding authors.

**Conflicts of Interest:** The authors declare no conflict of interest.

## References

1. Alt, V.; Giannoudis, P.V. Musculoskeletal infections—A global burden and a new subsection in Injury. *Injury* **2019**, *50*, 2152–2153. [CrossRef] [PubMed]
2. Rupp, M.; Walter, N.; Baertl, S.; Lang, S.; Lowenberg, D.W.; Alt, V. Terminology of bone and joint infection. *Bone Joint Res.* **2021**, *10*, 742–743. [CrossRef] [PubMed]

3. Zimmerli, W. Clinical practice. Vertebral osteomyelitis. *N. Engl. J. Med.* **2010**, *362*, 1022–1029. [CrossRef] [PubMed]
4. McHenry, M.C.; Easley, K.A.; Locker, G.A. Vertebral osteomyelitis: Long-term outcome for 253 patients from 7 Cleveland-area hospitals. *Clin. Infect. Dis.* **2002**, *34*, 1342–1350. [CrossRef] [PubMed]
5. Park, K.-H.; Kim, D.Y.; Lee, Y.-M.; Lee, M.S.; Kang, K.-C.; Lee, J.-H.; Park, S.Y.; Moon, C.; Chong, Y.P.; Kim, S.-H.; et al. Selection of an appropriate empiric antibiotic regimen in hematogenous vertebral osteomyelitis. *PLoS ONE* **2019**, *14*, e0211888. [CrossRef]
6. Lang, S.; Frömming, A.; Walter, N.; Freigang, V.; Neumann, C.; Loibl, M.; Ehrenschwender, M.; Alt, V.; Rupp, M. Is There a Difference in Clinical Features, Microbiological Epidemiology and Effective Empiric Antimicrobial Therapy Comparing Healthcare-Associated and Community-Acquired Vertebral Osteomyelitis? *Antibiotics* **2021**, *10*, 1410. [CrossRef]
7. Renz, N.; Haupenthal, J.; Schuetz, M.A.; Trampuz, A. Hematogenous vertebral osteomyelitis associated with intravascular device-associated infections—A retrospective cohort study. *Diagn. Microbiol. Infect. Dis.* **2017**, *88*, 75–81. [CrossRef]
8. Conan, Y.; Laurent, E.; Belin, Y.; Lacasse, M.; Amelot, A.; Mulleman, D.; Rosset, P.; Bernard, L.; Grammatico-Guillon, L. Large increase of vertebral osteomyelitis in France: A 2010–2019 cross-sectional study. *Epidemiol. Infect.* **2021**, *149*, e227. [CrossRef]
9. Grammatico, L.; Baron, S.; Rusch, E.; Lepage, B.; Surer, N.; Desenclos, J.C.; Besnier, J.M. Epidemiology of vertebral osteomyelitis (VO) in France: Analysis of hospital-discharge data 2002–2003. *Epidemiol. Infect.* **2008**, *136*, 653–660. [CrossRef]
10. Issa, K.; Diebo, B.G.; Faloon, M.; Naziri, Q.; Pourtaheri, S.; Paulino, C.B.; Emami, A. The Epidemiology of Vertebral Osteomyelitis in the United States From 1998 to 2013. *Clin. Spine Surg.* **2018**, *31*, E102–E108. [CrossRef]
11. Rupp, M.; Walter, N.; Pfeifer, C.; Lang, S.; Kerschbaum, M.; Krutsch, W.; Baumann, F.; Alt, V. The Incidence of Fractures Among the Adult Population of Germany-an Analysis From 2009 through 2019. *Dtsch. Arztebl. Int.* **2021**, *118*, 665–669. [CrossRef]
12. Kouijzer, I.J.E.; Scheper, H.; de Rooy, J.W.J.; Bloem, J.L.; Janssen, M.J.R.; van den Hoven, L.; Hosman, A.J.F.; Visser, L.G.; Oyen, W.J.G.; Bleeker-Rovers, C.P.; et al. The diagnostic value of 18F-FDG-PET/CT and MRI in suspected vertebral osteomyelitis—A prospective study. *Eur. J. Nucl. Med. Mol. Imaging* **2018**, *45*, 798–805. [CrossRef] [PubMed]
13. Raghavan, M.; Lazzeri, E.; Palestro, C.J. Imaging of Spondylodiscitis. *Semin. Nucl. Med.* **2018**, *48*, 131–147. [CrossRef] [PubMed]
14. Aagaard, T.; Roed, C.; Dahl, B.; Obel, N. Long-term prognosis and causes of death after spondylodiscitis: A Danish nationwide cohort study. *Infect. Dis.* **2016**, *48*, 201–208. [CrossRef]
15. Puth, M.-T.; Weckbecker, K.; Schmid, M.; Münster, E. Prevalence of multimorbidity in Germany: Impact of age and educational level in a cross-sectional study on 19,294 adults. *BMC Public Health* **2017**, *17*, 826. [CrossRef] [PubMed]
16. Iwata, E.; Scarborough, M.; Bowden, G.; McNally, M.; Tanaka, Y.; Athanasou, N.A. The role of histology in the diagnosis of spondylodiscitis: Correlation with clinical and microbiological findings. *Bone Joint J.* **2019**, *101-B*, 246–252. [CrossRef]
17. Lang, S.; Rupp, M.; Hanses, F.; Neumann, C.; Loibl, M.; Alt, V. Infektionen der Wirbelsäule: Pyogene Spondylodiszitis und implantatassoziierte vertebrale Osteomyelitis. *Unfallchirurg* **2021**, *124*, 489–504. [CrossRef]
18. Herren, C.; Höh, N. von der. Zusammenfassung der S2K-Leitlinie "Diagnostik und Therapie der Spondylodiszitis" (Stand 08/2020). *Die Wirbelsäule* **2021**, *5*, 18–20. [CrossRef]
19. Doutchi, M.; Seng, P.; Menard, A.; Meddeb, L.; Adetchessi, T.; Fuentes, S.; Dufour, H.; Stein, A. Changing trends in the epidemiology of vertebral osteomyelitis in Marseille, France. *New Microbes New Infect.* **2015**, *7*, 1–7. [CrossRef]
20. Lang, S.; Walter, N.; Schindler, M.; Baertl, S.; Szymski, D.; Loibl, M.; Alt, V.; Rupp, M. The Epidemiology of Spondylodiscitis in Germany: A Descriptive Report of Incidence Rates, Pathogens, In-Hospital Mortality, and Hospital Stays between 2010 and 2020. *J. Clin. Med.* **2023**, *12*, 3373. [CrossRef]
21. Vettivel, J.; Bortz, C.; Passias, P.G.; Baker, J.F. Pyogenic Vertebral Column Osteomyelitis in Adults: Analysis of Risk Factors for 30-Day and 1-Year Mortality in a Single Center Cohort Study. *Asian Spine J.* **2019**, *13*, 608–614. [CrossRef]
22. Zarrouk, V.; Gras, J.; Dubée, V.; de Lastours, V.; Lopes, A.; Leflon, V.; Allaham, W.; Guigui, P.; Fantin, B. Increased mortality in patients aged 75 years or over with pyogenic vertebral osteomyelitis. *Infect. Dis.* **2018**, *50*, 783–787. [CrossRef]
23. Yagdiran, A.; Otto-Lambertz, C.; Lingscheid, K.M.; Sircar, K.; Samel, C.; Scheyerer, M.J.; Zarghooni, K.; Eysel, P.; Sobottke, R.; Jung, N.; et al. Quality of life and mortality after surgical treatment for vertebral osteomyelitis (VO): A prospective study. *Eur. Spine J.* **2021**, *30*, 1721–1731. [CrossRef] [PubMed]
24. Bauer, M.; Gerlach, H.; Vogelmann, T.; Preissing, F.; Stiefel, J.; Adam, D. Mortality in sepsis and septic shock in Europe, North America and Australia between 2009 and 2019—Results from a systematic review and meta-analysis. *Crit. Care* **2020**, *24*, 239. [CrossRef]
25. Fleischmann, C.; Scherag, A.; Adhikari, N.K.J.; Hartog, C.S.; Tsaganos, T.; Schlattmann, P.; Angus, D.C.; Reinhart, K. Assessment of Global Incidence and Mortality of Hospital-treated Sepsis. Current Estimates and Limitations. *Am. J. Respir. Crit. Care Med.* **2016**, *193*, 259–272. [CrossRef] [PubMed]
26. Ma, S.; Evans, R.G.; Iguchi, N.; Tare, M.; Parkington, H.C.; Bellomo, R.; May, C.N.; Lankadeva, Y.R. Sepsis-induced acute kidney injury: A disease of the microcirculation. *Microcirculation* **2019**, *26*, e12483. [CrossRef]
27. Peerapornratana, S.; Manrique-Caballero, C.L.; Gómez, H.; Kellum, J.A. Acute kidney injury from sepsis: Current concepts, epidemiology, pathophysiology, prevention and treatment. *Kidney Int.* **2019**, *96*, 1083–1099. [CrossRef]
28. Mehta, R.L.; Bouchard, J.; Soroko, S.B.; Ikizler, T.A.; Paganini, E.P.; Chertow, G.M.; Himmelfarb, J. Sepsis as a cause and consequence of acute kidney injury: Program to Improve Care in Acute Renal Disease. *Intensive Care Med.* **2011**, *37*, 241–248. [CrossRef] [PubMed]

29. Dizier, S.; Forel, J.-M.; Ayzac, L.; Richard, J.-C.; Hraiech, S.; Lehingue, S.; Loundou, A.; Roch, A.; Guerin, C.; Papazian, L. Early Hepatic Dysfunction Is Associated with a Worse Outcome in Patients Presenting with Acute Respiratory Distress Syndrome: A Post-Hoc Analysis of the ACURASYS and PROSEVA Studies. *PLoS ONE* **2015**, *10*, e0144278. [CrossRef]
30. Strnad, P.; Tacke, F.; Koch, A.; Trautwein, C. Liver—Guardian, modifier and target of sepsis. *Nat. Rev. Gastroenterol. Hepatol.* **2017**, *14*, 55–66. [CrossRef]
31. Singer, M.; Deutschman, C.S.; Seymour, C.W.; Shankar-Hari, M.; Annane, D.; Bauer, M.; Bellomo, R.; Bernard, G.R.; Chiche, J.-D.; Coopersmith, C.M.; et al. The Third International Consensus Definitions for Sepsis and Septic Shock (Sepsis-3). *JAMA* **2016**, *315*, 801–810. [CrossRef] [PubMed]
32. Kang, S.-J.; Jang, H.-C.; Jung, S.-I.; Choe, P.G.; Park, W.B.; Kim, C.-J.; Song, K.-H.; Kim, E.S.; Kim, H.B.; Oh, M.-D.; et al. Clinical characteristics and risk factors of pyogenic spondylitis caused by gram-negative bacteria. *PLoS ONE* **2015**, *10*, e0127126. [CrossRef] [PubMed]
33. Husabø, G.; Nilsen, R.M.; Flaatten, H.; Solligård, E.; Frich, J.C.; Bondevik, G.T.; Braut, G.S.; Walshe, K.; Harthug, S.; Hovlid, E. Early diagnosis of sepsis in emergency departments, time to treatment, and association with mortality: An observational study. *PLoS ONE* **2020**, *15*, e0227652. [CrossRef]
34. van Belkum, A.; Bachmann, T.T.; Lüdke, G.; Lisby, J.G.; Kahlmeter, G.; Mohess, A.; Becker, K.; Hays, J.P.; Woodford, N.; Mitsakakis, K.; et al. Developmental roadmap for antimicrobial susceptibility testing systems. *Nat. Rev. Microbiol.* **2019**, *17*, 51–62. [CrossRef] [PubMed]
35. Lew, D.P.; Waldvogel, F.A. Osteomyelitis. *Lancet* **2004**, *364*, 369–379. [CrossRef] [PubMed]

**Disclaimer/Publisher's Note:** The statements, opinions and data contained in all publications are solely those of the individual author(s) and contributor(s) and not of MDPI and/or the editor(s). MDPI and/or the editor(s) disclaim responsibility for any injury to people or property resulting from any ideas, methods, instructions or products referred to in the content.

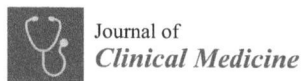

Article

# Cervical Spinal Epidural Abscess: Diagnosis, Treatment, and Outcomes: A Case Series and a Literature Review

Stamatios A. Papadakis [1,*], Margarita-Michaela Ampadiotaki [1], Dimitrios Pallis [1], Konstantinos Tsivelekas [1], Petros Nikolakakos [1], Labrini Agapitou [1] and George Sapkas [2]

[1] B' Orthopaedic Department, KAT General Hospital of Attica, 14561 Kifissia, Greece; marab.ortho@gmail.com (M.-M.A.); dimitrispallis99@gmail.com (D.P.); tsivelekaskonstantinos@gmail.com (K.T.); petros_nikolakakos@hotmail.com (P.N.); labrini.agapitou@gmail.com (L.A.)

[2] Orthopaedic Department, Metropolitan Hospital, 18547 Athens, Greece; gsapkas1@gmail.com

* Correspondence: sanpapadakis@gmail.com

**Abstract:** Although recent diagnostic and management methods have improved the prognosis of cervical epidural abscesses, morbidity and mortality remain significant. The purpose of our study is to define the clinical presentation of cervical spinal epidural abscess, to determine the early clinical outcome of surgical treatment, and to identify the most effective diagnostic and treatment approaches. Additionally, we analyzed studies regarding cervical epidural abscesses and performed a review of the literature. In this study, four patients with spinal epidural abscess were included. There were three men and one woman with a mean age of 53 years. Three patients presented with motor deficits, and one patient was diagnosed incidentally through spinal imaging. All the patients had fever, and blood cultures were positive. Staphylococcus aureus was the most common organism cultured from abscesses. All patients underwent a surgical procedure, and three patients recovered their normal neurological functions, but one remained with mild neurological disability that was resolved two years postoperatively. The mean follow-up period was 12 months, and no deaths occurred in this series. Furthermore, we identified 85 studies in the literature review and extracted data regarding the diagnosis and management of these patients. The timely detection and effective management of this condition are essential for minimizing its associated morbidity and mortality.

**Keywords:** cervical spinal epidural abscess; surgery; treatment; outcome

## 1. Introduction

Spinal epidural abscess (SEA) is an infection characterized by the accumulation of purulent material in the space between the dura mater and the osseoligamentous confines of the spinal canal [1,2]. It is an unusual disorder, and in a review carried out by Darouiche et al., the prevalence rate varied from 0.18 to 1.96 per 10,000 admissions in hospitals [3]. Despite recent improvements in the diagnosis and treatment of SEA, the mortality rate is still high, ranging from 4.6% to 31% [4].

Spinal epidural abscess has a peak incidence in the sixth and seventh decades of life [5]. When all large series are considered, male predominance is 2:1 [6]. Predisposing systemic conditions include diabetes mellitus, intravenous drug abuse, renal disease, alcoholism, HIV infection, malignancy, morbid obesity, long-term corticosteroid use, and septicemia [7,8]. Local conditions that predispose an individual to epidural space infection include recent spine trauma, spinal surgery, and intrathecal injection or catheter placement [9].

The responsible pathogens are identified through blood cultures or cultures taken during surgery. Of the microorganisms shown to be causative agents of spinal epidural abscesses, Staphylococcus aureus is the most prevalent [10]. The infection is often caused by Streptococcus species, which are the second most frequently isolated bacteria. Although less common in general, Gram-negative bacilli are frequently isolated from intravenous drug abusers [11]. Mycobacterium tuberculosis, fungal species, and parasitic organisms are rare causes of spinal epidural abscess, especially without associated vertebral osteomyelitis. In some patients, cultures are sterile, and the infecting organism cannot be identified. The mainstay of treatment for spinal epidural abscess is early diagnosis followed by surgical debridement and intravenous antibiotics [12].

Although detection can occur at any level of the spine, epidural abscess in the cervical spine is rare. The incidence of spinal epidural abscess affecting the cervical spine is observed in only 18% to 36% of SEA cases, which is lower than the occurrence in the lumbar or thoracic spine [6]. Despite its lower prevalence, cervical SEA is consistently associated with worse neurological functional outcomes and a higher risk of morbidity and mortality. These findings suggest that the cervical location presents a unique pathology compared to infections in the thoracic or lumbar regions, potentially influenced by factors such as dynamic motion and the presence of the cervical spinal cord [11].

The optimal treatment for cervical epidural abscesses remains controversial. Therefore, the purpose of our study is to define the clinical presentation of cervical spinal epidural abscess in a case series and to determine the early clinical outcome of surgical treatment. Also, we conducted a systematic review of the existing literature related to cervical epidural abscesses.

## 2. Materials and Methods

In this study, four patients with cervical spinal epidural abscess (CSEA) underwent surgical treatment in our department. There were three men and one woman. Their ages varied from 23 to 68 years, and the average age was 53 years.

Three patients presented with motor deficits, and one patient presented incidentally upon spinal imaging. Two patients had involvement of the anterior column of C2–C4, one patient had involvement of C1–C5, and another patient had involvement of C2–C5. All the patients had fever. The time between the appearance of clinical symptoms and surgical treatment was 14 days on average. The median time from admission to surgery was 72 h.

We identified predisposing factors to the development of the infection in two patients. Diabetes mellitus was present in one case and abuse of venous drugs in another.

The infectious agent was identified in all patients through cultures during surgery. Staphylococcus aureus was the predominant germ. Anteroposterior and lateral cervical spine radiographs and Gadolinium-enhanced magnetic resonance imaging (Gd-MRI) were performed in all patients (Figures 1 and 2). In all patients, the lesion was located in the anterior column.

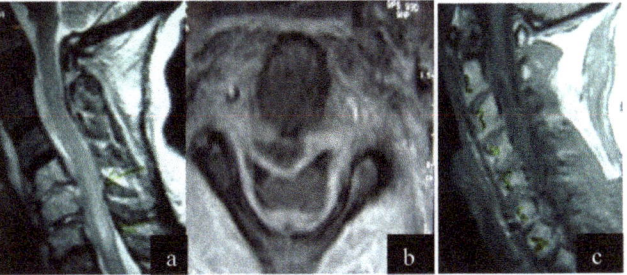

**Figure 1.** (**a**) Preoperative magnetic resonance imaging (MRI) sequence T2 lateral view. There is a cervical epidural abscess within the spinal canal below the posterior longitudinal ligament extending from C1 to C5, deformation of the signal of the spinal cord due to an inflammatory reaction. (**b**) Preoperative magnetic resonance imaging (MRI) sequence T2 axial view. The presence of a pathological cavity below the posterior longitudinal ligament is observed, causing compression of the thecal sac. (**c**) Preoperative magnetic resonance imaging (MRI) sequence T1 lateral view.

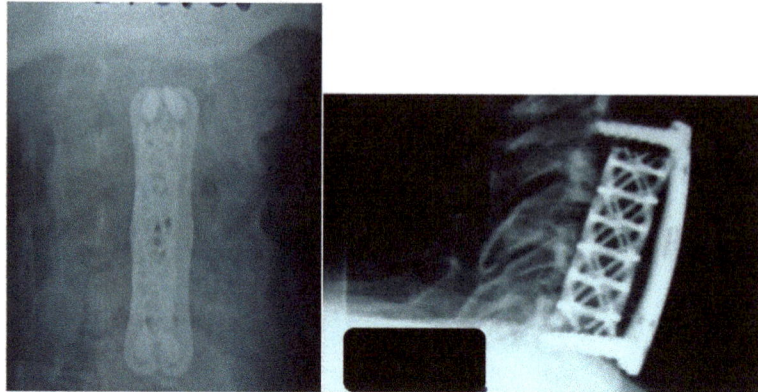

**Figure 2.** The patient underwent surgical intervention with decompression of the thecal sac. The first procedure was performed using an anterior approach, during which the affected vertebral bodies of C4 and C5 were removed and decompression of the thecal sac was carried out. A titanium cylinder was placed, and anterior stabilization was completed with a plate. Anteroposterior and lateral radiographs.

All patients underwent decompression under general anesthesia with partial or total corpectomy and fusion using an anterior or posterior approach, debridement, biopsy, and cultures (Figures 3 and 4). Postoperative immobilization with hard cervical orthosis was performed. Intravenous antibiotic therapy was used for 4–6 weeks.

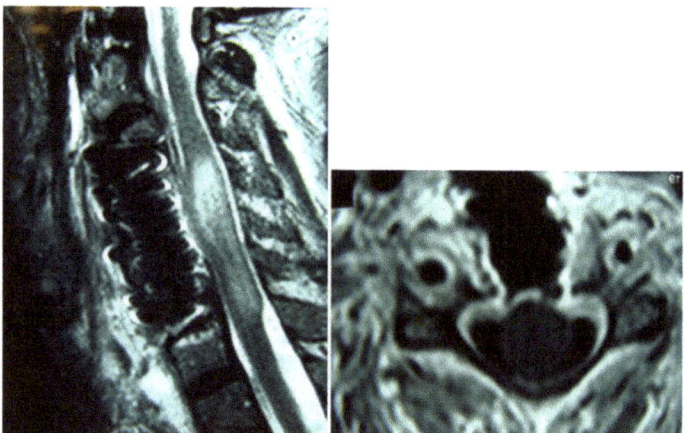

**Figure 3.** Postoperative magnetic resonance imaging, sagittal and axial views. The presence of a titanium mesh cage and dilation of the spinal cord sac are observed.

In addition, a literature review was conducted on the PubMed database, using the search terms "cervical epidural abscess" and "surgical treatment" up to December 2022. Two reviewers screened the initial search results and selected studies for review based on the following inclusion criteria: free full text, case reports and case series, English language, adult patients, and studies on humans. Studies were excluded from this review, due to the following exclusion criteria: no English language, full text unavailable, studies on animals, studies on pediatric patients, and inability to determine patients suffering from cervical abscesses from other locations in the same study.

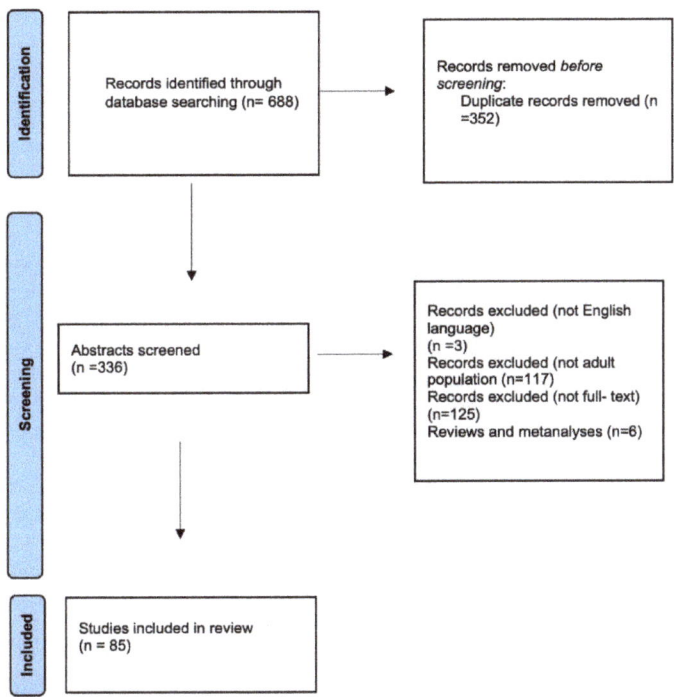

**Figure 4.** Literature search and flowchart.

The data that were abstracted from each study were: author, date of publication, total number of patients, gender, age, the level of abscess, pathogen, treatment, outcome, laboratory results, risk factors and previous history, and the presence of spondylodiscitis or an isolated epidural abscess.

## 3. Results

The mean follow-up period of our patients was 12 months (range: 8–18 months). All patients were included in the postoperative evaluation. Three out of the four patients returned to their previous functional status and daily activities fully three months after surgery. In one case, a neurologic deficit was persistent. The patient experienced bilateral upper limb numbness for two years postoperatively, along with muscle weakness graded at 4/5 on the left side and 3.5/5 on the right side. Full recovery was achieved two years postoperatively. Major complications were not observed in any of the patients. There were no deaths in this series, but two cases developed dysphagia, which was resolved without therapy after two weeks (Table 1).

The literature research initially revealed 688 articles related to the term "cervical epidural abscess". The full text was available for 211 studies; of those, 208 were written in English. There were 91 referred articles referring to the adult population. We then excluded reviews and metanalyses, and only case series and case reports were included. Thus, a total of 85 studies were included in this review.

**Table 1.** Data of our cases.

| Patients | Age | Gender | Level | Microorganism | Treatment | Symptoms | Outcome | Risk Factors |
|---|---|---|---|---|---|---|---|---|
| 1 | 23 | M | C2–C4 | Staphylococcus aureus | Debridement and fusion | Fever, pain, numbness, and muscle weakness bilaterally | Full recovery, dysphagia for 2 weeks postop | Abuse of venous drugs |
| 2 | 68 | M | C2–C4 | Staphylococcus aureus | Debridement and fusion | Fever, pain, numbness, and muscle weakness bilaterally | Full recovery | Diabetes mellitus |
| 3 | 56 | F | C1–C5 | Staphylococcus aureus | Debridement and fusion | Fever, pain, numbness, and muscle weakness bilaterally | Full recovery 2 years post op, muscle weakness | |
| 4 | 69 | M | C2–C5 | Staphylococcus aureus | Debridement and fusion | Incidentally upon spinal imaging | Full recovery, dysphagia for 2 weeks postop | |

The total number of patients included was 209—140 males and 69 females. The mean patient age was 56.2 years old, ranging from 23 to 87. Table 1 demonstrates the patients' features from each study. Regarding the level of abscess, it was more often observed at C1–C2 and at C5–C6. The most common pathogen was Staphylococcus aureus, observed in 100 cases (30 MRSA and 33 MSSA) (47.9%). Other pathogens that caused cervical abscesses were *Streptococcus* (5.7%), brucellosis (4.7%), *E. coli* (3.3%), *Pseudomonas* (1.9%), *Klebsiella* (1.4%), *Enterococcus*, *Proteus*, and *Mycobacterium tuberculosis*. The patients presented with symptoms including fever, neck pain, numbness, and weakness of the upper limbs. Twenty-five patients (11.9%) had no neurological deficit on admission, although nineteen had quadriparesis (9%). However, most of the patients underwent surgical management, such as corpectomy, fusion, drainage, and decompression, and only 14 patients received conservative treatment (6.6%). The most commonly mentioned risk factors were diabetes mellitus, drug abuse, renal disorder, previous surgical procedures, and dairy product consumption (Table 2).

Table 2. Literature review of published cases with cervical abscesses. (ps): present study.

| Author | Number of Patients | Age | Gender | Level | Microorganism | Treatment | Neurological Deficit Initially | Outcome | ESR/WBC/CRP |
|---|---|---|---|---|---|---|---|---|---|
| Frank et al. (1944) [13] | 1 | 43 | M | C2 | *Staph. aureus* | Hilton's method | Death from meningitis 15 w post | Death | Raised WBC |
| Leach et al. (1967) [14] | 1 | 49 | F | C1–C2 | *Staph. aureus* | Collar, antibiotics | No neurologic deficit | Full recovery 10 months | ESR = 36, WBC = 15 |
| Rimalovski et al. (1968) [15] | 1 | 48 | F | C2 | *Staph. aureus* | Penicillin, nitrofurantoine, staphcilin 3 months | No neurologic deficit | Death | WBC = 19.9 |
| Ahlback et al. (1970) [16] | 2 | (1) 44 (2) 43 | F M | (1) C1–C2 (2) C1–C2 | NA | (1) penicillin, streptomycin, tonsillectomy (2) cloxacillin, C1–C2 fusion | No neurologic deficit | (1) Cervical stiffness (2) Full recovery | (1) ESR = 50, WBC = 8 (2) ESR = 110, WBC = 7.9 |
| Vemireddi (1978) [17] | 1 | 58 | M | C1–C2 | *Staph. aureus* | Nafcillin, halo, dicloxacillin 3 m | Weakness in upper and lower right extremities | Cervical stiffness | WBC = 7.8, ESR = 74 |
| Venger et al. (1986) [18] | 1 | 29 | M | C2 | *Staph. aureus* | Halo, nafcillin | No neurologic deficit | Full recovery 6 m | WBC = 18, ESR = 50 |
| Zigler et al. (1987) [19] | 5 | (1) 62 (2) 66 (3) 67 (4) 56 (5) 72 | F M F F M | (1) C1–C2 (2) C1–C2 (3) C1–C2 (4) C1–C2 (5) C1–C2 | (1) *Staph. aureus* (2) *Staph. aureus* (3) *Staph. aureus* (4) *Pasteurella multocida* (5) *Staph. aureus* | (1) Oxacillin, posterior cervical fusion C1–C3 (2) Erythromycin, methicillin, halo cast, posterior cervical arthrodesis (3) Cervical traction, transoral biopsy and debridement of axis and atlas, oxacillin (4) Ampicillin, posterior fusion of occiput to axis (5) Oxacillin, posterior atlantoaxial arthrodesis, halo jacket | (1) Weakness in lower extremities (2) No neurological deficits (3) Hyperreflexia (4) Hyperreflexia (5) No neurological deficits | (1) Full recovery (2) Full recovery (3) Full recovery (4) Full recovery (5) Discomfort of the neck secondary to spondylosis | (1) WBC = 7.9 (2) WBC = 7.5, ESR = 108 (3) NA (4) WBC = 39, ESR = 105 |

Table 2. Cont.

| Author | Number of Patients | Age | Gender | Level | Microorganism | Treatment | Neurological Deficit Initially | Outcome | ESR/WBC/CRP |
|---|---|---|---|---|---|---|---|---|---|
| Bartels et al. (1990) [20] | 1 | 49 | M | C2–C7 | Staph. aureus | Lateral pharyngotomy to drain a large prevertebral abscess, antibiotics | No neurologic deficit | Full recovery | WBC 13.6 |
| Sebben et al. (1992) [21] | 1 | 59 | M | C2–C3 | Staph. aureus | Decompressive cervicotomy C2–C3 | | Good recovery | WBC = 8200, TKE = 100, CRP = 35 |
| Ruskin et al. (1992) [22] | 1 | 57 | M | C1–C2 | Staph. aureus, lactobacillus | Incision and drainage, imipenem | No neurologic deficit | Full recovery | WBC 17.6, ESR 90 |
| Keogh et al. (1992) [23] | 1 | 41 | M | C1–C2 | Staph. aureus | IV flucloxacillin and fusidic acid; transoral evacuation of extradural pus and excision of eroded odontoid peg; skull traction | No neurologic deficit | Complete resolution at 3 m f/u | WBC 17.9 |
| Azizi et al. (1995) [24] | 1 | 65 | M | Clivus-c1 | Na | Halo antibiotics | cranial nerve abnormalities | Residual abducens palsy | ESR = 132 |
| Sawada et al. (1996) [25] | 1 | 57 | M | C5–C6 | Staph. aureus | Discectomy | Quadriplegia | Good outcome | WBC = 6300, CRP = 6, ESR = 63 |
| Lam et al. (1996) [26] | 1 | 58 | M | C1–C2 | St aureus | Antibiotics | Bilateral weakness | Full recovery 9 m | ESR = 90, WBC = |
| Fukutake et al. (1998) [27] | 1 | 74 | M | C1–C2 | Streptococcus pn | Posterior fusion | Numbness of upper extremities | Full recovery 3 m | Esr 127, crp 31, wcc 21.5 |
| Weidau-Pazos et al. (1999) [28] | 2 | (1) 63 (2) 74 | M F | (1) C1–C2 (2) C1–C2 | (1) Staph. aureus (2) NA | (1) transoral decompression, hemilaminectomy (2) transoral decompression, halo, and posterior fusion | Paraparesis | Full recovery | (1) WBC = 13, ESR = 38 (2) WBC = 10, ESR = 85 |
| Anton et al. (1999) [29] | 1 | 75 | F | C1–C2 | Strept. viridians | Decompression, posterior fusion | quadriplegia | Limb weakness | NA |

Table 2. Cont.

| Author | Number of Patients | Age | Gender | Level | Microorganism | Treatment | Neurological Deficit Initially | Outcome | ESR/WBC/CRP |
|---|---|---|---|---|---|---|---|---|---|
| Suchomel et al. (2003) [30] | 3 | (1) 52 (2) 51 (3) 50 | M F M | (1) C1–C2 (2) C1–C2 (3) C1–C2 | (1) Staph. aureus (2) Staph. aureus (3) Staph. aureus | Decompression, posterior fusion, antibiotics 3 w | No neurologic deficit All | Full recovery | (1) ESR = 80 (2) WBC, ESR elevated (3) ESR = 90 |
| Haridas et al. (2003) [31] | 1 | 65 | M | C2 | Proteus mirabilis | Transoral decompression, posterior fusion | Upper motor neuron sign both lower extremities, Lhermitte sign (5 d) | Limb paralysis | |
| Yi et al. (2003) [32] | 1 | 39 | M | C5–C6 | NA | Laminectomy C5–C6 | Decreased upper and lower limb muscle power and bladder dysfunction (10 d) | Full recovery | |
| Ates et al. (2005) [33] | 1 | 42 | F | C3–C5 | Brucellosis | Anterior plate and iliac crest graft, doxycycline and rifampicin 3 months | Mild quadriparesis (3 m) | Full recovery | ESR = 80 |
| Burgess et al. (2005) [34] | 1 | | F | C2–C4 | MRSA | Laminectomy, dexamethasone, ceftriaxone, and vancomycin (26 h after admission) | Quadriplegia | Death | WBC = 11,400 |
| Moriya et al. (2005) [35] | 1 | 47 | M | C3–C5 | NA | Cefotaxime and piperacillin | Stiff deep reflexes in lower extremities (10 d) | Good outcome | NA |
| Paul et al. (2005) [36] | 1 | 54 | M | C2–C4 | Pseudomonas aeruginosa | Decompression, fusion, halo | No neurologic deficit | Neck pain | NA |
| Kulkarni et al. (2006) [37] | 1 | 56 | M | C4–C5 | Serratia marcescens | Decompression, iliac crest graft | No neurologic Deficit | Neck pain | ESR = 30, CRP = 1.1, WBC = 8 |
| Curry et al. (2007) [38] | 1 | 37 | F | C2–C3 | NA | Decompression, fusion | No neurologic deficit | Full recovery | WBC = 5.6, ESR = 68 |
| Jeon et al. (2007) [39] | 1 | 72 | M | C3–C4 | Eikenella corrodens | Corpectomy, ciprofloxacin | Right hemiparesis and left hypesthesia | Remaining right hemiparesis and left hypesthesia | CRP = 2, WBC = 12, ESR = 38 |
| Reid et al. (2007) [40] | 1 | 58 | M | C1–C2 | MRSA | Transoral decompression, posterior fusion | No neurologic deficit | Full recovery | WBC = 14, ESR = 109, CRP = 115 |

Table 2. Cont.

| Author | Number of Patients | Age | Gender | Level | Microorganism | Treatment | Neurological Deficit Initially | Outcome | ESR/WBC/CRP |
|---|---|---|---|---|---|---|---|---|---|
| Metcalfe et al. (2009) [41] | 1 | 62 | M | C6–C7 | *Candida* and *lactobacillus* | C6-C7 partial vertebrectomy, doxycycline, fluconazole | Weakness and pins and needles in both upper limbs, difficulty walking | Full Recovery 17 m | High CRP, IgA, IgG |
| Hantzidis et al. (2009) [42] | 1 | 65 | M | C5–C6 | Brucellosis | Cage, anterior plate Doxycycline and streptomycin 3 months | No neurologic deficit | Partial recovery, motor and sensory deficits C6 neurotome | |
| Fang et al. (2009) [43] | 1 | 31 | M | C4–C5 | *Staph. aureus* | Corpectomy, fusion, iliac crest graft | No neurologic deficit | Good outcome | 9800, 64 CRP = 4.5 |
| Ueda et al. (2009) [44] | 1 | 37 | M | C1 | *Streptococcus* spp | Antibiotics | No neurologic deficit | Full recovery | WBC = 20, CRP = 4.7 |
| Tamori et al. (2010) [45] | 1 | 80 | F | C5–C6 | *E. coli* | Decompression, drainage | Brown-Sequard syndrome | Paralysis of right upper limb | WBC = 1.2 CRP = 10 |
| Gezici et al. (2010) [46] | 1 | (1) 66 (2) 45 | M | C4–C5 C5–C7 | (1) NA (2) *Staph. aureus*, *Pseudomonas aeruginosa* | (1) Hemilaminectomy, facetectomy (2) Corpectomy, graft | Quadriparesis | Neurologic deficit | (1) Normal (2) WBC = 13, ESR = 136, CRP = 52 |
| Deshmukh (2010) [47] | 1 | 59 | F | C2–C3 C7–T1 | MRSA | Corpectomy, cervical collar | Quadriparesis | Full recovery | NA |
| Khoriati et al. (2012) [48] | 1 | 87 | M | C2 | NA | Occipitocervical fusion | No neurologic deficit | Good recovery | ESR = 91 |
| Ekici et al. (2012) [49] | 2 | (1) 61 (2) 63 | M F | (1) C4–C5 (2) C3–C4 | Brucellosis | (1) Decompression and discectomy without fusion, doxycycline, rifampicin for 3 months (2) Decompressive laminectomy, cage, doxycycline, Rifampicin for 3 months | (1) Weakness and hypoesthesia in upper limbs (2) Hypoesthesia in upper limbs | (1) Full recovery (2) Full recovery | (1) WBC = 8.7, CRP = 30.7, ESR = 32 (2) WBC = 7, CRP = 3.8, ESR = 12 |
| Lampropoulos et al. (2012) [50] | 1 | 70 | F | C4–C5 | Brucellosis | Streptomycin, doxycycline, rifampicin 4 m | No neurological deficits | Recovery | WBC = 6.1, ESR = 80, CRP = 8 |

Table 2. Cont.

| Author | Number of Patients | Age | Gender | Level | Microorganism | Treatment | Neurological Deficit Initially | Outcome | ESR/WBC/CRP |
|---|---|---|---|---|---|---|---|---|---|
| Soultanis et al. (2013) [51] | 1 | 53 | F | C3–C4 | *Enterococcus faecalis* | Decompression–fusion–antibiotics 9 w | Quadriparesis | Improvement | NA |
| Jensen et al. (2013) [52] | 9 | (5) 71 (6) 61 (7) 57 | F F M | (5) C4–C7 (6) C2–C3 (7) C3–C6 | *Strept. anginosus* NA *Staph. aureus* | Spondylodesis C3–C5 Spondylodesis and laminectomy Spondylodesis Antibiotics 3 months | Quadriparesis | Tetraplegia all | NA |
| Radulovic et al. (2013) [53] | 1 | 53 | F | C3–C4 | NA | Laminectomies C2–C4 | Quadriparesis | Quadriparesis initially, paresis of deltoid finally | WBC-18.7, ESR = 78 |
| O'neil et al. (2014) [54] | 1 | 64 | M | C4–C5 | *E. coli* | Discectomy and fusion | Poor balance, motor deficit | Initial poor balance, motor deficits, UTI Eventual improvement | WBC = 24, CRP = 79 |
| Giri et al. (2014) [55] | 1 | 49 | M | C5–C6 | MRSA | Decompression | No neurologic deficit | NA | ESR = 60, WBC = 2000, CRP = 9 |
| Alton et al. (2015) [56] | 62 | 23 (mean age) | 41 M 21 F | | MSSA (38.6%) MRSA (32.3%) Streptoococcus milleri (4.8%) Unknown (16.3%) | 56 treated surgically | 23 had neurologic deficit 39 no neurologic deficit | 17 remained with neurological deficit | CRP = 168, ESR = 77, WBC = 17 |
| Ghobrial et al. (2015) [57] | 40 | 53 (mean age) | 30 M 10 F | | MSSA (57.5%) MRSA (12.5%) *Pseudomonas* (5%) *Klebsiella* (2.5%) *E. coli* (2.5%) Negative (12.5%) | NA | NA | 6% complication rate | NA |

Table 2. Cont.

| Author | Number of Patients | Age | Gender | Level | Microorganism | Treatment | Neurological Deficit Initially | Outcome | ESR/WBC/CRP |
|---|---|---|---|---|---|---|---|---|---|
| Young et al. (2001) [58] | 6 | 41–74 | 5 M 1 F | NA | *Staph. aureus* | Anterior corpectomy and fusion | Quadriparesis | 4 ambulatory at last/2 quadriparesis | NA |
| Aranibar et al. (2015) [59] | 1 | 70 | F | C1–C2 | MRSA | Decompression, posterior fusion occipitocervically | Limb weakness | Limb weakness | NA |
| Kohlmann et al. (2015) [60] | 1 | 53 | F | C2–C5 | *E. coli* | Fusion and meropenem | No neurologic deficit | Good outcome | WBC-33, CRP = 163 |
| Ugarriza et al. (2005) [61] | 1 | 55 | M | C5–C7 | Brucellosis | Decompressive corpectomy and anterior fusion, rifampicin and doxycycline 8 weeks | NA | Full recovery | NA |
| Oh et al. (2015) [62] | 1 | 44 | M | C3–C4 | *Strept. viridans* | Ceftriaxone, gentamycin 12 w | No neurologic deficit | Full recovery | WBC = 12, ESR = 23, CRP = 24.9 |
| Zhang et al. (2017) [63] | 1 | 65 | F | C6–T8 | NA | Imipenem/cilastatin, famciclovir | No neurologic deficit | Full recovery | WBC = 24, ESR = 66, CRP = 193 |
| Lee et al. (2017) [64] | 1 | 49 | F | C3–C6 | *Staph. aureus* | Laminoplasty | Quadriparesis | Quadriplegia initially, Kyphotic deformity Good outcome | WBC = 23, ESR = 80, CRP = 114 |
| Li et al. (2017) [65] | 14 | 57.7 (mean age) | 9 M 5 F | C4– C5(4 patients C5– C6(5) C6– C7(3) | | Fusion and ilium bone graft | Quadriparesis | | ESR = 63, WBC = 16, CRP = 73 |
| Yang et al. (2017) [66] | 1 | 67 | F | C2–T1 | *Strept. intermedius* | Vancomycin, decompression | Numbness and weakness of right upper limb and lower limbs | Sensory abnormalities | WBC = 28 |
| Sakaguchi et al. (2017) [67] | 1 | 67 | M | C3–C7 | *E. coli* | Drainage and antibiotics | NA | Good outcome | WBC = 15, CRP = 28 |
| Kouki et al. (2017) [68] | 1 | 59 | M | C3–C5 | *Mycobacterium tuberculosis* | Laminectomy | Cervicobrachial neuralgia in the upper extremities and paresthesia (3 m) | NA | |

Table 2. Cont.

| Author | Number of Patients | Age | Gender | Level | Microorganism | Treatment | Neurological Deficit Initially | Outcome | ESR/WBC/CRP |
|---|---|---|---|---|---|---|---|---|---|
| McCann et al. (2018) [69] | 1 | 49 | M | C3–C4 | *Haemophilus parainfluenzae* | Decompression | No neurological deficit | Good outcome | WBC = 28, CRP = 16 |
| Noori et al. (2018) [70] | 1 | 29 | F | C3–T1 | *Pseud. aeruginosa* | Laminectomies and cefepime | No neurologic deficit | Good outcome | WBC = 9700 |
| Alyousef et al. (2018) [71] | 1 | 67 | M | C5–C7 | Brucellosis | Doxycycline, Aminoglycoside, Rifampicin 6 months | No neurologic deficit | Full recovery | WBC = 3.8, ESR = 55, CRP = 152 |
| Thomson et al. (2018) [72] | 1 | 66 | F | C1–T4 | *Staph. aureus* | Laminectomies, ceftriaxone | Mild quadriparesis | Full recovery | WBC = 20, CRP = 568 mg/dl |
| Yang et al. (2018) [66] | 1 | 67 | F | C5–C6 | *Strept. intermedius* | Surgical drainage and irrigation | Weakness in upper and lower extremities | Weakness in upper and lower extremities initially; afterwards, sensory deficit of left leg | WBC = 28 |
| La Fave et al. (2019) [73] | 1 | 45 | M | C1–C5 | MRSA | C2–C4 laminectomy | Quadriparesis | Persistent limb weakness | WBC = 17.6, |
| Roushan et al. (2019) [74] | 1 | 43 | M | C6–C7 | Brucellosis | Rifampicin, doxycycline, gentamycin for 4 months | bilateral hand paresthesia | Full recovery | WBC = 5.8, ESR = 62, CRP = 6 |
| Diyora et al. (2019) [75] | 1 | 30 | F | C2–C3 | MRSA and *Mycobacterium tuberculosis* | Decompressive laminectomy C2–C3, antibiotics 2 months | Hypotonia of upper and lower limbs | Full recovery | NA |
| Moustafa et al. (2019) [76] | 1 | 69 | M | C6–C7 | *E. coli* | Fusion and decompression | Upper- and lower-extremity weakness | Full recovery | ESR = 113, WBC = 24 |
| Zhang et al. (2019) [63] | 1 | 47 | M | C5–C6 | Brucellosis | Antibiotics | Incomplete limb paralysis | Good outcome | 7600, esr = 86, crp = 55 |

Table 2. Cont.

| Author | Number of Patients | Age | Gender | Level | Microorganism | Treatment | Neurological Deficit Initially | Outcome | ESR/WBC/CRP |
|---|---|---|---|---|---|---|---|---|---|
| Lukassen et al. (2019) [77] | 1 | 70 | F | C5–C6 | *Strept. intermedius* | Corpectomy, fusion | Upper limb paralysis | Good recovery, minor residual hypoesthesia | WBC = 19 |
| Noh et al. (2019) [78] | 1 | 58 | F | C5–C6 | *Staph. lugdunensis* | C5 corpectomy, Cefazolin, Rifampicin, Cephalexin 8 months | Deltoid weakness, Hoffman, Babinski | Full recovery | ESR= 57, CRP = 1.5 |
| Khan et al. (2020) [79] | 1 | 29 | M | C5 | Brucellosis | Corpectomy, cage, anterior fusion plate, Rifampicin, doxycycline for 3 months | Numbness of upper limbs | Full Recovery | NA |
| Sugimoto et al. (2020) [80] | 1 | 87 | M | C1–C2 | MRSA | Declined surgery, vancomycin 4 w | weakness of extremities | Good outcome (initially) | WBC = 6.4, CRP = 6 |
| Wu et al. (2020) [81] | 1 | 45 | F | C4–C7 | Anaerobic | meropenem, decompression –fusion | No neurologic deficit | Full recovery | CRP = 94, ESR = 17, WBC = 15 |
| Sati et al. (2021) [82] | 1 | 24 | M | C5–T3 | *Staph. aureus* | Hemilaminectomy | | Wheelchair, urinary catheter | CRP = 132, WBC = 10 |
| Richardson et al. (2021) [83] | 1 | 59 | M | C5–C7 | *Strept. intermedius* | Vancomycin, meropenem, clindamycin Laminectomy C5-C7 | Quadriparesis | Quadriplegia and necrotic fasciitis, death | WBC = 14.8 |
| Gennaro et al. (2021) [84] | 1 | (1) 56 (2) 55 | M M | (1) C4–C6 (2) C5–C7 | (1) *Staph. aureus* (2) MRSA | Decompressive laminectomy BOTH | Quadriparesis Quadriparesis | Quadriparesis BOTH | (1) CRP = 37, WBC = 14 (2) WBC = 11.7, CRP = 211 |
| Baghi et al. (2021) [85] | 1 | 22 | M | C5–C6 | Brucellosis | Doxycycline, aminoglycoside, surgical evaluation, rifampicin for 2 months | No neurologic deficit | Good outcome | WBC = 9.8, CRP= 51 |
| Lewis et al. (2023) [86] | 1 | 55 | F | C6–C7 | Neisseria | Fusion | No neurologic deficits | Good outcome | |

Table 2. Cont.

| Author | Number of Patients | Age | Gender | Level | Microorganism | Treatment | Neurological Deficit Initially | Outcome | ESR/WBC/CRP |
|---|---|---|---|---|---|---|---|---|---|
| Tomita et al. (2021) [87] | 1 | 79 | M | C6-C7 | *Klebsiella pneumoniae* | Ct-guided intervertebral drain | Weakness right arm | Good outcome | WBC = 4900, CRP = 3.6 |
| Ntinai et al. (2021) [88] | 1 | 71 | M | C2-C7 | *Klebsiella pneumoniae* | Drainage, ceftriaxone, ICU | Quadriparesis (2 w) Fever, cardiac arrest | Death | WBC = 21, |
| Lee et al. (2021) [64] | 1 | 50 | M | C3-C5 | *Streptococcus agalactiae* | Corpectomy, ampicillin, gentamycin 5 weeks | | Full recovery | WBC = 10, CRP = 1.2 |
| Herrera et al. (2022) [89] | 1 | 40 | M | C4-C5 | MRSA | Vancomycin, metronidazole, Cefepime. Decompression and fusion C4-C7 | Quadriparesis | Tetraplegia | ESR = 58, CRP= 4.1 WBC normal |
| Cao et al. (2022) [90] | 1 | 58 | M | C1-C7 | *Staph. aureus* | Decompression, ceftriaxone 5 weeks | Weakness in upper and lower limbs | Full recovery 6 m | NA |
| Abdelraheem et al. (2022) [91] | 1 | 51 | F | C5-C7 | *Pasteurella multocida* | Cervical corpectomy C6, cage and plate, ceftriaxone | Upper and lower limb weakness | Full recovery | ESR= 135, CRP = 202, WBC = 15 |
| Bara et al. (2022) [92] | 1 | 49 | M | C4-C5 | *Cutibacterium acnes* | Decompression C4-5, amoxicillin / clavulanic 6 weeks | Lost balance | Full recovery | Elevated |
| Shin et al. (2022) [93] | 1 | 75 | M | C6-T2 | *Staph. constellatus* | Decompression corpectomy, discectomy | Paraplegia | Improvement of symptoms, death at 1 year post op | WBC = 15, ESR= 120, CRP= 13 |
| Shafizad et al. (2022) [94] | 1 | 36 | M | C5-C6 | Brucellosis | C6 corpectomy, cage, anterior fusion | Weakness and hypoesthesia c5-C6 | Full recovery | WBC= 14,200, ESR= 33, CRP= 1.3 |
| Sapkas et al. (2023) (ps) | 4 | 53 | 3M 1F | C1-C5 | *Staph. aureus* | Decompression, fusion | Three patients presented with motor deficits, and one incidentally upon spinal imaging, fever | In one case, neurologic deficit remained | |

## 4. Discussion

Spinal epidural abscess is a rare condition that can result in significant morbidity and mortality if not diagnosed and treated in a timely manner [95]. The distinction between acute and chronic disease based on the presence of pyogenic abscess or granulation tissue formation is controversial among authors [96]. The disease can be classified into three phases: acute, subacute, and chronic, and the onset of symptoms usually occurs within hours to days but can also present with a more chronic course over weeks to months [97].

CSEA is most commonly caused by the hematogenous spread of bacteria from a localized infection elsewhere in the body, particularly the skin [97]. In some cases, the source of bacteremia is unknown. Local infections such as spondylitis or paravertebral abscess can also spread to the epidural space, while direct contamination from a penetrating wound or medical procedure can also be a cause of infection. Staphylococcus is the most commonly isolated organism in CSEA, as reported in earlier studies including our review which found it in 47.9% of cases [6]. The onset of symptoms in CSEA may be acute, subacute, or chronic, and can occur within hours to days or over weeks to months. Early diagnosis and prompt treatment are crucial to prevent high morbidity and mortality associated with SEA.

The incidence of spinal epidural abscess varies depending on the affected segment of the spine. While some authors report the lumbar spine as the most frequent site, others suggest a higher incidence in the thoracic segment. The cervical spine is the least commonly affected, with cases typically associated with spinal osteomyelitis [98]. In a study by Ghobrian et al, C4-C5 was the most common level of involvement in 59 patients with cervical spondylodiscitis who underwent surgical treatment, and they observed that the duration between symptom onset and surgery was a critical factor in the final outcome [57]. Patients with cervical epidural abscess often present with neck pain, fever, difficulty rotating the neck, and neurological deficits. Inflammatory markers such as WBC, ESR, and CRP can support diagnosis. Surgical treatment is strongly indicated in cases of conservative treatment failure, persistent symptoms, presence or deterioration of neurological deficits, spinal instability, abscess larger than 2.5 cm, ischemia or compression, deformities such as kyphosis or scoliosis, and sepsis [99]. In most studies included in the review, surgical treatment and debridement were the preferred options [100,101].

Differential diagnoses of an epidural abscess include spondylosis or degenerative disk syndromes, epidural hematoma, leptomeningeal carcinomatosis, metastatic disease to the spine, spinal cord hemorrhage or infarction, subdural hematoma or empyema, HIV-1-associated myelopathy, tropical myeloneuropathies, vitamin B-12-associated neurological diseases, and alcohol-related neuropathy [102]. Early surgical treatment is recommended over antibiotics alone, according to a study by Alton et al, which compared 62 patients with conservative treatment failure [56]. Tuberculous abscesses have a longer prodrome, frequently lack of leukocytosis and fever, and typically affect younger patients. CT-guided puncture is indicated if conservative treatment is being considered, although there is an additional risk of iatrogenic infection [103]. During the literature review, we found that patients with cervical spinal epidural abscesses due to brucellosis underwent conservative treatment with antibiotics without surgical intervention and achieved favorable outcomes [50,71,74,85].

Magnetic resonance imaging (MRI) is the preferred diagnostic tool for SEA due to its high sensitivity and specificity [7,18,23,26]. The typical MRI findings include a lesion with mass effect and hyper-intense signal on T1-weighted images, which enhances with Gadolinium injection and a nonhomogeneous and hyper-intense signal on T2-weighted images [104].

Surgical intervention is strongly indicated in cases of neural compression, spinal instability, or failure to obtain a satisfactory culture of the infecting organism [11,56]. The procedure typically involves a decompressive laminectomy, drainage of the abscess, and complete debridement of infected tissues. After surgery, patients are usually prescribed antimicrobial therapy for 4 to 6 weeks to prevent recurrence of the infection [11]. Timely diagnosis and management of spinal epidural abscess is critical for improving patient outcomes. Delayed diagnosis and treatment can lead to disease progression, exacerbation of neurological deficits, and increased mortality risk. Research has demonstrated that the duration between symptom onset and surgical intervention is a critical determinant of the final outcome [56]. Therefore, it is crucial to maintain a high level of suspicion regarding SEA in patients with risk factors and to promptly conduct appropriate diagnostic tests and start treatment.

Our patients presented with typical clinical symptoms, including neck pain, fever, and neurological deficits. Diagnosis was confirmed in all cases through magnetic resonance imaging (MRI). From the literature review, it is evident that surgical treatment is preferred in such cases. In two cases, we identified predisposing factors for the development of the infection. One patient had diabetes mellitus, while the other had a history of venous drug abuse.

Early diagnosis and treatment are critical for optimal outcomes in patients with CSEA. By identifying the factors that contribute to early diagnosis and appropriate management, healthcare providers can improve patient outcomes and reduce the risk of complications. This can include implementing screening protocols for high-risk patients, increasing awareness and education among healthcare providers, and promoting timely referral and consultation with specialists.

## 5. Conclusions

It is important to maintain a high index of suspicion for CSEA in patients with risk factors and relevant symptoms. Early diagnosis is crucial for a better prognosis and the most effective treatment is still immediate surgical drainage of the abscess combined with antibiotics. The limited number of studies in this review highlights the need for further research to establish stronger recommendations for the treatment of CSEA. Overall, timely diagnosis and management are critical in reducing the morbidity and mortality associated with this condition.

**Author Contributions:** Methodology, M.-M.A. and G.S.; formal analysis, D.P. and P.N.; investigation, G.S.; writing, M.-M.A., G.S. and L.A.; writing—review and editing, S.A.P. and K.T. All authors have read and agreed to the published version of the manuscript.

**Funding:** This research received no external funding.

**Institutional Review Board Statement:** Not applicable.

**Informed Consent Statement:** Not applicable.

**Data Availability Statement:** Not applicable.

**Conflicts of Interest:** The authors declare no conflict of interest.

## References

1. Bluman, E.M.; Palumbo, M.A.; Lucas, P.R. Spinal Epidural Abscess in Adults. *J. Am. Acad. Orthop. Surg.* **2004**, *12*, 155–163. [CrossRef] [PubMed]
2. Savage, K.; Holtom, P.D.; Zalavras, C.G. Spinal Epidural Abscess. Early Clinical Outcome in Patients Treated Medically. *Clin. Orthop. Relat. Res.* **2005**, *439*, 56–60. [CrossRef] [PubMed]
3. Darouiche, R.O.; Hamill, R.J.; Greenberg, S.B. Bacterial spinal epidural abscess. Review of 43 cases and literature survey. *Medicine* **1992**, *71*, 369–385. [CrossRef] [PubMed]
4. Maslen, D.R.; Jones, S.R.; Crislip, M.A.; Bracis, R.; Dworkin, R.J.; Flemming, J.E. Spinalepidural abscess: Optimizing patient care. *Arch. Intern. Med.* **1993**, *153*, 1713–1721. [CrossRef]
5. Danner, R.L.; Hartman, B.J. Update of spinal epidural abscess: 35 cases and review of the literature. *Rev. Infect. Dis.* **1987**, *9*, 265–274. [CrossRef]
6. Reihsaus, E.; Waldbaur, H.; Seeling, W. Spinal epidural abscess: A meta analysis of 915 patients. *Neurosurg. Rev.* **2000**, *23*, 175–205. [CrossRef]
7. Sillevis Smitt, P.; Tsafka, A.; van den Bent, M.; de Bruin, H.; Hendriks, W.; Vecht, C.; Teng-van de Zande, F. Spinal epidural abscess complicating chronic epidural analgesia in 11 cancer patients: Clinical findings and magnetic resonance imaging. *J. Neurol.* **1999**, *246*, 815–820. [CrossRef] [PubMed]

8. Still, J.M.; Abramson, R.; Law, E.J. Development of an epidural abscess following staphylococcal septicemia in an acutely burned patient: Case report. *J. Trauma* **1995**, *38*, 958–959. [CrossRef]
9. Byers, K.; Axelrod, P.; Michael, S.; Rosen, S. Infections complicating tunneled intraspinal catheter systems used to treat chronic pain. *Clin. Infect. Dis.* **1995**, *21*, 403–408. [CrossRef] [PubMed]
10. Veljanoski, D.; Tonna, I.; Barlas, R.; Abdel-Fattah, A.R.; Almoosawy, S.A.; Bhatt, P. Spinal infections in the north-east of Scotland: A retrospective analysis. *Ann. R. Coll. Surg. Engl.* **2023**, *105*, 428–433. [CrossRef] [PubMed]
11. Epstein, N. Diagnosis, and Treatment of Cervical Epidural Abscess and/or Cervical Vertebral Osteomyelitis with or without Retropharyngeal Abscess; A Review. *Surg. Neurol. Int.* **2020**, *11*, 160. [CrossRef]
12. Tsantes, A.G.; Papadopoulos, D.V.; Vrioni, G.; Sioutis, S.; Sapkas, G.; Benzakour, A.; Benzakour, T.; Angelini, A.; Ruggieri, P.; Mavrogenis, A.F. World Association Against Infection in Orthopedics And Trauma W A I O T Study Group On Bone And Joint Infection Definitions. Spinal Infections: An Update. *Microorganisms* **2020**, *8*, 476. [CrossRef]
13. Al-Hourani, K.; Al-Aref, R.; Mesfin, A. Upper Cervical Epidural Abscess in Clinical Practice: Diagnosis and Management. *Global Spine J.* **2016**, *6*, 383–393. [CrossRef] [PubMed]
14. Leach, R.E.; Robert, E.; Goldstein, H. Howard; Younger, Donna. Osteomyelitis of the Odontoid Process: A Case Report. *J. Bone Jt. Surg.* **1967**, *49*, 369–371. [CrossRef]
15. Rimalovski, A.B.; Aronson, S.M. Abscess of medulla oblongata associated with osteomyelitis of odontoid process. Case report. *J. Neurosurg.* **1968**, *29*, 97–101. [CrossRef] [PubMed]
16. Ahlbäck, S.; Collert, S. Destruction of the Odontoid Process Due to Atlanto-Axial Pyogenic Spondylitis. *Acta Radiol.* **1970**, *10*, 394–400. [CrossRef]
17. Vemireddy, N. Osteomyelitis of cervical spine. *Orthopaed Rev.* **1978**, *7*, 109–114.
18. Venger, B.H.; Musher, D.M.; Brown, E.W.; Baskin, D.S. Isolated C-2 osteomyelitis of hematogenous origin: Case report and literature review. *Neurosurgery* **1986**, *18*, 461–464. [CrossRef]
19. Zigler, J.E.; Bohlman, H.H.; Robinson, R.A.; Riley, L.H.; Dodge, L.D. Pyogenic osteomyelitis of the occiput, the atlas, and the axis. A report of five cases. *J. Bone Joint Surg. Am.* **1987**, *69*, 1069–1073. [CrossRef]
20. Bartels, J.W.; Brammer, R.E. Cervical osteomyelitis with prevertebral abscess formation. *Otolaryngol. Head. Neck Surg.* **1990**, *102*, 180–182. [CrossRef] [PubMed]
21. Sebben, A.L.; Graells, X.S.; Benato, M.L.; Santoro, P.G.; Kulcheski, Á.L. High cervical spine spondylodiscitis management and literature review. *Rev. Assoc. Med. Bras.* **2017**, *63*, 18–20. [CrossRef] [PubMed]
22. Ruskin, J.; Shapiro, S.; McCombs, M.; Greenberg, H.; Helmer, E. Odontoid osteomyelitis. An unusual presentation of an uncommon disease. *West. J. Med.* **1992**, *156*, 306–308.
23. Keogh, S.; Crockard, A. Staphylococcal infection of the odontoid peg. *Postgrad. Med. J.* **1992**, *68*, 51–54. [CrossRef] [PubMed]
24. Azizi, S.A.; Fayad, P.B.; Fulbright, R.; Giroux, M.L.; Waxman, S.G. Clivus and cervical spinal osteomyelitis with epidural abscess presenting with multiple cranial neuropathies. *Clin. Neurol. Neurosurg.* **1995**, *97*, 239–244. [CrossRef]
25. Sawada, M.; Iwamura, M.; Hirata, T.; Sakai, N. Cervical discitis associated with spinal epidural abscess caused by methicillin-resistant staphylococcus aureus. *Neurol. Med. Chir.* **1996**, *36*, 40–44. [CrossRef] [PubMed]
26. Lam, C.H.; Ethier, R.; Pokrupa, R. Conservative therapy of atlantoaxial osteomyelitis. A case report. *Spine* **1996**, *21*, 1820–1823. [CrossRef]
27. Fukutake, T.; Kitazaki, H.; Hattori, T. Odontoid osteomyelitis complicating pneumococcal pneumonia. *Eur. Neurol.* **1998**, *39*, 126–127.
28. Wiedau-Pazos, M.; Curio, G.; Grüsser, C. Epidural abscess of the cervical spine with osteomyelitis of the odontoid process. *Spine* **1999**, *24*, 133–136. [CrossRef]
29. Anton, K.; Christoph, R.; Cornelius, F.M. Osteomyelitis and pathological fracture of the axis. Case illustration. *J. Neurosurg.* **1999**, *90*, 162.
30. Suchomel, P.; Buchvald, P.; Barsa, P.; Lukas, R.; Soukup, T. Pyogenic osteomyelitis of the odontoid process: Single stage decompression and fusion. *Spine* **2003**, *28*, 239–244. [CrossRef]
31. Haridas, A.; Walsh, D.C.; Mowle, D.H. Polymicrobial Osteomyelitis of the Odontoid Process with Epidural Abscess: Case Report and Review of Literature. *Skull Base* **2003**, *13*, 107–111. [CrossRef] [PubMed]
32. Yi, H.J.; Oh, S.H.; Kwon, O.J.; Kim, H. Cervical epidural abscess secondary to aorto-duodenal fistula: A case report. *J. Korean Med. Sci.* **2003**, *18*, 116–119. [CrossRef] [PubMed]
33. Ates, O.; Cayli, S.R.; Koçak, A.; Kutlu, R.; Onal, R.E.; Tekiner, A. Spinal epidural abscess caused by brucellosis. Two case reports. *Neurol. Med. Chir.* **2005**, *45*, 66–70. [CrossRef] [PubMed]
34. Burgess, C.M.; Wolverson, A.S.; Dale, M.T. Cervical epidural abscess: A rare complication of intravenous cannulation. *Anaesthesia* **2005**, *60*, 605–608. [CrossRef]
35. Moriya, M.; Kimura, T.; Yamamoto, Y.; Abe, K.; Sakoda, S. Successful treatment of cervical spinal epidural abscess without surgery. *Intern. Med.* **2005**, *44*, 1110. [CrossRef]
36. Paul, C.A.; Kumar, A.; Raut, V.V.; Garhnam, A.; Kumar, N. Pseudomonas cervical osteomyelitis with retropharyngeal abscess: An unusual complication of otitis media. *J. Laryngol. Otol.* **2005**, *119*, 816–818. [CrossRef]
37. Kulkarni, A.G.; Hee, H.T. Adjacent level discitis after anterior cervical discectomy and fusion (ACDF): A case report. *Eur. Spine J.* **2006**, *15*, 559–563. [CrossRef]

38. Curry, J.M.; Cognetti, D.M.; Harrop, J.; Boon, M.S.; Spiegel, J.R. Cervical discitis and epidural abscess after tonsillectomy. *Laryngoscope* **2007**, *117*, 2093–2096. [CrossRef]
39. Jeon, S.H.; Han, D.C.; Lee, S.G.; Park, H.M.; Shin, D.J.; Lee, Y.B. Eikenella corrodens cervical spinal epidural abscess induced by a fish bone. *J. Korean Med. Sci.* **2007**, *22*, 380–382. [CrossRef]
40. Reid, P.J.; Holman, P.J. Iatrogenic pyogenic osteomyelitis of C1 and C2 treated with transoral decompression and delayed occipitocervical arthrodesis. Case report. *J. Neurosurg. Spine* **2007**, *7*, 664–668. [CrossRef]
41. Metcalfe, S.; Morgan-Hough, C. Cervical epidural abscess and vertebral osteomyelitis following non-traumatic oesophageal rupture: A case report and discussion. *Eur. Spine J.* **2009**, *18*, 224–227. [CrossRef] [PubMed]
42. Hantzidis, P.; Papadopoulos, A.; Kalabakos, C.; Boursinos, L.; Dimitriou, C.G. Brucella cervical spondylitis complicated by spinal cord compression: A case report. *Cases J.* **2009**, *2*, 6698. [CrossRef] [PubMed]
43. Fang, W.K.; Chen, S.H.; Huang, D.W.; Huang, K.C. Post-traumatic Osteomyelitis with Spinal Epidural Abscess of Cervical Spine in a Young Man with No Predisposing Factor. *J. Chin. Med. Assoc.* **2009**, *72*, 210–213. [CrossRef] [PubMed]
44. Ueda, Y.; Kawahara, N.; Murakami, H.; Matsui, T.; Tomita, K. Pyogenic osteomyelitis of the atlas: A case report. *Spine* **2009**, *20*, 34. [CrossRef]
45. Tamori, Y.; Takahashi, T.; Suwa, H.; Ohno, K.; Nishimoto, Y.; Nakajima, S.; Asada, M.; Kita, T.; Tsutsumi, M. Cervical epidural abscess presenting with Brown-Sequard syndrome in a patient with type 2 diabetes. *Intern. Med.* **2010**, *49*, 1391–1393. [CrossRef]
46. Gezici, A.R.; Ergün, R. Cervical epidural abscess in haemodialysis patients by catheter related infection: Report of two cases. *J. Korean Med. Sci.* **2010**, *25*, 176–179. [CrossRef]
47. Deshmukh, V.R. Midline trough corpectomies for the evacuation of an extensive ventral cervical and upper thoracic spinal epidural abscess. *J. Neurosurg. Spine* **2010**, *13*, 229–233. [CrossRef]
48. Khoriati, A.; Kitson, J.; Deol, R.S. Cervical spinal abscess: An insidious presentation and unusual pathology. *Ann. R. Coll. Surg. Engl.* **2012**, *94*, 184–185. [CrossRef]
49. Ekici, M.A.; Ozbek, Z.; Gökoğlu, A.; Menkü, A. Surgical management of cervical spinal epidural abscess caused by Brucella melitensis: Report of two cases and review of the literature. *J. Korean Neurosurg. Soc.* **2012**, *51*, 383–387. [CrossRef]
50. Lampropoulos, C.; Kamposos, P.; Papaioannou, I.; Niarou, V. Cervical epidural abscess caused by brucellosis. *BMJ Case Rep.* **2012**, *2012*, bcr2012007070. [CrossRef]
51. Soultanis, K.C.; Sakellariou, V.I.; Starantzis, K.A.; Stavropoulos, N.A.; Papageloupoulos, P.J. Insidious Onset of Tetraparesis due to Cervical Epidural Abscess from *Enterococcus faecalis*. *Case Rep. Med.* **2013**, *2013*, 513920. [CrossRef]
52. Jensen, E.C.; Rosted, A. Tuberkuløs spondylit med psoasabsces hos en ung mand uden indvandrerbaggrund [*Tuberculous spondylitis* with a psoas abscess in a young man without an immigrant background]. *Ugeskr. Laeger.* **2002**, *164*, 4937–4938.
53. Radulovic, D.; Vujotic, L. Cervical spinal epidural abscess after oesophagoscopy. *Eur. Spine J.* **2013**, *22*, 369–372. [CrossRef]
54. O'Neill, S.C.; Baker, J.F.; Ellanti, P.; Synnott, K. Cervical epidural abscess following an *Escherichia coli* urinary tract infection. *BMJ Case Rep.* **2014**, *2014*, bcr2013202078. [CrossRef] [PubMed]
55. Giri, U.; Thavalathil, B.C.; Varghese, R. Vertebral osteomyelitis in an immunosuppressed patient with rheumatoid arthritis. *BMJ Case Rep.* **2014**, *2014*, bcr2014206944. [CrossRef]
56. Alton, T.B.; Patel, A.R.; Bransford, R.J.; Bellabarba, C.; Lee, M.J.; Chapman, J.R. Is there a difference in neurologic outcome in medical versus early operative management of cervical epidural abscesses? *Spine J.* **2015**, *15*, 10–17. [CrossRef] [PubMed]
57. Ghobrial, G.M.; Beygi, S.; Viereck, M.J.; Maulucci, C.M.; Sharan, A.; Heller, J.; Jallo, J.; Prasad, S.; Harrop, J.S. Timing in the surgical evacuation of spinal epidural abscesses. *Neurosurg. Focus* **2014**, *37*, E1. [CrossRef]
58. Young, W.F.; Weaver, M.; Snyder, B.; Narayan, R. Reversal of tetraplegia in patients with cervical osteomyelitis--epidural abscess using anterior debridement and fusion. *Spinal Cord* **2001**, *39*, 538–540. [CrossRef] [PubMed]
59. Aranibar, R.J.; Del Monaco, D.C.; Gonzales, P. Anterior Microscopic Transtubular (MITR) Surgical Approach for Cervical Pyogenic C1-2 Abscess: A Case Report. *Int. J. Spine Surg.* **2015**, *9*, 56. [CrossRef]
60. Kohlmann, R.; Nefedev, A.; Kaase, M.; Gatermann, S.G. Community-acquired adult *Escherichia coli* meningitis leading to diagnosis of unrecognized retropharyngeal abscess and cervical spondylodiscitis: A case report. *BMC Infect. Dis.* **2015**, *15*, 567. [CrossRef]
61. Ugarriza, L.F.; Porras, L.F.; Lorenzana, L.M.; Rodríguez-Sánchez, J.A.; García-Yagüe, L.M.; Cabezudo, J.M. Brucellar spinal epidural abscesses. Analysis of eleven cases. *Br. J. Neurosurg.* **2005**, *19*, 235–240. [CrossRef] [PubMed]
62. Oh, J.S.; Shim, J.J.; Lee, K.S.; Doh, J.W. Cervical epidural abscess: Rare complication of bacterial endocarditis with *Streptococcus viridans*: A case report. *Korean J. Spine* **2015**, *12*, 22–25. [CrossRef] [PubMed]
63. Zhang, J.H.; Wang, Z.L.; Wan, L. Cervical epidural analgesia complicated by epidural abscess: A case report and literature review. *Medicine* **2017**, *96*, e7789. [CrossRef] [PubMed]
64. Lee, J.M.; Heo, S.Y.; Kim, D.K.; Jung, J.P.; Park, C.R.; Lee, Y.J.; Kim, G.S. Quadriplegia after Mitral Valve Replacement in an Infective Endocarditis Patient with Cervical Spine Spondylitis. *Korean J. Thorac. Cardiovasc. Surg.* **2021**, *54*, 218–220. [CrossRef]
65. Li, H.; Chen, Z.; Yong, Z.; Li, X.; Huang, Y.; Wu, D. Emergency 1-stage anterior approach for cervical spine infection complicated by epidural abscess. *Medicine* **2017**, *96*, e7301. [CrossRef] [PubMed]
66. Yang, C.S.; Zhang, L.J.; Sun, Z.H.; Yang, L.; Shi, F.D. Acute prevertebral abscess secondary to intradiscal oxygen-ozone chemonucleolysis for treatment of a cervical disc herniation. *J. Int. Med. Res.* **2018**, *46*, 2461–2465. [CrossRef] [PubMed]

67. Sakaguchi, A.; Ishimaru, N.; Ohnishi, H.; Kawamoto, M.; Takagi, A.; Yoshimura, S.; Kinami, S.; Sakamoto, S. Retropharyngeal abscess with cervical discitis and vertebral osteomyelitis caused by Escherichia coli in a patient with liver cirrhosis. *Infez. Med.* **2017**, *25*, 169–173.
68. Kouki, S.; Landolsi, M.; Ben Lassoued, M.; Gharsallah, I. Uncommon cause of cervicobrachial neuralgia: Epidural abscess complicating tuberculous arthritis. *BMJ Case Rep.* **2017**, *2017*, bcr2017219458. [CrossRef]
69. McCann, N.; Barakat, M.F.; Schafer, F. An aggressive form of *Haemophilus parainfluenzae* infective endocarditis presenting with limb weakness. *BMJ Case Rep.* **2018**, *2018*, bcr-2017.
70. Noori, S.A.; Gungor, S. Spinal epidural abscess associated with an epidural catheter in a woman with complex regional pain syndrome and selective IgG3 deficiency: A case report. *Medicine* **2018**, *97*, e13272. [CrossRef]
71. Alyousef, M.; Aldoghaither, R. First case of cervical epidural abscess caused by brucellosis in Saudi Arabia: A case report and literature review. *Cases* **2018**, *12*, 107–111. [CrossRef]
72. Thomson, C. Spinal cord compression secondary to epidural abscess: The importance of prompt diagnosis and management. *Case Rep.* **2018**, *2018*, bcr2017220694. [CrossRef]
73. LaFave, J.; Bramante, R. Upper Cervical Epidural Abscess Resulting in Respiratory Compromise After Lumbar Steroid Injection. *J. Emerg. Med.* **2019**, *57*, 66–69. [CrossRef]
74. Roushan, M.R.; Ebrahimpour, S.; Afshar, Z.M.; Babazadeh, A. Cervical Spine Spondylitis with an Epidural Abscess in a Patient with Brucellosis: A Case Report. *J. Crit. Care Med.* **2019**, *9*, 103–106. [CrossRef]
75. Diyora, B.; Patil, S.; Bhende, B.; Patel, M.; Dhall, G.; Nayak, N. Concurrent Spinal Epidural Tubercular and Pyogenic Abscess of Cervical Spine without Bony Involvement. *J. Neurosci. Rural. Pract.* **2019**, *10*, 374–378. [CrossRef]
76. Moustafa, A.; Kheireldine, R.; Khan, Z.; Alim, H.; Khan, M.S.; Alsamman, M.A.; Youssef, E. Cervical Spinal Osteomyelitis with Epidural Abscess following an Escherichia coli Urinary Tract Infection in an Immunocompetent Host. *Case Rep. Infect. Dis.* **2019**, *16*, 5286726. [CrossRef]
77. Lukassen, J.; Aalbers, M.W.; Coppes, M.H.; Groen, R. Cervical spondylodiscitis following cricopharyngeal botulinium toxin injection. *Eur. Ann. Otorhinolaryngol. Head. Neck Dis.* **2019**, *136*, 313–316. [CrossRef]
78. Noh, T.; Zervos, T.M.; Chen, A.; Chedid, M. Treatment of a Staphylococcus lugdunensis cervical epidural abscess. *BMJ Case Rep.* **2019**, *12*, e227449. [CrossRef]
79. Khan, M.M.; Babu, R.A.; Iqbal, J.; Batas, S.N.; Raza, A. Cervical Epidural Abscess due to Brucella Treated with Decompression and Instrumentation: A Case Report and Review of Literature. *Asian J. Neurosurg.* **2020**, *15*, 440–444. [CrossRef]
80. Sugimoto, H.; Hayashi, T.; Nakadomari, S.; Sugimoto, K. Delayed diagnosis of an upper cervical epidural abscess masked due to crowned dens syndrome. *BMJ Case Rep.* **2020**, *20*, 13. [CrossRef]
81. Wu, B.; He, X.; Peng, B.G. Pyogenic discitis with an epidural abscess after cervical analgesic discography: A case report. *World J. Clin. Cases.* **2020**, *8*, 2318–2324. [CrossRef] [PubMed]
82. Sati, W.O.; Haddad, M.; Anjum, S. A Case of Spinal Epidural Abscess Presenting with Horner Syndrome. *Cureus* **2021**, *13*, e14541. [CrossRef]
83. Richardson, C.; Wattenbarger, S. A case report of quadriplegia and acute stroke from tracking retropharyngeal and epidural abscess complicated by necrotizing fasciitis. *J. Am. Coll. Emerg. Physicians Open* **2021**, *2*, e12524. [CrossRef]
84. Gennaro, N.; Bonifacio, C.; Corato, M.; Milani, D.; Politi, L.S. Quadriparesis caused by retropharyngeal and epidural abscess in COVID-19 patients. *Neurol. Sci.* **2021**, *42*, 1683–1685. [CrossRef]
85. Baghi, M.A.; Al-Aani, F.K.; Rahil, A.; Ayari, B. Brucellar cervical epidural abscess—A rare cause of neck pain. *Cases* **2021**, *24*, e01101. [CrossRef] [PubMed]
86. Fox-Lewis, A.; Luan, K.; Hopkins, C. Neisseria gonorrhoeae cervical spine epidural abscess requiring spinal decompression and instrumented fusion. *J. Infect. Chemother.* **2023**, *29*, 527–529. [CrossRef]
87. Tomita, K.; Matsumoto, T.; Kamono, M.; Miyazaki, K.; Hasebe, T. CT fluoroscopy-guided percutaneous intervertebral drain insertion for cervical pyogenic spondylodiscitis. *Diagn. Interv. Radiol.* **2021**, *27*, 269–271. [CrossRef]
88. Nitinai, N.; Punpichet, M.; Nasomsong, W. Fatal Cervical Spinal Epidural Abscess and Spondylodiscitis Complicated with Rhombencephalitis Caused by Klebsiella pneumoniae: A Case Report and Literature Review. *Cureus* **2021**, *2*, 13. [CrossRef]
89. Herrera, D.; Acosta-Rullan, J.M.; Fox, D.; Concepcion, L.; Hughes, J. Quadriplegia from cervical osteomyelodiscitis with vertebral collapse: A case report. *Clin. Case Rep.* **2022**, *10*, e6591. [CrossRef]
90. Cao, J.; Fang, J.; Shao, X.; Shen, J.; Jiang, X. Case Report: A case of cervical spinal epidural abscess combined with cervical paravertebral soft tissue abscess. *Front. Surg.* **2022**, *9*, 967806. [CrossRef]
91. Abdelraheem, M.; Mohamed, Y.; Houlihan, E.; Murray, O. Treatment of Pasteurella multocida Cervical Epidural Abscess. *Cureus.* **2022**, *14*, e25507. [CrossRef]
92. Bara, G.A.; Thissen, J. Cervical epidural abscess due to implantation of a spinal cord stimulation lead. *Clin. Case Rep.* **2022**, *10*, e05931. [CrossRef]
93. Shin, K.E. Epidural abscess formation after chemoradiation therapy for esophageal cancer: A case report and literature review. *Medicine* **2022**, *101*, e29426. [CrossRef]
94. Shafizad, M.; Ehteshami, S.; Shojaei, H.; Jalili Khoshnoud, R. Cervical spine epidural abscess caused by brucellosis: A case report and literature review. *Clin. Case Rep.* **2022**, *10*, e05644. [CrossRef] [PubMed]

95. Tang, H.J.; Lin, H.J.; Liu, Y.C.; Li, C.-M. Spinal Epidural Abscess. Experience with 46 Patients and Evaluation of Prognostic Factors. *J. Infect.* **2002**, *45*, 76–81. [CrossRef] [PubMed]
96. Curling, D.O., Jr.; Gower, W.; McWhorten, J.M. Changing concepts in spinal epidural abscess: A report of 29 cases. *Neurosurgery* **1990**, *27*, 185–192. [CrossRef] [PubMed]
97. Browder, J.; Meyers, R. Infections of the spinal epidural space: An aspect of vertebral osteomyelitis. *Am. J. Sur.* **1987**, *37*, 4–26. [CrossRef]
98. Krauss, W.E.; McCormick, P.C. Infections of the dural spaces. *Neurosurg. Clin. N. Am.* **1992**, *3*, 421–433. [CrossRef]
99. Saeed, K.; Esposito, S.; Ascione, T.; Bassetti, M.; Bonnet, E.; Carnelutti, A.; Chan, M.; Lye, D.C.; Cortes, N.; Dryden, M.; et al. International Society of Antimicrobial Chemotherapy (ISAC) Bone and Skin & Soft Tissue Infections Working Group. Hot topics on vertebral osteomyelitis from the International Society of Antimicrobial Chemotherapy. *Int. J. Antimicrob. Agents* **2019**, *54*, 125–133.
100. Turner, A.; Zhao, L.; Gauthier, P.; Chen, S.; Roffey, D.M.; Wai, E.K. Management of cervical spine epidural abscess: A systematic review. *Ther. Adv. Infect. Dis.* **2019**, *6*, 2049936119863940. [CrossRef]
101. Bagley, C.A.; Dudukovich, K.J.; Wolinsky, J.P.; Gokaslan, Z.L. Surgical management of lumbosacral spinal epidural abscess. *Operat Tech. Neurosurg.* **2005**, *7*, 206–221. [CrossRef]
102. Marais, S.; Roos, I.; Mitha, A.; Mabusha, S.J.; Patel, V.; Bhigjee, A.I. Spinal Tuberculosis: Clinicoradiological Findings in 274 Patients. *Clin. Infect. Dis.* **2018**, *67*, 89–98. [CrossRef]
103. Inamasu, J.; Shizu, N.; Tsutsumi, Y.; Hirose, Y. Infected epidural hematoma of the lumbar spine associated with invasive pneumococcal disease. *Asian J. Neurosurg.* **2015**, *10*, 58. [CrossRef]
104. Gupta, N.; Kadavigere, R.; Malla, S.; Bhat, S.N.; Saravu, K. Differentiating tubercular from pyogenic causes of spine involvement on Magnetic Resonance Imaging. *Infez. Med.* **2023**, *31*, 62–69.

**Disclaimer/Publisher's Note:** The statements, opinions and data contained in all publications are solely those of the individual author(s) and contributor(s) and not of MDPI and/or the editor(s). MDPI and/or the editor(s) disclaim responsibility for any injury to people or property resulting from any ideas, methods, instructions or products referred to in the content.

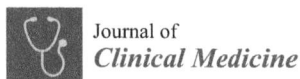 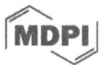

Article

# Diagnostic Sensitivity of Blood Culture, Intraoperative Specimen, and Computed Tomography-Guided Biopsy in Patients with Spondylodiscitis and Isolated Spinal Epidural Empyema Requiring Surgical Treatment

Mido Max Hijazi [1,*], Timo Siepmann [2], Alexander Carl Disch [3], Uwe Platz [3], Tareq A. Juratli [1], Ilker Y. Eyüpoglu [1] and Dino Podlesek [1]

[1] Department of Neurosurgery, Division of Spine Surgery, Technische Universität Dresden, Faculty of Medicine, and University Hospital Carl Gustav Carus, Fetscherstrasse 74, 01307 Dresden, Germany; tareq.juratli@ukdd.de (T.A.J.); ilker.eyuepoglu@ukdd.de (I.Y.E.); dino.podlesek@ukdd.de (D.P.)

[2] Department of Neurology, Technische Universität Dresden, Faculty of Medicine, and University Hospital Carl Gustav Carus, Fetscherstrasse 74, 01307 Dresden, Germany; timo.siepmann@ukdd.de

[3] Department of Orthopedics and Traumatology, Technische Universität Dresden, Faculty of Medicine, and University Hospital Carl Gustav Carus, Fetscherstrasse 74, 01307 Dresden, Germany; alexander.disch@ukdd.de (A.C.D.); uwe.platz@ukdd.de (U.P.)

* Correspondence: mido.hijazi@ukdd.de; Tel.: +49-1799847820

**Abstract:** Background: the successful treatment of spondylodiscitis (SD) and isolated spinal epidural empyema (ISEE) depends on early detection of causative pathogens, which is commonly performed either via blood cultures, intraoperative specimens, and/or image-guided biopsies. We evaluated the diagnostic sensitivity of these three procedures and assessed how it is influenced by antibiotics. Methods: we retrospectively analyzed data from patients with SD and ISEE treated surgically at a neurosurgery university center in Germany between 2002 and 2021. Results: we included 208 patients (68 [23–90] years, 34.6% females, 68% SD). Pathogens were identified in 192 cases (92.3%), including 187 (97.4%) pyogenic and five (2.6%) non-pyogenic infections, with Gram-positive bacteria accounting for 86.6% (162 cases) and Gram-negative for 13.4% (25 cases) of the pyogenic infections. The diagnostic sensitivity was highest for intraoperative specimens at 77.9% (162/208, $p = 0.012$) and lowest for blood cultures at 57.2% (119/208) and computed tomography (CT)-guided biopsies at 55.7% (39/70). Blood cultures displayed the highest sensitivity in SD patients (SD: 91/142, 64.1% vs. ISEE: 28/66, 42.4%, $p = 0.004$), while intraoperative specimens were the most sensitive procedure in ISEE (SD: 102/142, 71.8% vs. ISEE: 59/66, 89.4%, $p = 0.007$). The diagnostic sensitivity was lower in SD patients with ongoing empiric antibiotic therapy (EAT) than in patients treated postoperatively with targeted antibiotic therapy (TAT) (EAT: 77/89, 86.5% vs. TAT: 53/53, 100%, $p = 0.004$), whereas no effect was observed in patients with ISEE (EAT: 47/51, 92.2% vs. TAT: 15/15, 100%, $p = 0.567$). Conclusions: in our cohort, intraoperative specimens displayed the highest diagnostic sensitivity especially for ISEE, whereas blood cultures appear to be the most sensitive for SD. The sensitivity of these tests seems modifiable by preoperative EAT in patients with SD, but not in those with ISEE, underscoring the distinct differences between both pathologies.

**Keywords:** spondylodiscitis; isolated spinal epidural empyema; diagnostic sensitivity; blood culture; intraoperative specimen; computed tomography-guided biopsy

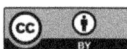

## 1. Introduction

Spondylodiscitis (SD) and isolated spinal epidural empyema (ISEE) are common types of primary spinal infections that are challenging to treat [1–3]. The reported incidence in the literature is five to six cases per 100,000 patient-years, but recent data suggests a higher incidence of 30/250,000 [4]. ISEE is an isolated infection of the epidural space with the accumulation of purulent substance without a concurrent SD, while SD refers to a primary infection of the intervertebral disc with secondary osteomyelitis of the adjacent endplates that occasionally occurs with epidural empyema [5,6].

Standardized treatment guidelines for SD and ISEE are currently lacking [7,8]. Surgical treatment followed by conservative management with antibiotic therapy takes several weeks and months for patients to recover. However, inadequate antibiotic therapy during this period can increase patient morbidity [9]. Reliable diagnostics including pathogen detection with antibiogram resistogram are indispensable for infection treatment. Three procedures are available for isolating causative pathogens, including blood cultures, intraoperative specimens, and computed tomography (CT)-guided biopsies.

Some studies suggest that blood cultures can yield early positive results due to hematogenous spreading of the infection, in particular in patients with SD [10]. To minimize a contamination, blood cultures need to be withdrawn from two or three different sites [11]. At least three pairs of blood cultures (aerobic and anaerobic culture medium) should be collected before the initiation of antibiotic therapy, irrespective of febrile temperatures [12]. This allows the isolation of a causative pathogen in up to 37.5% of cases [13].

Intraoperative sampling on site of the infectious focus is considered the most sensitive and specific method for pathogen detection [14]. CT-guided biopsy is an additional option to isolate pathogens, especially in cases when abscess formations such as psoas abscesses are visible on diagnostic imaging. However, the sensitivity of each procedure is limited when performed alone, whereas a combination of these procedures can increase the likelihood of successful pathogen detection [15,16].

In case of severe infections, empirical antibiotic therapy (EAT) is usually initiated preoperatively and then switched to targeted antibiotic therapy (TAT) after the causative pathogen has been identified, based on resistogram. Other cases are initially managed with TAT according to the resistogram [4].

A few studies have reported on the diagnostic sensitivity of these three procedures for SD and ISEE [12,17]. However, the impact of ongoing EAT on pathogen detection in SD and ISEE has not been thoroughly addressed. Therefore, this retrospective study aims to assess the diagnostic sensitivity of the three procedures and evaluate the influence of prior EAT on outcomes.

## 2. Materials and Methods

### 2.1. Study Design and Patient Data

A retrospective observational study was performed on a cohort of 208 consecutive patients with SD and ISEE who underwent surgical treatment at our neurosurgery department from 2002 to 2021. All surgically treated patients with SD or ISEE aged over 18 years and without intradural infection were included. The study was approved by the local ethics committee of Dresden university hospital (Reference number BO-EK-17012022). Patient data were identified and extracted via review of electronic medical records using the ORBIS system (ORBIS, Dedalus, Bonn, Germany) and neuroimaging files through the IMPAX system (IMPAX, Impax Asset Management Group plc, London, UK). Detailed demographic, clinical, radiological, laboratory and microbiological analyses were evaluated between groups.

### 2.2. Clinical Management

The diagnosis of SD or ISEE was obtained according to the Clinical Practice Guidelines for the diagnosis and treatment of native vertebral osteomyelitis in Adults of the Infectious Diseases Society of America (IDSA) [18]. Primary treatment was conservative with intravenous antibiotics in a conservative external or internal clinic, whereas the patient was referred to our clinic if surgical treatment was required, e.g., in cases with neurological deficits, spinal instability, or epidural abscess. Our cohort of 187 patients included surgical ISEE or SD patients with primary immediate indication for open surgery. Depending on disease severity, surgical therapy involved abscess evacuation, dorsal decompression with/without dorsal interbody fusion, ventral debridement with anterior cervical discectomy and fusion (ACDF), or vertebral body replacement. Surgical decision making was based on clinical experience and several defined radiographic signs. Patients undergoing spinal instrumentation had preoperative CT scans to assess bony integrity.

Patients with ISEE were treated with abscess evacuation with/without drainage or ACDF for abscesses ventral to the cervical spinal cord. Patients with SD underwent either abscess evacuation or/and instrumentation for instability, deformity, and pain-related immobility. In case of psoas abscess, drainage was performed CT-guided.

SD patients with a spinal epidural abscess without deformity underwent decompression with removal of the abscess and vertebral disc with/without dorsal interbody fusion. If the vertebral body height reduction was less than 50%, dorsal decompression with interbody fusion was performed first, and optionally with secondary ventral debridement with vertebral body replacement. In cases where vertebral body reduction was more than 50%, dorsal decompression with instrumentation followed by vertebral body replacement was performed.

*2.3. Antibiotic Therapy*

Each patient received either TAT or EAT, depending on the clinical condition at the time of admission and as recommended by the local infectious disease department. Our cohort included many patients with known infection who were already treated with antibiotics externally and presented to our clinic for surgical treatment. If antibiotics were continued or discontinued for less than 48 h, we defined this condition as being under ongoing antibiotic therapy and called this group EAT, whereas patients without antibiotic therapy or with an antibiotic-free period of more than 2 days formed the TAT group. EAT was switched to TAT after the identification of the pathogen. Intravenous antibiotic therapy was switched to oral antibiotics after approximately 4 weeks, and the total duration of antibiotic therapy was approximately 8 weeks.

*2.4. Methods for Pathogen Detection*

Blood cultures were preferably collected from all patients before starting antibiotic therapy, using three pairs of blood cultures at two or three different peripheral sites (aerobic and anaerobic media) for microbiological assessment. Some patients presented to our clinic in a septic condition with ongoing antibiotic therapy, thus blood culture collection in an antibiotic-free period was not possible, nor was antibiotic suspension justifiable in this case.

Intraoperatively obtained tissue was placed in Schaedler boullions (bioMérieux, Nürtingen, Germany) directly in the operating room and these were then sent to our institute of medical microbiology and virology for analysis. There, the boullions were first incubated at 37 degrees and examined for turbidity after 48 h. Once turbidity was detected, the culture suspension was plated out on Columbia Blood Agar (bioMérieux, Nürtingen, Germany) and HCB Agar (bioMérieux, Nürtingen, Germany). Aerobic culture growth was checked for the first time after 24 h and anaerobic culture growth after another 48 h.

CT-guided biopsy was performed exclusively in case of psoas abscess by the neuroradiologists or radiologists, whereas paravertebral dorsal abscesses and epidural empyema were managed during open surgery. All patients received a pre-interventional contrast-enhanced MRI of the spine and an additional CT for planning. A psoas abscess was always observed on contrast-enhanced MRI of the spine and classified by the neuroradiologist or radiologist as a formation with fluid-equivalent signal intensity and biopsy-worthy formation. An abscess was defined as iso- or hypointense on T1-weighted images, with fluid-equivalent signal intensity on T2-weighted images, and with edge enhancement on contrast-enhanced T1-weighted fat-saturated images [19]. Our cohort did not include CT-guided biopsy of disc, vertebral body, dorsal paravertebral abscess, or epidural abscess. The approach was chosen based on anatomic considerations and the predominant site of the infective lesions. The liquefied contents of the abscess were aspirated and sent for microbiological examination; in addition, a sample was fixed in formalin for pathohistological analysis. In our study, 128 patients (61.5%) were diagnosed with psoas abscess, of which 70 patients (54.7%) were tappable, 50 patients had SD, and 20 had ISEE. Following CT-guided sampling, all patients received a suction-irrigation drainage system from which samples were collected two times daily, and the abscess cavity was also irrigated with gentamycin or vancomycin two times daily, depending on the resistogram. After obtaining three pathogen-free results from the suction-irrigation drainage samples, the drainage was removed.

### 2.5. Microbiological Assessment

Bacteria with high to moderate pathogenic potential that are unlikely to present as contaminants, such as methicillin-susceptible staphylococcus aureus (MSSA), were deemed significant if they were detected in at least one culture. However, potentially low pathogenic bacteria, e.g., cutibacterium, were only considered clinically significant if they were identified in at least two independent cultures. Cases with negative microbiologic results, but with clear clinical and radiographic evidence of SD or ISEE, were classified as positive with non-identified pathogens.

### 2.6. Case Presentation

This following figure presented a case from our series showing our clinical management of spondylodiscitis (Figure 1).

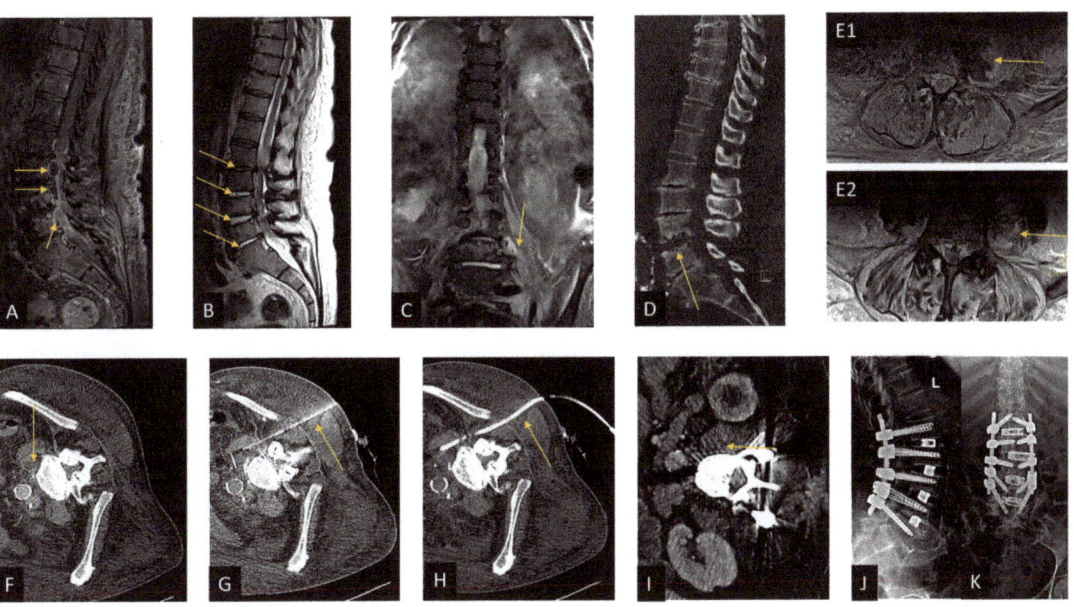

**Figure 1.** Case presentation demonstrating CT-guided biopsy and surgical management in spondylodiscitis. This figure shows a patient from our cohort who suffered from spondylodiscitis with concomitant spinal epidural empyema and psoas abscess left; the 74-year-old patient was pretreated externally with calculated antibiotics (ceftriaxone, flucloxacillin, and metronidazole) and had paraparesis of the legs and sepsis; risk factors were a BMI greater than 35 kg/m and diabetes mellitus with chronic malum perforans pedis. Blood cultures were initially obtained from two different peripheral regions, followed immediately with microsurgical decompression with abscess evacuation and application of a suction-irrigation drainage system. CT-guided drainage of the psoas abscess was performed on the first postoperative day, whereas *Staphelococcus aureus* was detected only in blood

culture and subsequently treated with flucloxacillin and rifampicin. Due to increasing bone destruction, transforaminal lumbar interbody fusion (TLIF) was performed at L1/L2, L2/L3, L3/4, and L4/L5 level. The patient was moved from the intensive care unit to the normal ward and mobilized at ward level. (**A**) Preoperative sagittal T1-weighted fat-saturated contrast-enhanced MRI image of the lumbar spine shows the epidural abscess in the spinal canal at L2–L4 level, marked with arrows. (**B**) Preoperative sagittal T2-weighted MRI image, arrows show spondylodiscitis at L1/L2, L2/L3, L3/L4, and L4/L5 level. (**C**) preoperative coronal T2-weighted short-tau inversion recovery (T2w-STIR) MRI image, arrow shows a psoas abscess on the left. (**D**) Preoperative sagittal reformated CT image, arrow shows bone destruction mainly at the level of L4/L5. (**E1**) Preoperative axial T1-weighted fat-saturated contrast-enhanced MRI image, arrow shows psoas abscess. (**E2**) Preoperative axial T2-weighted fat-saturated MRI image with arrow pointing to psoas abscess on the left. (**F–H**): Illustration of CT-guided puncture of a left psoas abscess in three steps in an axial CT image. (**F**) Planning CT, (**G**) needle puncture, and (**H**) insertion of a suction-irrigation drain. Partially imaged central venous catheter in the iliac vein (**G**,**H**). (**I**) Postoperative axial CT image showing the regreening of the psoas abscess after draining the abscess. (**J**,**K**) A postoperative lateral (**J**) and anteroposterior (**K**) radiograph after performing TLIF spondylodesis from L1 to L5.

### 2.7. Statistical Analysis

Data were statistically analyzed with the SPSS software package (SPSS Statistics 28, IBM, Armonk, New York, NY, USA). Descriptive statistics were used, and categorical variables were adjusted by Fisher exact tests or chi-square tests where appropriate. Numerical variables were analyzed with Mann-Whitney U tests. A binomial test was also used. All statistical tests were two-sided, and a value $p < 0.05$ was considered statistically significant. The sensitivity of a method was calculated as follows: S = true positive/(true positive + false negative) [20].

## 3. Results

### 3.1. Demographics and Baseline Characteristics

We enrolled 208 patients (males: 136, 65.4% vs. females: 72, 34.6%, $p < 0.001$) aged 68 [23–90] y, median [interquartile range] with SD (142, 68.3%) and ISEE (66, 31.7%). Intraoperative specimens and blood cultures were obtained in all cases, while computed tomography (CT)-guided biopsies were performed in 70 tappable cases (54.7%) of 128 patients with psoas abscess (61.5%). A causative pathogen was isolated in 192 cases (92.3%), of which 187 cases (97.4%) presented a pyogenic pathogen and five cases (2.4%) a non-pyogenic pathogen. Gram-positive pathogens were detected in 162 of 187 cases (86.6%), whereas a Gram-negative pathogen was identified in only 25 cases (13.4%). Empiric antibiotic therapy (EAT) was initiated preoperatively in 140 patients (67.3%) and switched following pathogen detection, whereas targeted antibiotic therapy (TAT) was started postoperatively according to resistogram in 68 patients (32.7%). Twelve patients (6%) died due to the disease and its complications (Table 1).

Ages, sex, diabetes mellitus, immunosuppression, and obesity are the most known risk factors in SD and ISEE. In our cohort, diabetes mellitus was observed in 70 patients (37.4%), while 59 patients (31.6%) had a BMI (body mass index) over 30 kg/m$^2$ and 27 patients (14.4%) were immunosuppressed.

Primary sources of infection were identified in 137 patients (73.3%); however, infections resulting directly from surgical spine procedures were not included in this study. We identified 37 skin infections (19.8), 17 infections after epidural application (9.1%), 16 respiratory tract infections (8.6%), nine gastrointestinal tract infections (4. 8%), 13 urinary tract infections (7.0%), eight port-associated infections (4.3%), six retropharyngeal and prevertebral infections (3.2%), 22 foreign body-associated infections (11.8%), three endocarditis of prosthetic valves (1, 6%), five odontogenic infections (2.7%), one infection attributable to immunodeficiency (0.5%), while in 50 patients (26.7%) the cause of infection remained unclear.

**Table 1.** Baseline characteristics.

| Baseline Characteristics | N = 208 | Percentage |
|---|---|---|
| Male | 136 | 65.4% |
| Female | 72 | 34.6% |
| Age | 68 [23–90] y * | - |
| Spondylodiscitis | 142 | 68.3% |
| Isolated spinal epidural empyema | 66 | 31.7% |
| Surgery | 208 | 100% |
| Blood cultures | 208 | 100% |
| Psoas abscess | 128 | 61.5% |
| CT-guided biopsy of Psoas | 70/128 | 54.7% |
| Known causative pathogens | 192 | 92.3% |
| Unknown causative pathogens | 16 | 7.7% |
| Pyogenic spinal infection | 187/192 | 97.4% |
| Non-pyogenic spinal infection | 5/192 | 2.6% |
| Gram-positive pathogens | 162/187 | 86.6% |
| Gram-negative pathogens | 25/187 | 13.4% |
| Empiric antibiotic therapy | 140 | 67.3% |
| Targeted antibiotic therapy | 68 | 32.7% |
| Duration of intravenous antibiotics | 4 [3–6] w * | - |
| Duration of antibiotics | 8 [6–12] w * | - |
| Death | 12 | 5.8% |

CT: computer tomography, *: median [interquartile range].

### 3.2. Diagnostic Sensitivity of Procedures

The highest sensitivity of pathogen detection was achieved using intraoperative specimens (162/208, 77.9%), followed by blood cultures (119/208, 57.2%) and being lowest at CT-guided biopsies (39/70, 55.7%, $p = 0.012$). The diagnostic sensitivity was 92.3% (192/208) for all procedures combined (Figure 2).

### 3.3. Diagnostic Sensitivity in SD and ISEE

Blood cultures demonstrated significantly higher diagnostic sensitivity for SD than for ISEE (SD: 91/142, 64.1% vs. ISEE: 28/66, 42.4%, $p = 0.004$). In contrast, the diagnostic sensitivity of intraoperative specimens was significantly higher in ISEE than in SD (SD: 102/142, 71.8% vs. ISEE: 59/66, 89.4%, $p = 0.007$). On the other hand, no difference in the sensitivity of CT-guided biopsy between both groups was observed (SD: 28/50, 56.0% vs. ISEE: 11/20, 55.0%, $p = 1.0$) (Figure 3).

### 3.4. Sensitivity under Ongoing Empiric Antibiotic Therapy

The diagnostic sensitivity of all three procedures combined was significantly higher in SD patients with postoperative TAT than in SD patients with EAT (EAT: 77/89, 86.5% vs. TAT: 53/53, 100%, $p = 0.004$). No such effect was observed in patients with ISEE (EAT: 47/51, 92.2% vs. TAT: 15/15, 100%, $p = 0.567$). Blood cultures, intraoperative specimens and CT-guided biopsies showed no significant difference in SD and ISEE in terms of sensitivity to the timing of antibiotic administration (Table 2). Intraoperative specimen showed the best diagnostic sensitivity in all groups (TAT-SD: 81.1%, TAT-ISEE: 86.7%, EAT-SD: 67.4%, and EAT-ISEE: 90.2%).

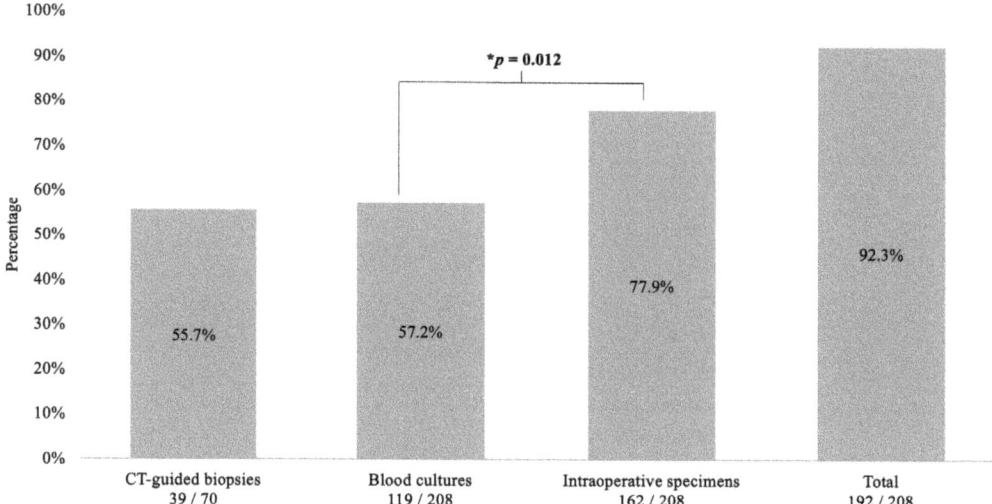

**Figure 2.** Sensitivity of blood culture, intraoperative specimen, and CT-guided biopsy. This figure shows the diagnostic sensitivity of the three procedures in combination and alone. The best results are obtained when all diagnostic procedures are used together, and the best individual result is achieved with intraoperative specimens, which are significantly more effective than blood cultures (77.9% vs. 57.2%, $p = 0.012$). * Binomial test. CT: computed tomography.

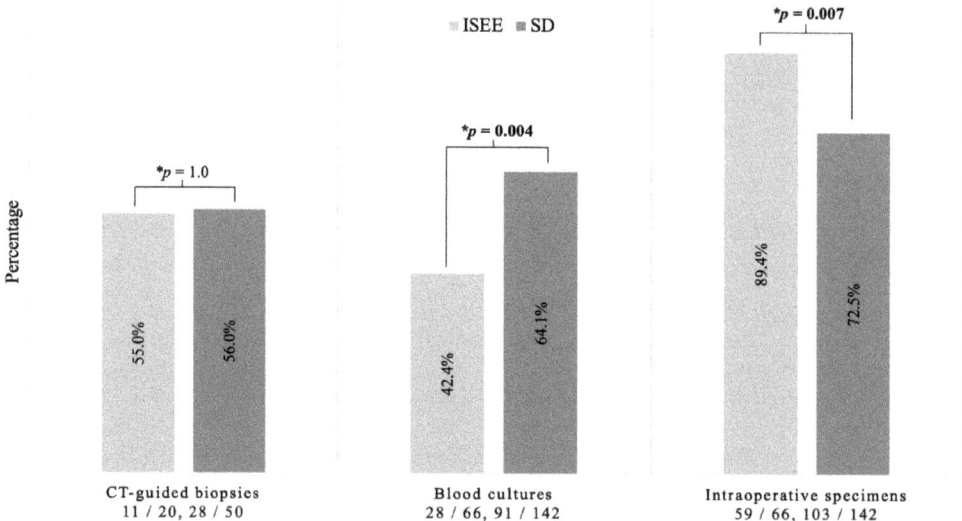

**Figure 3.** Diagnostic sensitivity in spondylodiscitis and isolated spinal epidural empyema. This figure shows the significant difference between both groups, especially in blood cultures ($p = 0.004$) and intraoperative specimens ($p = 0.007$). No difference was found between both groups concerning CT-guided biopsies. * Fisher exact test. ISEE: isolated spinal epidural empyema SD: spondylodiscitis, CT: computed tomography.

### 3.5. Sensitivity of Single Procedure in SD and ISEE Patient Treated with EAT or TAT

The pathogen could always be isolated in the SD- and ISEE-TAT groups, with blood culture, intraoperative specimen, and CT-guided biopsy as single procedure showing no significant difference between SD and ISEE. In contrast, we observed a difference between the SD- and ISEE-EAT groups. The diagnostic sensitivity of blood culture alone was higher in the SD-EAT than in the ISEE-EAT (SD-EAT: 14/89, 18.2% vs. ISEE-EAT: 1/51, 2.1%, $p = 0.010$). The ISEE-EAT group showed better sensitivity than SD-EAT for intraoperative specimen (SD-EAT: 19/89, 24.7% vs. ISEE-EAT: 24/51, 51.1%, $p = 0.002$). CT-guided biopsy revealed no difference between the two groups (SD-EAT: 2/89, 2.6% vs. ISEE-EAT: 0/51, 0.0%, $p = 0.534$) (Table 3).

Table 2. Diagnostic sensitivity under ongoing empiric antibiotic therapy.

| Infection Subgroup | All Three Procedures | Blood Cultures | Intraoperative Specimens | CT-Guided Biopsies |
|---|---|---|---|---|
| SD with TAT | 53/53 (100%) | 35/53 (66.0%) | 43/53 (81.1%) | 11/22 (50%) |
| SD with ongoing EAT | 77/89 (86.5%) | 56/89 (62.9%) | 60/89 (67.4%) | 17/28 (66.7%) |
| $p$-value * | **0.004** | 0.722 | 0.084 | 0.568 |
| ISEE with TAT | 15/15 (100%) | 7/15 (46.7%) | 13/15 (86.7%) | 4/5 (80%) |
| ISEE with ongoing EAT | 47/51 (92.2%) | 21/51 (41.2%) | 46/51 (90.2%) | 7/15 (46.7%) |
| $p$-value * | 0.567 | 0.771 | 0.653 | 0.319 |

ISEE: isolated spinal epidural empyema, SD: spondylodiscitis, CT: computer tomography, EAT: empiric antibiotic therapy, TAT: targeted antibiotic therapy, *: Fisher exact test. Bold values are significant results ($p < 0.05$) as indicated in the methods.

Table 3. Diagnostic sensitivity of single procedures in SD and ISEE patient treated with EAT or TAT.

| Procedure of Pathogen Detection | TAT | | | EAT | | |
|---|---|---|---|---|---|---|
| | SD | ISEE | $p$-Value * | SD | ISEE | $p$-Value * |
| Exclusively blood culture | 8/53 (15.1) | 2/15 (13.3) | 1.0 | 14/89 (18.2%) | 1/51 (2.1%) | **0.010** |
| Exclusively intraoperative specimens | 15/53 (28.3) | 7/15 (46.7%) | 0.218 | 19/89 (24.7%) | 24/51 (51.1%) | **0.002** |
| Exclusively CT-guided Biopsy | 0/53 (0.0%) | 0/15 (0.0%) | — | 2/89 (2.6%) | 0/51 (0.0%) | 0.534 |
| More than one procedure | 30/53 (56.6%) | 6/15 (40.0%) | 0.380 | 42/89 (54.5%) | 22/51 (46.8%) | 0.725 |
| Unknown pathogens | 0 | 0 | | 12 | 4 | |

ISEE: isolated spinal epidural empyema, SD: spondylodiscitis, CT: computer tomography, EAT: empiric antibiotic therapy, TAT: targeted antibiotic therapy, *: Fisher exact test. Bold values are significant results ($p < 0.05$) as indicated in the methods.

*3.6. The First Result of Detected Pathogen in SD and ISEE Treated with EAT or TAT*

The first result of pathogen detection from blood culture, intraoperative specimen, and CT-guided biopsy showed no significant differences between SD and ISEE treated with TAT, but pathogens were always detected. The result of the first pathogen isolation in the EAT group was different between ISEE and SD. Blood culture in SD (SD-EAT: 50/89, 64.9% vs. ISEE-EAT: 18/51, 38.3%) and intraoperative specimen in ISEE (SD-EAT: 24/89, 31.2% vs. ISEE-EAT: 28/51, 59.6%, $p = 0.008$) played the most important role. CT-guided biopsy showed no differences between the two groups (SD-EAT: 3/89, 3.9% vs. ISEE-EAT: 1/51, 2.1%) (Table 4).

*3.7. The role of Each Procedure in Pathogen Detection in Both Entities*

To determine which procedure as stand-alone was able to detect the most pathogens, we analyzed pathogen detection for all procedures in both subgroups, considering each procedure separately and in combination with others.

**Table 4.** The first result of detected pathogen in SD and ISEE treated with EAT or TAT.

| Procedure of First Pathogen Detection | TAT | | | EAT | | |
|---|---|---|---|---|---|---|
| | SD | ISEE | *p*-Value * | SD | ISEE | *p*-Value * |
| Blood culture | 31/53 (58.5%) | 6/15 (40%) | | 50/89 (64.9%) | 18/51 (38.3%) | |
| Intraoperative specimens | 21/53 (39.6%) | 8/1 (53.3%) | 0.340 | 24/89 (31.2%) | 28/51 (59.6%) | **0.008** |
| CT-guided Biopsy | 1/53 (1.9%) | 1/15 (6.7%) | | 3/89 (3.9%) | 1/51 (2.1%) | |
| Unknown pathogens | 0 | 0 | | 12 | 4 | |

ISEE: isolated spinal epidural empyema, SD: spondylodiscitis, CT: computer tomography, EAT: empiric antibiotic therapy, TAT: targeted antibiotic therapy, *: Fisher exact test. Bold values are significant results ($p < 0.05$) as indicated in the methods.

### 3.7.1. Spondylodiscitis

A quarter of pathogens were detected exclusively by intraoperative specimens (34/130, 26.2%), while 16.9% (22/130) were identified solely by blood cultures ($p < 0.142$). Only 1.5% (2/130) were detected by CT-guided biopsy. Over half of the pathogens (72/130, 55.4%) were found in more than one procedure (Figure 4).

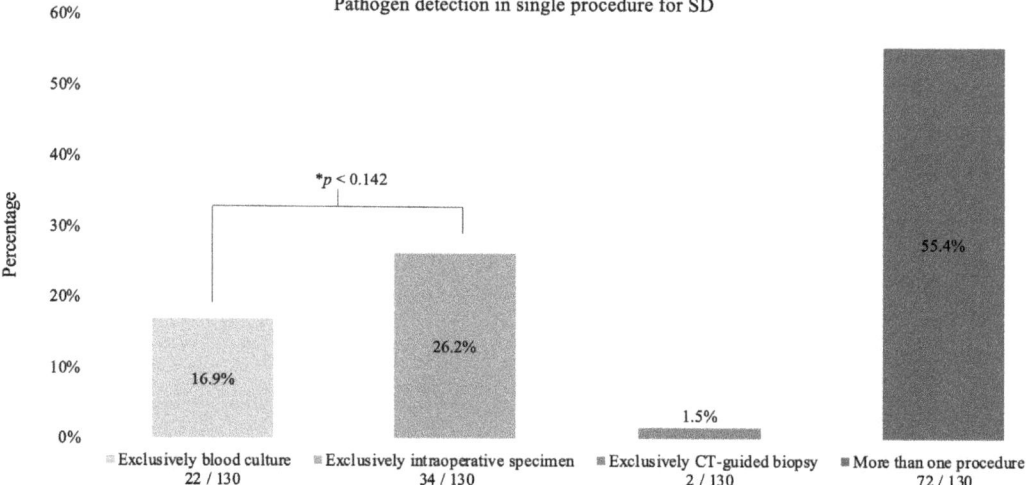

**Figure 4.** Pathogen detection in spondylodiscitis. This diagram shows in which procedures pathogens were detected in spondylodiscitis patients. There were 142 patients in total. Pathogens were detected in 130 patients. * Binomial test.

### 3.7.2. Isolated Spinal Epidural Empyema

Half of the pathogens (31/62, 50%) were exclusively detected by intraoperative specimens, while only 4.5% (3/62) were detected by blood cultures ($p < 0.001$) and none were detected by CT-guided biopsy. Less than half of the pathogens were detected in more than one procedure (28/62, 45.2%) (Figure 5).

### 3.8. The First Result of Antibiogram and Resistogram from All Procedures

The time required to detect pathogens in blood cultures from blood and for intraoperative specimens from pus, tissue, or bone is different. In clinical practice, the results of all procedures (CT-guided biopsy, intraoperative specimen, and blood culture) are not available at the same time to the physician performing the procedure, however, the first result is the most important and provides the antibiogram and resistogram for initiating and switching antibiotic therapy. In this context, the comparison between intraoperative specimen and blood culture is relevant, since both procedures were performed on the same day in our center. There is a predicted delay in CT-guided biopsy, which was usually performed one or two days after surgery.

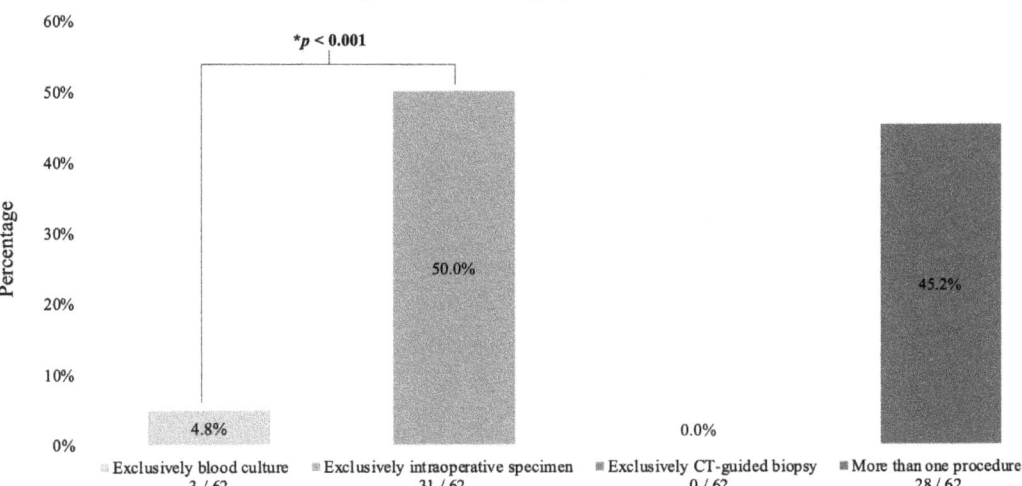

**Figure 5.** Pathogen detection in isolated spinal epidural empyema. This figure demonstrates the procedures used to detect the pathogens in epidural empyema patients. In total, there were 66 patients. Pathogens were detected in 62 patients. * Binomial test.

3.8.1. Spondylodiscitis

The first results were obtained in 62.3% (n = 81) from blood cultures, in 34.6% from intraoperative specimens (n = 45) and in 3.1% (n= 4) from CT-guided biopsies ($p < 0.001$) (Figure 6).

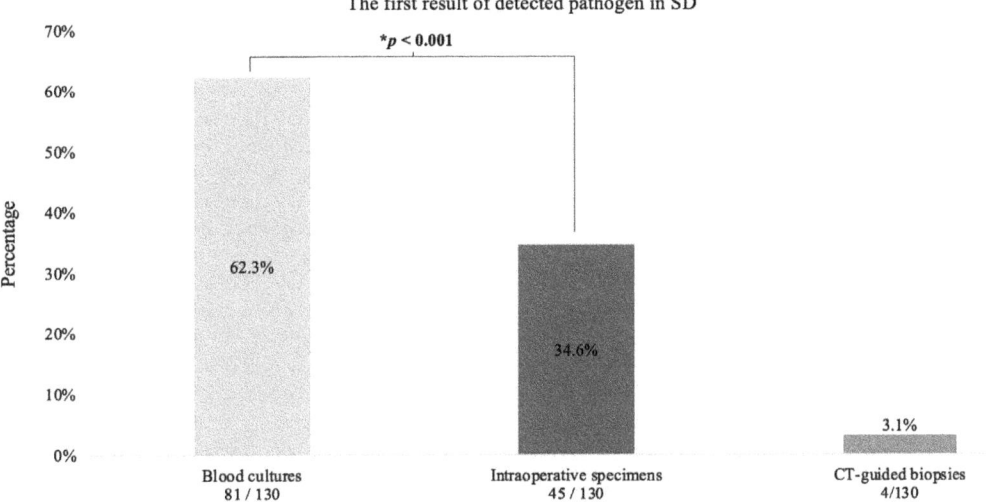

**Figure 6.** The first result of detected pathogen in spondylodiscitis. This diagram shows the first result of detected pathogen in Spondylodiszitis (SD) patients. * Binomial test.

### 3.8.2. Isolated Spinal Epidural Empyema

The first results (36 cases) were obtained from intraoperative specimens in 58.1%, from blood cultures in 38.7% (n = 24) and from CT-guided biopsies in 3.2% (n = 2) ($p < 0.001$) (Figure 7).

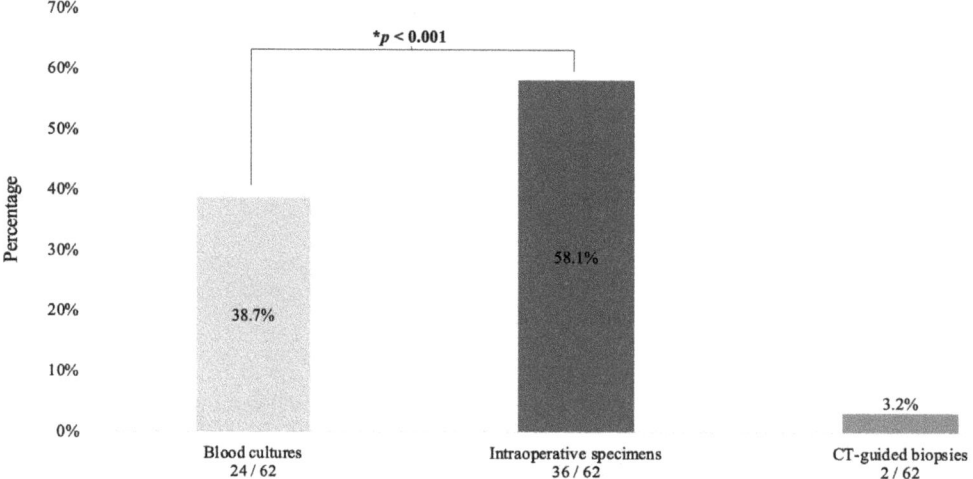

**Figure 7.** The first result of detected pathogen in isolated spinal epidural empyema. This diagram reveals the first pathogen detection in isolated spinal epidural empyema (ISEE) patients. * Binomial test.

## 4. Discussion

The main finding of our retrospective observational study is that intraoperative specimens demonstrate the highest diagnostic sensitivity for ISEE, whereas blood cultures show superior sensitivity in detecting pathogens in patients with SD. Interestingly, ongoing antibiotic treatment only affected the sensitivity of these tests in SD patients, with no significant effect on diagnostic yield in ISEE.

Consistent with previous studies, male patients were diagnosed with SD and ISEE twice as often as females in our cohort [5,16]. Gram-positive pathogens were identified in 86.6% of pyogenic infections, which is in line with the literature data ranging from 74 to 82% [21–23]. Our antibiotic management was based on the IDSA guidelines [18]. The mortality rate in our cohort was 6%, which is comparable to previous studies [16]. Moreover, our pathogen detection rate of 92.3% using all three diagnostic procedures combined is in accordance with the results of previous observational studies that detected pathogens in 67% and 100% of cases [4,16,24,25]. Authors have reported divergent diagnostic sensitivity of blood culture, image-guided biopsy, and intraoperative specimen for SD and ISEE (Table 5) [4,12,16,17,25–36].

The diagnostic sensitivity of blood cultures in SD and ISEE patients varies widely from 30% to 78% according to previously published reports [12,16,17,24–28,30–40]. However, a systematic review of 14 clinical retrospective studies found that blood cultures routinely obtained in 91% of cases had an average sensitivity of 58%, which is consistent with our results (57.2%) [16]. The diagnostic sensitivity of image-guided biopsy ranges from 44.1% to 82.5% and can be increased by using different techniques such as X-ray or CT for sampling and different sites such as psoas, disc, or vertebral body [12,17,24,25,29,36–39]. Consistent with this spectrum, we were able to detect a pathogen with CT-guided biopsies from psoas abscess in 55.7% of cases.

**Table 5.** References on sensitivity of blood culture, intraoperative specimen, image-guided biopsy.

| Author | Blood Culture | Image-Guided Biopsy | Intraoperative Specimen |
| --- | --- | --- | --- |
| Vettivel et al. [37] | 37 (48.7%) | 30/40 (75%) * | |
| Heuer et al. [38] | 145/307 (47%) | 213/307 (64%) * | |
| Widdrington et al. [25] | 40/78 (51%) | 21/29 (72%) | 25/38 (66%) |
| Hasan et al. [39] | 17/40 (42.5%) | 33/40 (82.5%) | NR |
| Stangenberg et al. [34] | 97/182 (53.3%) | NR | 134/202 (66.3%) |
| Nolla et al. [12] | 46/64 (63.4%) | 11/21 (52%) | 15/20 (75%) |
| Colmenero et al. [28] | 52/152 (34.2%) | NR | NR |
| Pigrau et al. [40] | 71/91 (78%) | NR | NR |
| McHenry et al. [17] | 156/255 (61.2%) | 86/124 (69.4%) | 88/113 (77.9%) |
| Patzakis et al. [33] | 13/26 (50%) | NR | NR |
| Zarrouk et al. [36] | 14/29 (48.3%) | 11/15 (73.4%) | NR |
| Carragee et al. [27] | 66/111 (59.5%) | NR | NR |
| Ledermann et al. [30] | 25/41 (61%) | NR | NR |
| Bateman et al. [26] | 23/52 (44.2%) | NR | 24/32 (75%) |
| Torda et al. [35] | 10/16 (62.5%) | NR | NR |
| Osenbach et al. [32] | 12/40 (30%) | NR | NR |
| Hadjipavlou et al. [29] | NR | 19/26 (73.1%) | 25/40 (62.5%) |
| Nather et al. [31] | 5/9 (55.6%) | NR | 14/16 (87.5%) |
| Current study | 119/208 (57%) | 39/70 (56%) | 162/208 (78%) |

NR: not reported. *: The authors did not distinguish between image-guided biopsy and intraoperative specimen.

Intraoperative specimens yielded the best results in the literature ranging from 59.6% to 87.5% [12,17,24–26,29,31,34,37,38]. Similarly, using this procedure, we were able to detect a pathogen in 77.9% of patients.

Data on the diagnostic sensitivity of all procedures in SD and ISEE are limited in the literature. The diagnostic sensitivity of blood cultures and intraoperative specimens differed between SD and ISEE. Blood culture sensitivity was higher in SD, whereas intraoperative specimen sensitivity was higher in ISEE. This supports the assumption that SD is mainly a hematogenous dissemination, whereas ISEE is a local encapsulated mass with pus or inflammatory tissue, which can ideally be reached by intraoperative sampling.

Previous studies have shown that blood cultures can detect pathogens in 57.2% of cases, with even higher rates up to 70% in antibiotic-naive patients [4,12,16]. In our study, the sensitivity of all three methods was significantly lower in SD patients under ongoing EAT than in SD patients without antibiotics, whereas the sensitivity in ISEE showed no significant difference in relation to antibiotic therapy.

The diagnostic sensitivity of the stand-alone procedure showed no differences between SD and ISEE when the patient was treated with TAT, whereas the EAT group differed in terms of blood culture as the most sensitive stand-alone procedure in SD and intraoperative specimen in ISEE. Our study also showed the same results in terms of the first result of pathogen detection in SD and ISEE patients treated with TAT or EAT.

In our cohort, pathogen detection in ISEE was higher in intraoperative specimens exclusively compared with blood cultures (50% versus 5%), demonstrating the importance of surgical sampling in ISEE. This was not significant in SD. The first decisive result of pathogen detection in SD patients was achieved in 62.3% of cases by blood culture and in 58.1% of cases of ISEE by the intraoperative specimen in our study. Therefore, blood cultures in SD and intraoperative samples in ISEE seem to be of the highest importance to allow the administration of targeted antibiotics.

CT-guided biopsy was performed only in the psoas abscess but not in the disc compartment in SD or in the epidural empyema in ISEE, where infectious processes usually occur, which may have influenced our results. The results of a CT-guided biopsy for pathogen detection varies and depends on the examination technique, the examiner, patient collective, and the specimen being collected. Numerous other factors, including laboratory parameters (C-reactive protein > 50 mg/L), CT features (nonsclerotic endplate erosions), and magnetic resonance criteria (paravertebral/epidural abscess formation), appeared to be associated with positive pathogen detection [41].

For specific anatomic structures, such as the psoas, CT-guided biopsy with drainage is essential because of the percutaneous minimally invasive technique and success rate in targeting, as well as the low complication rate. In addition, CT-guided biopsy is an essential procedure in patients without instability or neurologic deficits due to the avoidance of surgery with potential complications despite the anesthetic and healing disruption risks. The above demonstrates how important CT-guided biopsy is for the treatment of SD and ISEE. The poorly presented results of CT-guided biopsy in this study compared with blood culture and intraoperative specimen may be influenced by the selective surgical patient, timing of the procedure, and anatomic structure of the collection (psoas abscess only). Nevertheless, this study demonstrated favorable diagnostic sensitivity for CT-guided biopsy compared with the existing literature, which suggested a successful pathogen detection rate ranging from 28.1% to 57.1% [42,43], and provided a novel comparison of all three procedures with limitations.

*Limitations and Strengths of This Study*

This study has inherent limitation due to its retrospective nature. However, our findings provide valuable insights into the diagnostic sensitivity of blood cultures, intraoperative specimens, and CT-guided biopsies and serve a basis for prospective research. The monocentric design of our study limits the generalizability of our observations. Nevertheless, our cohort of SD and ISEE patients underwent comprehensive phenotyping, including, detailed demographic, clinical, radiological, laboratory and microbiological assessments, which enhances the internal validity of our data. To confirm our findings and assess their external validity, well-designed multicentric studies are needed, preferably in a prospective interventional setting [44].

## 5. Conclusions

To achieve the best diagnostic sensitivity for causative pathogens, all procedures are essential, particularly intraoperative specimens and blood cultures. Intraoperative specimens yielded the highest single result, followed by blood cultures. However, blood cultures remain crucial due to their non-invasive nature. Blood cultures are crucial for identifying pathogens in SD, while intraoperative specimens are essential for isolating pathogens in ISEE.

Blood cultures play the most important role in pathogen identification in SD, while intraoperative specimens are leading in the description of pathogens in ISEE. Without surgical intervention, nearly half of the pathogens in ISEE patients cannot be detected. This study reveals that the combined diagnostic procedures have lower sensitivity in SD patients with ongoing EAT, but not in ISEE patients.

**Author Contributions:** M.M.H.: conceptualization, methodology, software, validation, formal analysis, investigation, resources, data curation, writing—original draft preparation, project administration, and funding acquisition. I.Y.E., T.A.J., D.P., A.C.D., U.P., T.S. and M.M.H.: writing—review and editing, visualization, and supervision. All authors have read and agreed to the published version of the manuscript.

**Funding:** This research received no external funding.

**Institutional Review Board Statement:** The study was conducted in accordance with the Declaration of Helsinki and approved by the Institutional Review Board of the local ethics committee at the University Hospital Dresden (protocol code: BO-EK-17012022, January 2022).

**Informed Consent Statement:** Patient consent was waived due to the retrospective, anonymous character of this study.

**Data Availability Statement:** The original contributions presented in the study are included in the article, further inquiries can be directed to the corresponding author.

**Acknolegdment:** We would like to thank Gabriele Schackert and Kay Engellandt for their support.

**Conflicts of Interest:** The authors declare no conflict of interest.

# References

1. Butler, J.S.; Shelly, M.J.; Timlin, M.; Powderly, W.G.; O'Byrne, J.M. Nontuberculous pyogenic spinal infection in adults: A 12-year experience from a tertiary referral center. *Spine* **2006**, *31*, 2695–2700. [CrossRef] [PubMed]
2. Frangen, T.M.; Kalicke, T.; Gottwald, M.; Andereya, S.; Andress, H.J.; Russe, O.J.; Muller, E.J.; Muhr, G.; Schinkel, C. Die operative Therapie der Spondylodiszitis. *Unfallchirurg* **2006**, *109*, 743–753. [CrossRef]
3. Tsiodras, S.; Falagas, M.E. Clinical assessment and medical treatment of spine infections. *Clin. Orthop. Relat. Res.* **2006**, *444*, 38–50. [CrossRef] [PubMed]
4. Herren, C.; Jung, N.; Pishnamaz, M.; Breuninger, M.; Siewe, J.; Sobottke, R. Spondylodiscitis: Diagnosis and Treatment Options. *Dtsch. Arztebl. Int.* **2017**, *114*, 875–882. [CrossRef] [PubMed]
5. Zarghooni, K.; Rollinghoff, M.; Sobottke, R.; Eysel, P. Treatment of spondylodiscitis. *Int. Orthop.* **2012**, *36*, 405–411. [CrossRef] [PubMed]
6. Rosc-Bereza, K.; Arkuszewski, M.; Ciach-Wysocka, E.; Boczarska-Jedynak, M. Spinal epidural abscess: Common symptoms of an emergency condition. A case report. *Neuroradiol. J.* **2013**, *26*, 464–468. [CrossRef]
7. Quack, V.; Hermann, I.; Rath, B.; Dietrich, K.; Spreckelsen, C.; Luring, C.; Arbab, D.; Mueller, C.A.; Shousha, M.; Clusmann, H.; et al. Current treatment strategies for spondylodiscitis in surgical clinics in Germany. *Z. Orthop. Unfall* **2014**, *152*, 577–583. [CrossRef]
8. Rustemi, O.; Raneri, F.; Alvaro, L.; Gazzola, L.; Beggio, G.; Rossetto, L.; Cervellini, P. Single-approach vertebral osteosynthesis in the treatment of spinal osteolysis by spondylodiscitis. *Neurosurg. Focus.* **2019**, *46*, E9. [CrossRef]
9. Decker, S.; Schroder, B.M.; Stubig, T.; Sehmisch, S. Common infectious challenges of the thoracic and lumbar spine: Spondylodiscitis and postoperative wound infection. *Unfallchirurg* **2022**, *125*, 33–40. [CrossRef]
10. Cunha, B.A. Osteomyelitis in elderly patients. *Clin. Infect. Dis.* **2002**, *35*, 287–293. [CrossRef]
11. Nagashima, H.; Tanishima, S.; Tanida, A. Diagnosis and management of spinal infections. *J. Orthop. Sci.* **2018**, *23*, 8–13. [CrossRef] [PubMed]
12. Nolla, J.M.; Ariza, J.; Gomez-Vaquero, C.; Fiter, J.; Bermejo, J.; Valverde, J.; Escofet, D.R.; Gudiol, F. Spontaneous pyogenic vertebral osteomyelitis in nondrug users. *Semin. Arthritis Rheum.* **2002**, *31*, 271–278. [CrossRef]
13. Nickerson, E.K.; Sinha, R. Vertebral osteomyelitis in adults: An update. *Br. Med. Bull.* **2016**, *117*, 121–138. [CrossRef] [PubMed]
14. Pingel, A. Spondylodiscitis. *Z. Orthop. Unfall* **2021**, *159*, 687–703. [CrossRef] [PubMed]
15. Fleege, C.; Wichelhaus, T.A.; Rauschmann, M. Systemic and local antibiotic therapy of conservative and operative treatment of spondylodiscitis. *Orthopade* **2012**, *41*, 727–735. [CrossRef] [PubMed]
16. Mylona, E.; Samarkos, M.; Kakalou, E.; Fanourgiakis, P.; Skoutelis, A. Pyogenic vertebral osteomyelitis: A systematic review of clinical characteristics. *Semin. Arthritis Rheum.* **2009**, *39*, 10–17. [CrossRef]
17. McHenry, M.C.; Easley, K.A.; Locker, G.A. Vertebral osteomyelitis: Long-term outcome for 253 patients from 7 Cleveland-area hospitals. *Clin. Infect. Dis.* **2002**, *34*, 1342–1350. [CrossRef]
18. Berbari, E.F.; Kanj, S.S.; Kowalski, T.J.; Darouiche, R.O.; Widmer, A.F.; Schmitt, S.K.; Hendershot, E.F.; Holtom, P.D.; Huddleston, P.M., 3rd; Petermann, G.W.; et al. Executive Summary: 2015 Infectious Diseases Society of America (IDSA) Clinical Practice Guidelines for the Diagnosis and Treatment of Native Vertebral Osteomyelitis in Adults. *Clin. Infect. Dis.* **2015**, *61*, 859–863. [CrossRef]
19. Chandnani, V.P.; Beltran, J.; Morris, C.S.; Khalil, S.N.; Mueller, C.F.; Burk, J.M.; Bennett, W.F.; Shaffer, P.B.; Vasila, M.S.; Reese, J.; et al. Acute experimental osteomyelitis and abscesses: Detection with MR imaging versus CT. *Radiology* **1990**, *174*, 233–236. [CrossRef]
20. Parikh, R.; Mathai, A.; Parikh, S.; Chandra Sekhar, G.; Thomas, R. Understanding and using sensitivity, specificity and predictive values. *Indian. J. Ophthalmol.* **2008**, *56*, 45–50. [CrossRef]
21. Bernard, L.; Dinh, A.; Ghout, I.; Simo, D.; Zeller, V.; Issartel, B.; Le Moing, V.; Belmatoug, N.; Lesprit, P.; Bru, J.P.; et al. Antibiotic treatment for 6 weeks versus 12 weeks in patients with pyogenic vertebral osteomyelitis: An open-label, non-inferiority, randomised, controlled trial. *Lancet* **2015**, *385*, 875–882. [CrossRef] [PubMed]
22. Fragio Gil, J.J.; Gonzalez Mazario, R.; Salavert Lleti, M.; Roman Ivorra, J.A. Vertebral osteomyelitis: Clinical, microbiological and radiological characteristics of 116 patients. *Med. Clin.* **2020**, *155*, 335–339. [CrossRef]

23. Kehrer, M.; Pedersen, C.; Jensen, T.G.; Hallas, J.; Lassen, A.T. Increased short- and long-term mortality among patients with infectious spondylodiscitis compared with a reference population. *Spine J.* **2015**, *15*, 1233–1240. [CrossRef] [PubMed]
24. Pola, E.; Taccari, F.; Autore, G.; Giovannenze, F.; Pambianco, V.; Cauda, R.; Maccauro, G.; Fantoni, M. Multidisciplinary management of pyogenic spondylodiscitis: Epidemiological and clinical features, prognostic factors and long-term outcomes in 207 patients. *Eur. Spine J.* **2018**, *27*, 229–236. [CrossRef] [PubMed]
25. Widdrington, J.D.; Emmerson, I.; Cullinan, M.; Narayanan, M.; Klejnow, E.; Watson, A.; Ong, E.L.C.; Schmid, M.L.; Price, D.A.; Schwab, U.; et al. Pyogenic Spondylodiscitis: Risk Factors for Adverse Clinical Outcome in Routine Clinical Practice. *Med. Sci.* **2018**, *6*, 96. [CrossRef] [PubMed]
26. Bateman, J.L.; Pevzner, M.M. Spinal osteomyelitis: A review of 10 years' experience. *Orthopedics* **1995**, *18*, 561–565. [CrossRef]
27. Carragee, E.J. Pyogenic vertebral osteomyelitis. *J. Bone Joint Surg. Am.* **1997**, *79*, 874–880. [CrossRef] [PubMed]
28. Colmenero, J.D.; Jimenez-Mejias, M.E.; Sanchez-Lora, F.J.; Reguera, J.M.; Palomino-Nicas, J.; Martos, F.; Garcia de las Heras, J.; Pachon, J. Pyogenic, tuberculous, and brucellar vertebral osteomyelitis: A descriptive and comparative study of 219 cases. *Ann. Rheum. Dis.* **1997**, *56*, 709–715. [CrossRef]
29. Hadjipavlou, A.G.; Mader, J.T.; Necessary, J.T.; Muffoletto, A.J. Hematogenous pyogenic spinal infections and their surgical management. *Spine* **2000**, *25*, 1668–1679. [CrossRef]
30. Ledermann, H.P.; Schweitzer, M.E.; Morrison, W.B.; Carrino, J.A. MR imaging findings in spinal infections: Rules or myths? *Radiology* **2003**, *228*, 506–514. [CrossRef]
31. Nather, A.; David, V.; Hee, H.T.; Thambiah, J. Pyogenic vertebral osteomyelitis: A review of 14 cases. *J. Orthop. Surg.* **2005**, *13*, 240–244. [CrossRef]
32. Osenbach, R.K.; Hitchon, P.W.; Menezes, A.H. Diagnosis and management of pyogenic vertebral osteomyelitis in adults. *Surg. Neurol.* **1990**, *33*, 266–275. [CrossRef] [PubMed]
33. Patzakis, M.J.; Rao, S.; Wilkins, J.; Moore, T.M.; Harvey, P.J. Analysis of 61 cases of vertebral osteomyelitis. *Clin. Orthop. Relat. Res.* **1991**, *264*, 178–183. [CrossRef]
34. Stangenberg, M.; Mende, K.C.; Mohme, M.; Kratzig, T.; Viezens, L.; Both, A.; Rohde, H.; Dreimann, M. Influence of microbiological diagnosis on the clinical course of spondylodiscitis. *Infection* **2021**, *49*, 1017–1027. [CrossRef] [PubMed]
35. Torda, A.J.; Gottlieb, T.; Bradbury, R. Pyogenic vertebral osteomyelitis: Analysis of 20 cases and review. *Clin. Infect. Dis.* **1995**, *20*, 320–328. [CrossRef]
36. Zarrouk, V.; Feydy, A.; Salles, F.; Dufour, V.; Guigui, P.; Redondo, A.; Fantin, B. Imaging does not predict the clinical outcome of bacterial vertebral osteomyelitis. *Rheumatology* **2007**, *46*, 292–295. [CrossRef]
37. Vettivel, J.; Bortz, C.; Passias, P.G.; Baker, J.F. Pyogenic Vertebral Column Osteomyelitis in Adults: Analysis of Risk Factors for 30-Day and 1-Year Mortality in a Single Center Cohort Study. *Asian Spine J.* **2019**, *13*, 608–614. [CrossRef]
38. Heuer, A.; Strahl, A.; Viezens, L.; Koepke, L.G.; Stangenberg, M.; Dreimann, M. The Hamburg Spondylodiscitis Assessment Score (HSAS) for Immediate Evaluation of Mortality Risk on Hospital Admission. *J. Clin. Med.* **2022**, *11*, 660. [CrossRef]
39. Hasan, G.A.; Raheem, H.Q.; Qutub, M.; Wais, Y.B.; Katran, M.H.; Shetty, G.M. Management of Pyogenic Spondylodiscitis Following Nonspinal Surgeries: A Tertiary Care Center Experience. *Int. J. Spine Surg.* **2021**, *15*, 591–599. [CrossRef] [PubMed]
40. Pigrau, C.; Almirante, B.; Flores, X.; Falco, V.; Rodriguez, D.; Gasser, I.; Villanueva, C.; Pahissa, A. Spontaneous pyogenic vertebral osteomyelitis and endocarditis: Incidence, risk factors, and outcome. *Am. J. Med.* **2005**, *118*, 1287. [CrossRef]
41. Braun, A.; Germann, T.; Wunnemann, F.; Weber, M.A.; Schiltenwolf, M.; Akbar, M.; Burkholder, I.; Kauczor, H.U.; Rehnitz, C. Impact of MRI, CT, and Clinical Characteristics on Microbial Pathogen Detection Using CT-Guided Biopsy for Suspected Spondylodiscitis. *J. Clin. Med.* **2019**, *9*, 32. [CrossRef]
42. Michel, S.C.; Pfirrmann, C.W.; Boos, N.; Hodler, J. CT-guided core biopsy of subchondral bone and intervertebral space in suspected spondylodiskitis. *AJR Am. J. Roentgenol.* **2006**, *186*, 977–980. [CrossRef] [PubMed]
43. Rieneck, K.; Hansen, S.E.; Karle, A.; Gutschik, E. Microbiologically verified diagnosis of infectious spondylitis using CT-guided fine needle biopsy. *APMIS* **1996**, *104*, 755–762. [CrossRef] [PubMed]
44. Spieth, P.M.; Kubasch, A.S.; Penzlin, A.I.; Illigens, B.M.; Barlinn, K.; Siepmann, T. Randomized controlled trials—A matter of design. *Neuropsychiatr. Dis Treat.* **2016**, *12*, 1341–1349. [CrossRef] [PubMed]

**Disclaimer/Publisher's Note:** The statements, opinions and data contained in all publications are solely those of the individual author(s) and contributor(s) and not of MDPI and/or the editor(s). MDPI and/or the editor(s) disclaim responsibility for any injury to people or property resulting from any ideas, methods, instructions or products referred to in the content.

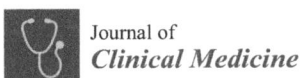

Article

# The Epidemiology of Spondylodiscitis in Germany: A Descriptive Report of Incidence Rates, Pathogens, In-Hospital Mortality, and Hospital Stays between 2010 and 2020

Siegmund Lang [1,*], Nike Walter [1], Melanie Schindler [1], Susanne Baertl [1,2], Dominik Szymski [1], Markus Loibl [3], Volker Alt [1] and Markus Rupp [1]

[1] Department for Trauma Surgery, University Medical Center Regensburg, Franz-Josef-Strauss-Allee 11, 93053 Regensburg, Germany
[2] Centrum für Muskuloskeletale Chirurgie, Universitätsmedizin Berlin, Charitéplatz1, 10117 Berlin, Germany
[3] Department of Spine Surgery, Schulthess Clinic Zurich, Lenghalde 2, 8008 Zurich, Switzerland
* Correspondence: siegmund.lang@ukr.de; Tel.: +49-941944-6805

**Abstract:** Background: Spondylodiscitis can lead to significant morbidity and mortality. Understanding its up-to-date epidemiological characteristics and trends is important to improve patient care. Methods: This study analyzed trends in the incidence rate of spondylodiscitis cases in Germany between 2010 and 2020, as well as the pathogens, in-hospital mortality rate, and length of hospital stay. Data were obtained from the Federal Statistical Office and the Institute for the Hospital Remuneration System database. The ICD-10 codes "M46.2-", "M46.3-" and "M46.4-" were evaluated. Results: The incidence rate of spondylodiscitis increased to 14.4/100,000 inhabitants, with 59.6% cases occurring in patients 70 years or older and affecting mainly the lumbar spine (56.2%). Absolute case numbers increased from 6886 by 41.6% to 9753 in 2020 (IIR = 1.39, 95% CI 0.62–3.08). Staphylococci and *Escherichia coli* were the most coded pathogens. The proportion of resistant pathogens was 12.9%. In-hospital mortality rates increased to a maximum of 64.7/1000 patients in 2020, intensive care unit treatment was documented in 2697 (27.7%) cases, and the length of stay per case was 22.3 days. Conclusion: The sharply increasing incidence and in-hospital mortality rate of spondylodiscitis highlights the need for patient-centered therapy to improve patient outcomes, especially in the geriatric, frail population, which is prone to infectious diseases.

**Keywords:** spondylodiscitis; mortality; pathogens; antimicrobial resistance; epidemiology; geriatric population

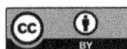

## 1. Introduction

Musculoskeletal infections represent a major challenge in orthopedic and trauma surgery [1]. Infections of the spine caused by pyogenic bacteria without prior surgery or implant insertion involving the intervertebral disc and vertebral bodies are referred to as (pyogenic) spondylodiscitis [2]. Patients suffering from spondylodiscitis commonly need to be hospitalized [3–6]. Insidious courses, especially in infections with low virulent pathogens, often lead to delayed diagnosis, which can be associated with high morbidity and mortality [7]. In this context, the significance of infections with coagulase-negative staphylococci (CONS) must be increasingly emphasized [8–10]. Even after completing treatment, patients tend to suffer relevant impairment in quality of life [11]. Epidemiological studies have observed rising incidence rates of spondylodiscitis in Europe, indicating an ongoing challenge for stakeholders in healthcare systems [12–14]. In general, the treatment of elderly patients, who are especially prone to infections, will keep gaining importance for musculoskeletal surgeons [15]. On the one hand, increasing numbers of comorbidities of an aging population can be assumed as potential reasons for this development [16,17].

Conversely, advancements in imaging technology have led to improved diagnostic capabilities, resulting in an increased number of documented cases of spondylodiscitis [18,19]. Lastly, the standardization in pathogen identification methods has emerged and most likely further contributed to the detection of spondylodiscitis [20,21]. Up-to-date diagnostic and therapeutic measurements in spondylodiscitis treatment recently have been summarized [22,23]. Nevertheless, considerable heterogeneity in reports on the epidemiology of spondylodiscitis persists, analyses of nationwide databases are sparse and the rate of in-hospital mortality remains to be elucidated [12,14,24,25].

Therefore, the aim of this study was (1) to determine the epidemiological characteristics of pyogenic spondylodiscitis and the development of the nationwide incidence in adults from 2010 through 2020. (2) The second aim was to provide a comprehensive overview of the pathogens documented as concomitant diagnoses in 2020. (3) Lastly, we aimed to analyze the development of the in-hospital mortality rate, duration of hospitalization and proportion of cases which required intensive care unit (ICU) treatment between 2010 and 2020.

## 2. Materials and Methods

### 2.1. Federal Statistical Office of Germany (Destatis)

Data consisting of annual codes of the tenth version of the International Statistical Classification of Diseases and Related Health Problems (ICD-10) diagnosis codes from German medical institutions between 2010 and 2020 were provided by the Federal Statistical Office of Germany (Destatis). The total number of spondylodiscitis cases was quantified by adding ICD-10 codes "M46.2-", "M46.3-" and "M46.4-" and analyzed as a function of sex and age in 10-year increments for patients older than 20 years between 2010 and 2020. Incidence rates were calculated based on Germany's historical population aged 20 years or older provided by Destatis. Here, the number of inhabitants in each of the 16 German federal states was considered by year of birth for each year of the period 2010 through 2020. The deadline of each year was December 31. Incidence rate ratios (IIR) with the corresponding 95% confidence interval (CI) and percentage changes were calculated by dividing the incidence in 2020 by the incidence of the preceding year for all spondylodiscitis cases. Changes in the incidence rate ratios were determined relative to the year 2010. Furthermore, Destatis provided the number of in-hospital deaths and number of hospitalization days for spondylodiscitis cases during the observation period.

### 2.2. Institute for the Hospital Remuneration System (InEK GmbH)

In accordance with Section 17b of the German Hospital Financing Act, a universal, performance-based, and flat-rate remuneration system has been introduced for general hospital services. The basis for this is the German Diagnosis Related Groups system (G-DRG system), whereby each inpatient case of treatment is remunerated through a corresponding DRG lump sum payment. The InEK GmbH provides detailed data on the main diagnoses (based on ICD-10 codes), age and sex distribution, length of hospital stays, reasons for discharge (including "death"), number of intensive care unit (ICU) cases and coded concomitant diagnoses (based on ICD-10 codes) (22). The InEK browser enables analysis back to the year 2019. The following comprehensive analysis was made only for the year 2020. Based on the ICD-10 codes for spondylodiscitis, as listed above, data for total case numbers, numbers of pathogens coded as concomitant diagnoses, number of in-hospital deaths, and the number of cases with ICU treatment were extracted. Informed Consent and Investigational Review Board (IRB) approval was not required for this study as it used data from anonymous, de-identified, administrative databases.

## 3. Results

### 3.1. The Development of the Nationwide Incidence of Spondylodiscitis from 2010 to 2020

In total 95,075 in-hospital spondylodiscitis cases were registered between 2010 and 2020. In 2010, a total number of 6886 cases were listed in Germany, constituting an annual incidence of 10.4 cases per 100,000 inhabitants (95% CI 10.1–10.6). In the following years, the incidence rose steadily, resulting in a maximum of 14.8 cases per 100,000 inhabitants (95% CI 14.5–15.1) in 2019. In 2020, the number slightly decreased to an incidence of 14.4 per 100,000 inhabitants (95% CI 14.1–14.7). Compared to the year 2010, absolute case numbers increased by 41.6% (IIR 1.39, 95% CI 0.62–3.08). Of all the cases analyzed, the majority (59.6%) occurred in patients aged 70 years or older. Male patients constituted 58.2% of the cohort. In 2020, the male/female ratio was 1.5. No relevant changes in the male/female ratios were observed in the 11 years period (Table 1, Figure 1). The proportion of patients 70 years or older increased from 54.4% in 2010 to 62.2% in 2020 (Table 1, Figure 2). In 2020, most frequently, spondylodiscitis was present in the lumbar spine (56.2%), followed by the thoracic spine (18.3%), and the cervical spine (6.7%). Spondylodiscitis with multiple foci was documented in 2.2% of the cases (Figure 3).

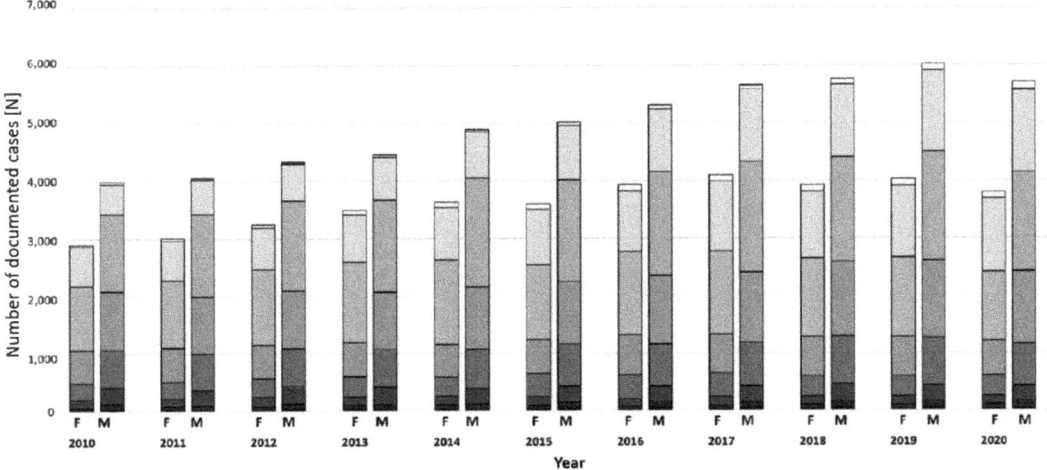

**Figure 1.** Age and gender distribution of Spondylodiscitis cases between 2010 through 2020 in absolute numbers.

**Table 1.** Historic development of spondylodiscitis diagnoses between 2010 and 2020.

| Year | Total Number | German Population 20 Years or Older | Change in Total Numbers (Relative to 2010) | Incidence per 100,000 Inhabitants | Incidence Relative to the Preceding Year | Incidence Rate Ratio Relative to the Preceding Year [95% CI] | Ratio of Female/Male | Ratio Aged ≤70 Years/ >70 Years |
|---|---|---|---|---|---|---|---|---|
| 2010 | 6886 | 66,549,975 | - | 10.4 [10.1–10.6] | - | - | 42/58 | 46/54 |
| 2011 | 7067 | 65,398,514 | 2.6% | 10.6 [10.4–10.9] | 2% | 1.02 [0.44–2.41] | 43/57 | 44/56 |
| 2012 | 7582 | 65,665,069 | 10.1% | 11.4 [11.3–11.9] | 7% | 1.07 [0.47–2.48] | 43/57 | 43/57 |
| 2013 | 7946 | 65,943,867 | 15.4% | 12.2 [11.8–12.4] | 7% | 1.07 [0.48–2.39] | 44/56 | 41/59 |
| 2014 | 8519 | 66,677,665 | 23.7% | 13.0 [12.6–13.2] | 7% | 1.07 [0.49–2.34] | 43/57 | 39/61 |
| 2015 | 8618 | 67,097,676 | 25.2% | 13.1 [12.7–13.2] | 1% | 1.01 [0.47–2.17] | 42/58 | 40/60 |
| 2016 | 9243 | 67,440,230 | 34.2% | 13.9 [13.4–14.0] | 6% | 1.06 [0.50–2.26] | 43/57 | 40/60 |
| 2017 | 9749 | 67,540,025 | 41.6% | 14.5 [14.1–14.7] | 4% | 1.04 [0.50–2.18] | 42/58 | 38/62 |
| 2018 | 9677 | 67,724,921 | 40.5% | 14.3 [14.0–14.6] | −1% | 0.99 [0.48–2.06] | 40/60 | 40/60 |
| 2019 | 10,035 | 67,864,036 | 45.7% | 14.8 [14.5–15.1] | 3% | 1.03 [0.50–2.14] | 40/60 | 39/61 |
| 2020 | 9753 | 67,820,457 | 41.6% | 14.4 [14.1–14.7] | −3% | 0.97 [0.62–3.08] | 40/60 | 38/62 |

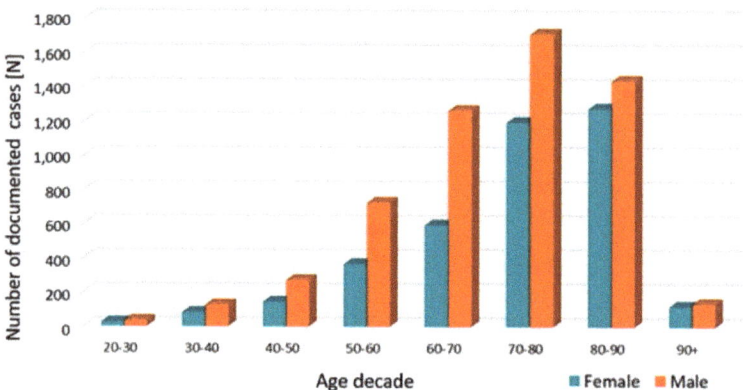

**Figure 2.** Age and gender distribution of spondylodiscitis cases in 2020 in absolute numbers.

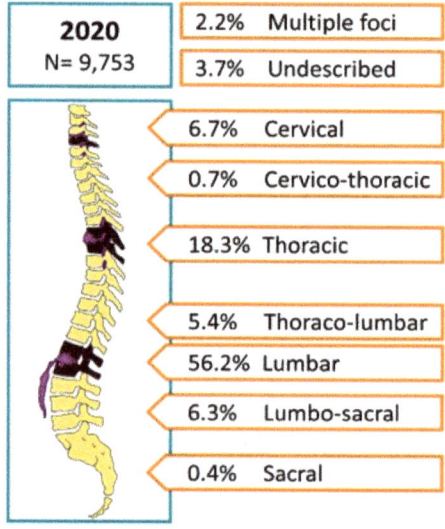

**Figure 3.** The distribution of spondylodiscitis by anatomical location of 9753 InEK cases in 2020 (designed with Inkscape and Microsoft PowerPoint).

*3.2. Pathogens Codes in Spondylodiscitis Cases in 2020*

Pathogens were coded for as concomitant diagnosis in 7589 cases (77.8%) in 2020. It could not be differentiated if these pathogens were exclusively causative for spondylodiscitis. In most cases "other/unspecified staphylococci" were documented (27.1%), followed by *E. coli* and other Enterobacterales (22.4%), *Staphylococcus aureus* (*S. aureus*) (19.4%) and streptococci (17.8%). *Pseudomonas* spp. and other non-fermenters were documented in 5.2% of the cases (Table 2). In 12.9% of cases where pathogens were identified, codes indicating resistance to antimicrobial drugs were applied. The most commonly identified resistant pathogen was *Enterococcus faecium* with resistance against glycopeptide antibiotics (U80.30; 2.8% of all cases), followed by methicillin-resistant *S. aureus* (U80.00; MRSA; 1.9%), and 3MRGN *E. coli* (U81.20; 1.6%). Overall, Gram-positive pathogens made up 65.0% of all resistant pathogens.

**Table 2.** Pathogens documented as concomitant diagnosis of spondylodiscitis cases in 2020 (sorted by frequency).

| ICD-10 Code | Pathogen (Coded as Concomitant Diagnosis) | Number of Cases | Percentage of Cases with Pathogen | Cumulative Percentage | Stratified Pathogens |
|---|---|---|---|---|---|
| B95.7 | Other staphylococci. | 1258 | 16.6% | | |
| A49.0 | Staphylococcal infection of unspecified location. | 722 | 9.5% | 27.1% | Other/unspecified staphylococci |
| B95.8 | Unspecified staphylococci. | 78 | 1.0% | | |
| B96.2 | *Escherichia coli* (*E. coli*) and other Enterobacterales. | 1702 | 22.4% | 22.4% | *E. coli* and Enterobacterales |
| B95.6 | *S.s aureus*. | 1472 | 19.4% | 19.4% | *S. aureus* |
| B95.2 | Streptococci, group D, and enterococci. | 840 | 11.1% | | |
| B95.48 | Other specified streptococci. | 310 | 4.1% | | |
| B95.1 | Streptococcus, group B. | 94 | 1.2% | | |
| B95.5 | Unspecified streptococci. | 46 | 0.6% | 17.8% | Streptococci |
| B95.3 | Streptococcus pneumoniae. | 19 | 0.3% | | |
| B95.41 | Streptococcus, group C. | 17 | 0.2% | | |
| B95.42 | Streptococci, group G. | 16 | 0.2% | | |
| B95.0 | Streptococcus, group A. | 11 | 0.1% | | |
| B96.5 | *Pseudomonas* and other nonfermenters. | 395 | 5.2% | 5.2% | *Pseudomonas* and other nonfermenters |
| B95.91 | Other specified Gram-positive, anaerobic, non-spore-forming pathogens. | 243 | 3.2% | 4.8% | Other Gram-positive pathogens |
| B95.90 | Other specified Gram-positive aerobic pathogens. | 124 | 1.6% | | |
| B96.8 | Other specified bacteria. | 114 | 1.5% | | |
| B96.6 | *Bacteroides fragilis* and other Gram-negative anaerobes. | 64 | 0.8% | | |
| B96.7 | *Clostridium perfringens* and other Gram-positive, spore-forming anaerobes. | 26 | 0.3% | 3.2% | Other |
| B98.0 | *Helicobacter pylori* (*H. pylori*). | 20 | 0.3% | | |
| B96.3 | Haemophilus and Moraxella. | 18 | 0.2% | | |

### 3.3. In-Hospital Mortality Rate, Hospitalization and ICU Treatment

The in-hospital mortality rate in spondylodiscitis cases increased from 45.6 per 1000 patients (95% CI 40.6–50.6) to a maximum of 64.7 per 1000 patients (95% CI 59.6–69.7) in 2020. The absolute number of in-hospital deaths rose by 101.0% from $n = 314$ in 2010 to $n = 631$ in 2020 (Table 3). The total number of inpatient treatment days in 2010 was 173,581, corresponding to a calculated hospital length of stay of 25.2 days per case. By 2020, the total number of hospital days increased to 217,416 (+25.3%). Given the increasing number of spondylodiscitis cases, the calculated hospital length of stay per case was 22.3 days in 2020. The maximum number of hospital days was recorded in 2019 at 230,093 days (22.9 days per case). In 2020, ICU treatment was documented in 2697 (27.7%) spondylodiscitis cases. The mortality rate of ICU cases was 165.0 per 1000 patients. Among spondylodiscitis patients who received treatment in an ICU, 72.5% were aged 65 years or older. The percentage ratio of male to female patients was 63/37. The mean hospitalization time of ICU cases was calculated to be $31.3 \pm 26.6$ days in 2020.

Table 3. Historic development of in-hospital deaths of spondylodiscitis cases between 2010 and 2020.

| Year | Total Number | German Population Aged 20 Years or Older | Change in Total Numbers (Relative to 2010) | In-Hospital Mortality Rate per 1.000 Patients [95% CI] | Incidence Rate Ratio Relative to the Preceding Year [95% CI] |
|---|---|---|---|---|---|
| 2010 | 314 | 6886 | - | 45.6 [40.6–50.6] | 1.0 [0.6–1.4] |
| 2011 | 307 | 7067 | −2.2% | 43.4 [38.6–48.3] | 1.0 [0.6–1.5] |
| 2012 | 314 | 7582 | 0.0% | 41.4 [36.8–46.0] | 1.2 [0.8–1.8] |
| 2013 | 393 | 7946 | 25.2% | 49.5 [44.6–54.3] | 1.0 [0.7–1.4] |
| 2014 | 409 | 8519 | 30.3% | 48.0 [43.4–52.7] | 1.2 [0.8–1.7] |
| 2015 | 478 | 8618 | 52.2% | 55.5 [50.5–60.4] | 1.0 [0.7–1.5] |
| 2016 | 513 | 9243 | 63.4% | 55.5 [50.7–60.3] | 1.1 [0.8–1.6] |
| 2017 | 596 | 9749 | 89.8% | 61.1 [56.2–66.0] | 1.0 [0.7–1.4] |
| 2018 | 577 | 9677 | 83.8% | 59.6 [54.8–64.5] | 1.0 [0.7–1.4] |
| 2019 | 585 | 10,035 | 86.3% | 58.3 [53.6–63.0] | 1.1 [0.8–1.6] |
| 2020 | 631 | 9753 | 101.0% | 64.7 [59.6–69.7] | 1.4 [1.0–2.1] |

## 4. Discussion

As a main finding of this cross-sectional study, we report a significant increase of spondylodiscitis cases in the adult German population by 41.6% between 2010 and 2020. While studies relying on data from single hospitals may yield skewed results, the findings presented here are based on nationwide reports from the largest country of the European Union. The study provides a comprehensive, historical overview of the age and gender distribution, in-hospital mortality rate, and hospitalization time of spondylodiscitis cases. It further presents the coded pathogens, anatomical site of infection, and characteristics of cases treated in an ICU in 2020.

### 4.1. The Development of the Nationwide Incidence of Spondylodiscitis between 2010 and 2020

Increasing rates of spondylodiscitis cases have been reported by several authors during the last decades [12–14,26]. The majority of reports on pyogenic spondylodiscitis introduce an estimated incidence of 0.2 to 2.4/100,000 per annum, mostly based on the analysis of Grammatico et al. from 2002 to 2003 [13]. Most recently, Conan et al. reported an increase in spondylodiscitis incidence from 6.1/100,000 in 2010 to 11.3/100,000 (+46%) in 2019 based on a French nationwide database, including 42,105 hospitalized patients [14]. Similarly, the current study demonstrated an increase in the spondylodiscitis incidence in the adult German population of 41.6% during the 11-year study period including 95,075 spondylodiscitis cases; the incidence was 14.4 per 100,000 inhabitants in 2020. Consistent with the literature, the male-to-female ratio was 1.5 in 2020, and the analysis demonstrated no relevant change in the sex distribution during the 11-year observation period [13,14]. It must be assumed that an improvement and better availability of CT and MRI diagnostics may have contributed to a higher detection rate of spinal infections, comparable to the trend in vertebral insufficiency fractures [27]. The enhanced awareness and recognition of spondylodiscitis among healthcare professionals could also lead to more accurate and timely diagnoses, resulting in a higher reported incidence [22]. However, it can be assumed that an important reason for the rising incidence is the aging population, which suffers from an increasing number of comorbidities [9,16]. The increasing prevalence of risk factors, such as diabetes mellitus, obesity, and immunosuppression, which predispose individuals to infections including spondylodiscitis has been underlined by Kremers et al., who demonstrated a significant increase in osteomyelitis cases in their population-based study on 760 incident cases [28]. Mavrogenis et al. presumed that a rise in the susceptible population and improved diagnosis capabilities have increased the reported incidence of the disease in recent years [29]. This thesis is underlined by the reported age distribution in the current study; of all cases, 59.6% were 70 years or older. We demonstrated that the proportion of patients aged 70 years or older increased from 54.4% in 2010 to 62.2%. Furthermore, the growing number of invasive spinal procedures and interventions, such as spinal instrumentation surgeries, may be associated with a higher risk of postoperative or interventional spondylodiscitis, and consequently contribute to the observed increase in overall cases [30,31]. Interestingly, the incidence rate of spondylodiscitis decreased from 2019 to 2020 by 2.7%, against the identified rising trend in the previous years. Bearing in mind the decimating effect on the hospitalization rates in orthopedic and trauma surgery, it can be hypothesized that the COVID-19 pandemic may have contributed to this development [32,33].

*4.2. Pathogens*

Contradictory to the body of literature, we found staphylococci other than *S. aureus* to be identified most frequently, followed by *E. coli* and Enterobacterales. The high prevalence of other staphylococci suggested a high share of CONS. This is in line with recent reports on the growing importance of the role of healthcare-associated infections, in particular device-associated bloodstream infections for the etiology of spondylodiscitis [9,34]. Kim et al. demonstrated in a retrospective review of 586 culture-confirmed spondylodiscitis case an age-dependent prevalence of causative pathogens. *S. aureus* was more common in patients aged <60 years (53.7%), whereas Gram-negative bacteria were more common in patients aged 60 years or older (30.9%, vs. 14.7% in patients aged <60 years) [35]. They further showed an association between Gram-negative pathogens in patients with liver cirrhosis and solid tumors [35]. Interestingly, *S. aureus* was only documented in 19.4% of cases with identified pathogens. This contradicts the vast majority of literature, reporting *S. aureus* as the most common causative pathogen in around 50% of spondylodiscitis cases [24,36]. Notable, Conan et al. reported comparable pathogen prevalence in their up-to-date, nationwide study; all staphylococci accounted for 55.0% of pathogens (46.5% in our results), Gram-negative pathogens for 21.1% (22.4%) and streptococci for 10.2% (17.8%) [14]. This may suggest increasing importance of Gram-negative pathogens and CONS, mirroring the epidemiological development towards older, frail patients. Reports on (multi-resistant) pathogens in spinal and musculoskeletal disease vary widely, and they depend on the socio-economic and geographical background of the cohort. In the current study, codes for pathogens with resistance against antimicrobial drugs were applied in 12.9% of cases with identified pathogens. [37–39]. The most common resistant pathogen was *Enterococcus faecium* with resistance against glycopeptide antibiotics, second was methicillin-resistant *S. aureus* and third 3MRGN *E. coli*. This distribution is concordant with the recent development of pathogen resistance in Germany, where *Enterococcus faecium* shows rising resistance rates against Vancomycin [40]. In contrast, the rates of 3MRGN *E. coli* and MRSA are decreasing [40]. The rise in antibiotic-resistant pathogens could contribute in the complexity of spondylodiscitis treatment, potentially leading to increased morbidity and mortality rates [26,41].

It must be pointed out that the coding quality for pathogens is usually low. Furthermore, it could not be differentiated if the pathogens documented as a concomitant diagnosis in the InEK database were causative for spondylodiscitis in the current analysis, which therefore must be interpreted carefully.

*4.3. In-Hospital Mortality Rate, Hospitalization Time and ICU Treatment*

Following the Europe-wide trend [42], the average length of stay of spondylodiscitis patients decreased from 25.2 days in 2010 to 22.3 days in 2020. Thisstill f exceeds the mean length of stay of 8.7 days of all hospitalized patients in Germany in 2020 by far [42]. We demonstrated an increase in the in-hospital mortality rate from 45.6 per 1000 patients to a maximum of 64.7 per 1000 patients in 2020, a 101.0% increase in the total number. The high proportion of 27.7% of cases treated in the ICU, with a mortality rate of 165.0 per 1000 patients, highlights the severity of the disease. In a recent retrospective cohort study on 155 patients with pyogenic vertebral osteomyelitis, we found an in-hospital mortality rate of 12.9% [8]. Even higher mortality rates are reported in the mid-to-long-term follow-up in the literature; Yagdiran et al. reported a 1- and 2-year mortality rate of 20% and 23%, respectively [6]. Vettivel et al. reported a mortality rate of 5.2% at 30 days and 22.3% at one year in a single-center study on 76 patients with pyogenic vertebral osteomyelitis. The high incidence of the concomitant disease is likely a major factor in the risk of mortality in the elderly population that is susceptible to developing spondylodiscitis. Kehrer et al. showed a 1-year mortality rate of 20% in a cohort of 298 patients [43]. They claimed that the main factors associated with short-term mortality were severe neurologic deficits at the time of admission, epidural abscess and comorbidities [43]. In a nationwide Danish study Aagaard et al. found that spondylodiscitis patients have increased long-term mortality, mainly due to comorbidities, particularly substance abuse [17]. The current study did not consider concomitant diagnoses or treatment aspects as factors influencing mortality rates. In addition, the data sources do not allow for an evaluation outside the inpatient sector. Potential risk and protective factors for spondylodiscitis mortality remain to be investigated nationwide.

*4.4. Strengths and Limitations*

An outstanding characteristic of this epidemiological evaluation is that the analysis is based on registry data consisting of ICD-10 diagnosis codes from all German medical institutions showing the development of the incidence rate of spondylodiscitis over eleven years. The main limitation of this study is that it represents a purely descriptive report and thus, a lack of statistical analysis beyond incidence rate ratios and corresponding 95% confidence intervals must be acknowledged. Only inpatient data were available. In addition, correct coding cannot be assured. A detailed annual analysis was conducted only for the primary diagnoses because the InEK data browser only enables analysis of concomitant diagnoses back to 2019. Furthermore, this analysis does not provide information on the treatment modalities such as surgery or antimicrobial therapy. Our data source does not provide these details, but their relevance in understanding spondylodiscitis management must be emphasized. Future studies should consider these aspects to provide a more comprehensive view of the condition and its treatment.

## 5. Conclusions

Between 2010 and 2020 the incidence rate of hospitalized spondylodiscitis cases increased notably to 14.4 per 100,000 adult inhabitants in Germany. This trend primarily affected elderly men. It is important to consider that factors such as an aging population, more frequent medical interventions and improved diagnostic techniques could have contributed to the rising incidence. Despite advances in treatment strategies, the average in-hospital mortality increased during the observation period and the rate of ICU treatments was high. The epidemiological trend observed in this study is consistent with nationwide developments. It is crucial to emphasize the need for patient-centered therapy, specifically tailored to the elderly and frail population, while taking into account the evolving spectrum of pathogens. Further research is needed to understand the underlying causes of this increase in incidence and to optimize treatment and preventive strategies for spondylodiscitis.

**Author Contributions:** Conceptualization, S.L., N.W. and M.R.; data curation, S.L. and D.S.; formal analysis, S.L., N.W., M.S. and D.S.; investigation, S.L., M.S., D.S. and M.R.; methodology, S.L., N.W. and S.B.; project administration, S.L.; resources, S.L.; supervision, S.L., M.L., V.A. and M.R.; validation, S.L., N.W. and M.L.; visualization, S.B.; writing—original draft, S.L. and M.R.; writing—review and editing, S.L., N.W., M.S., S.B., D.S., M.L., V.A. and M.R.. All authors have read and agreed to the published version of the manuscript.

**Funding:** This research received no external funding.

**Institutional Review Board Statement:** Methods were carried out following local data privacy guidelines and ethical regulations. As only anonymized data from a national, open-access databank were evaluated no approval of the local ethic committee was necessary: Informed Consent and Investigational Review Board (IRB) was not required for this study as it used data from an anonymous, de-identified, administrative database.

**Informed Consent Statement:** Patient consent was waived as only anonymized data from a national, open-access databank. No studies on humans or animals were conducted by the authors for this paper.

**Data Availability Statement:** All data presented in this study are available on demand from the corresponding author.

**Acknowledgments:** We thank the Federal Statistical Office of Germany (Destatis) for their support of this work.

**Conflicts of Interest:** The authors declare no conflict of interest.

# References

1. Alt, V.; Giannoudis, P.V. Musculoskeletal infections—A global burden and a new subsection in Injury. *Injury* **2019**, *50*, 2152–2153. [CrossRef] [PubMed]
2. Rupp, M.; Walter, N.; Baertl, S.; Lang, S.; Lowenberg, D.W.; Alt, V. Terminology of bone and joint infection. *Bone Jt. Res.* **2021**, *10*, 742–743. [CrossRef] [PubMed]
3. Zimmerli, W. Vertebral Osteomyelitis. *N. Engl. J. Med.* **2010**, *362*, 1022–1029. [CrossRef] [PubMed]
4. Akiyama, T.; Chikuda, H.; Yasunaga, H.; Horiguchi, H.; Fushimi, K.; Saita, K. Incidence and risk factors for mortality of vertebral osteomyelitis: A retrospective analysis using the Japanese diagnosis procedure combination database. *BMJ Open* **2013**, *3*, e002412. [CrossRef]
5. Loibl, M.; Stoyanov, L.; Doenitz, C.; Brawanski, A.; Wiggermann, P.; Krutsch, W.; Nerlich, M.; Oszwald, M.; Neumann, C.; Salzberger, B.; et al. Outcome-related co-factors in 105 cases of vertebral osteomyelitis in a tertiary care hospital. *Infection* **2014**, *42*, 503–510. [CrossRef]
6. Yagdiran, A.; Otto-Lambertz, C.; Lingscheid, K.M.; Sircar, K.; Samel, C.; Scheyerer, M.J.; Zarghooni, K.; Eysel, P.; Sobottke, R.; Jung, N.; et al. Quality of life and mortality after surgical treatment for vertebral osteomyelitis (VO): A prospective study. *Eur. Spine J.* **2021**, *30*, 1721–1731. [CrossRef]
7. McHenry, M.C.; Easley, K.A.; Locker, G.A. Vertebral osteomyelitis: Long-term outcome for 253 patients from 7 Cleveland-area hospitals. *Clin. Infect. Dis. Off. Publ. Infect. Dis. Soc. Am.* **2002**, *34*, 1342–1350. [CrossRef]
8. Lang, S.; Frömming, A.; Walter, N.; Freigang, V.; Neumann, C.; Loibl, M.; Ehrenschwender, M.; Alt, V.; Rupp, M. Is There a Difference in Clinical Features, Microbiological Epidemiology and Effective Empiric Antimicrobial Therapy Comparing Healthcare-Associated and Community-Acquired Vertebral Osteomyelitis? *Antibiotics* **2021**, *10*, 1410. [CrossRef]
9. Renz, N.; Haupenthal, J.; Schuetz, M.A.; Trampuz, A. Hematogenous vertebral osteomyelitis associated with intravascular device-associated infections—A retrospective cohort study. *Diagn. Microbiol. Infect. Dis.* **2017**, *88*, 75–81. [CrossRef]
10. Park, K.-H.; Kim, D.Y.; Lee, Y.-M.; Lee, M.S.; Kang, K.-C.; Lee, J.-H.; Park, S.Y.; Moon, C.; Chong, Y.P.; Kim, S.H.; et al. Selection of an appropriate empiric antibiotic regimen in hematogenous vertebral osteomyelitis. *PLoS ONE* **2019**, *14*, e0211888. [CrossRef]
11. Lang, S.; Walter, N.; Froemming, A.; Baertl, S.; Szymski, D.; Alt, V.; Rupp, M. Long-term patient-related quality of life outcomes and ICD-10 symptom rating (ISR) of patients with pyogenic vertebral osteomyelitis: What is the psychological impact of this life-threatening disease? *Eur. Spine J.* **2023**, *Online ahead of print.* [CrossRef]
12. Issa, K.; Diebo, B.G.; Faloon, M.; Naziri, Q.; Pourtaheri, S.; Paulino, C.B.; Emami, A. The Epidemiology of Vertebral Osteomyelitis in the United States From 1998 to 2013. *Clin. Spine Surg.* **2018**, *31*, E102–E108. [CrossRef] [PubMed]
13. Grammatico, L.; Baron, S.; Rusch, E.; Lepage, B.; Surer, N.; Desenclos, J.C.; Besnier, J.M. Epidemiology of vertebral osteomyelitis (VO) in France: Analysis of hospital-discharge data 2002–2003. *Epidemiol. Infect.* **2008**, *136*, 653–660. [CrossRef] [PubMed]
14. Conan, Y.; Laurent, E.; Belin, Y.; Lacasse, M.; Amelot, A.; Mulleman, D.; Rosset, P.; Bernard, L.; Grammatico-Guillon, L. Large increase of vertebral osteomyelitis in France: A 2010–2019 cross-sectional study. *Epidemiol. Infect.* **2021**, *149*, e227. [CrossRef] [PubMed]
15. Rupp, M.; Walter, N.; Pfeifer, C.; Lang, S.; Kerschbaum, M.; Krutsch, W.; Baumann, F.; Alt, V. The Incidence of Fractures Among the Adult Population of Germany–an Analysis From 2009 through 2019. *Dtsch. Arztebl. Int.* **2021**, *118*, 665–669. [CrossRef]
16. Puth, M.-T.; Weckbecker, K.; Schmid, M.; Münster, E. Prevalence of multimorbidity in Germany: Impact of age and educational level in a cross-sectional study on 19,294 adults. *BMC Public Health* **2017**, *17*, 826. [CrossRef]
17. Aagaard, T.; Roed, C.; Dahl, B.; Obel, N. Long-term prognosis and causes of death after spondylodiscitis: A Danish nationwide cohort study. *Infect. Dis.* **2016**, *48*, 201–208. [CrossRef]
18. Raghavan, M.; Lazzeri, E.; Palestro, C.J. Imaging of Spondylodiscitis. *Semin. Nucl. Med.* **2018**, *48*, 131–147. [CrossRef]
19. Kouijzer, I.J.E.; Scheper, H.; de Rooy, J.W.J.; Bloem, J.L.; Janssen, M.J.R.; van den Hoven, L.; Hosman, A.J.; Visser, L.G.; Oyen, W.J.; Bleeker-Rovers, C.P.; et al. The diagnostic value of 18F-FDG-PET/CT and MRI in suspected vertebral osteomyelitis—A prospective study. *Eur. J. Nucl. Med. Mol. Imaging* **2018**, *45*, 798–805. [CrossRef]

20. EUCAST: AST of Bacteria n.d. Available online: https://www.eucast.org/ast_of_bacteria/ (accessed on 8 November 2021).
21. Iwata, E.; Scarborough, M.; Bowden, G.; McNally, M.; Tanaka, Y.; Athanasou, N.A. The role of histology in the diagnosis of spondylodiscitis: Correlation with clinical and microbiological findings. *Bone Jt. J.* **2019**, *101–B*, 246–252. [CrossRef]
22. Herren, C.; von der Höh, N.; der Leitlinienkommission der Deutschen Wirbelsäulengesellschaft, N. Zusammenfassung der S2K-Leitlinie "Diagnostik und Therapie der Spondylodiszitis" (Stand 08/2020). *Die Wirbelsäule* **2021**, *5*, 18–20. [CrossRef]
23. Lang, S.; Rupp, M.; Hanses, F.; Neumann, C.; Loibl, M.; Alt, V. Infektionen der Wirbelsäule. *Unfallchirurg* **2021**, *124*, 489–504. [CrossRef]
24. Doutchi, M.; Seng, P.; Menard, A.; Meddeb, L.; Adetchessi, T.; Fuentes, S.; Dufour, H.; Stein, A. Changing trends in the epidemiology of vertebral osteomyelitis in Marseille, France. *N. Microbes N. Infect.* **2015**, *7*, 1–7. [CrossRef]
25. Petkova, A.S.; Zhelyazkov, C.B.; Kitov, B.D. Spontaneous Spondylodiscitis—Epidemiology, Clinical Features, Diagnosis and Treatment. *Folia Med.* **2017**, *59*, 254–260. [CrossRef] [PubMed]
26. Kehrer, M.; Pedersen, C.; Jensen, T.G.; Lassen, A.T. Increasing incidence of pyogenic spondylodiscitis: A 14-year population-based study. *J. Infect.* **2014**, *68*, 313–320. [CrossRef] [PubMed]
27. Graul, I.; Vogt, S.; Strube, P.; Hölzl, A. Significance of Lumbar MRI in Diagnosis of Sacral Insufficiency Fracture. *Glob. Spine J.* **2021**, *11*, 1197–1201. [CrossRef] [PubMed]
28. Kremers, H.M.; Nwojo, M.E.; Ransom, J.E.; Wood-Wentz, C.M.; Melton, L.J.; Huddleston, P.M. Trends in the epidemiology of osteomyelitis: A population-based study, 1969 to 2009. *J. Bone Jt. Surg.* **2015**, *97*, 837–845. [CrossRef]
29. Mavrogenis, A.F.; Megaloikonomos, P.D.; Igoumenou, V.G.; Panagopoulos, G.N.; Giannitsioti, E.; Papadopoulos, A.; Papagelopoulos, P.J. Spondylodiscitis revisited. *EFORT Open Rev.* **2017**, *2*, 447–461. [CrossRef]
30. Friedly, J.; Standaert, C.; Chan, L. Epidemiology of Spine Care: The Back Pain Dilemma. *Phys. Med. Rehabil. Clin. N. Am.* **2010**, *21*, 659–677. [CrossRef]
31. Heck, V.J.; Klug, K.; Prasse, T.; Oikonomidis, S.; Klug, A.; Himpe, B.; Egenolf, P.; Lenz, M.; Eysel, P.; Scheyerer, M.J. Projections from Surgical Use Models in Germany Suggest a Rising Number of Spinal Fusions in Patients 75 Years and Older Will Challenge Healthcare Systems Worldwide. *Clin. Orthop. Relat. Res.* **2023**, Online ahead of print. [CrossRef]
32. Blum, P.; Putzer, D.; Liebensteiner, M.C.; Dammerer, D. Impact of the COVID-19 Pandemic on Orthopaedic and Trauma Surgery—A Systematic Review of the Current Literature. *Vivo* **2021**, *35*, 1337–1343. [CrossRef] [PubMed]
33. Wähnert, D.; Colcuc, C.; Beyer, G.; Kache, M.; Komadinic, A.; Vordemvenne, T. Effects of the first lockdown of the COVID-19 pandemic on the trauma surgery clinic of a German Level I Trauma Center. *Eur. J. Trauma Emerg. Surg.* **2021**, *48*, 841–846. [CrossRef] [PubMed]
34. Pigrau, C.; Rodríguez-Pardo, D.; Fernández-Hidalgo, N.; Moretó, L.; Pellise, F.; Larrosa, M.-N.; Puig, M.; Almirante, B. Health care associated hematogenous pyogenic vertebral osteomyelitis: A severe and potentially preventable infectious disease. *Medicine* **2015**, *94*, e365. [CrossRef] [PubMed]
35. Kim, D.Y.; Kim, U.J.; Yu, Y.; Kim, S.-E.; Kang, S.-J.; Jun, K.-I.; Kang, C.K.; Song, K.H.; Choe, P.G.; Kim, E.S.; et al. Microbial Etiology of Pyogenic Vertebral Osteomyelitis According to Patient Characteristics. *Open Forum Infect Dis.* **2020**, *7*, ofaa176. [CrossRef]
36. Mylona, E.; Samarkos, M.; Kakalou, E.; Fanourgiakis, P.; Skoutelis, A. Pyogenic vertebral osteomyelitis: A systematic review of clinical characteristics. *Semin. Arthritis Rheum.* **2009**, *39*, 10–17. [CrossRef]
37. Park, K.-H.; Chong, Y.P.; Kim, S.-H.; Lee, S.-O.; Choi, S.-H.; Lee, M.S.; Jeong, J.Y.; Woo, J.H.; Kim, Y.S. Clinical characteristics and therapeutic outcomes of hematogenous vertebral osteomyelitis caused by methicillin-resistant Staphylococcus aureus. *J. Infect.* **2013**, *67*, 556–564. [CrossRef]
38. Dudareva, M.; Hotchen, A.J.; Ferguson, J.; Hodgson, S.; Scarborough, M.; Atkins, B.L.; McNally, M.A. The microbiology of chronic osteomyelitis: Changes over ten years. *J. Infect.* **2019**, *79*, 189–198. [CrossRef]
39. Cassini, A.; Högberg, L.D.; Plachouras, D.; Quattrocchi, A.; Hoxha, A.; Simonsen, G.S.; Colomb-Cotinat, M.; Kretzschmar, M.E.; Devleesschauwer, B.; Cecchini, M.; et al. Attributable deaths and disability-adjusted life-years caused by infections with antibiotic-resistant bacteria in the EU and the European Economic Area in 2015: A population-level modelling analysis. *Lancet Infect. Dis.* **2019**, *19*, 56–66. [CrossRef]
40. Ärzteblatt DÄG Redaktion Deutsches. Antibiotikaresistenzen: Ein heterogenes Bild. Deutsches Ärzteblatt 2020. Available online: https://www.aerzteblatt.de/archiv/211751/Antibiotikaresistenzen-Ein-heterogenes-Bild (accessed on 24 November 2021).
41. Murray, C.J.L.; Ikuta, K.S.; Sharara, F.; Swetschinski, L.; Aguilar, G.R.; Gray, A.; Han, C.; Bisignano, C.; Rao, P.; Wool, E.; et al. Global burden of bacterial antimicrobial resistance in 2019: A systematic analysis. *Lancet* **2022**, *399*, 629–655. [CrossRef]
42. Hospital Discharges and Length of Stay Statistics n.d. Available online: https://ec.europa.eu/eurostat/statistics-explained/index.php?title=Hospital_discharges_and_length_of_stay_statistics (accessed on 6 November 2022).
43. Kehrer, M.; Pedersen, C.; Jensen, T.G.; Hallas, J.; Lassen, A.T. Increased short- and long-term mortality among patients with infectious spondylodiscitis compared with a reference population. *Spine J.* **2015**, *15*, 1233–1240. [CrossRef]

**Disclaimer/Publisher's Note:** The statements, opinions and data contained in all publications are solely those of the individual author(s) and contributor(s) and not of MDPI and/or the editor(s). MDPI and/or the editor(s) disclaim responsibility for any injury to people or property resulting from any ideas, methods, instructions or products referred to in the content.

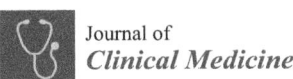 

*Review*

# Intramedullary Spinal Cord Abscess with Concomitant Spinal Degenerative Diseases: A Case Report and Systematic Literature Review

Redwan Jabbar [1,†], Bartosz Szmyd [1,†], Jakub Jankowski [1], Weronika Lusa [1,2], Agnieszka Pawełczyk [1], Grzegorz Wysiadecki [3], R. Shane Tubbs [4,5,6,7,8], Joe Iwanaga [4,6] and Maciej Radek [1,*]

1. Department of Neurosurgery, Spine and Peripheral Nerves Surgery, Medical University of Lodz, 90-549 Lodz, Poland
2. Department of Clinical Chemistry and Biochemistry, Medical University of Lodz, 90-419 Lodz, Poland
3. Department of Normal and Clinical Anatomy, Chair of Anatomy and Histology, Medical University of Lodz, Żeligowskiego 7/9, 90-752 Lodz, Poland
4. Department of Neurosurgery, Tulane Center for Clinical Neurosciences, Tulane University School of Medicine, New Orleans, LA 70112, USA
5. Department of Neurosurgery and Ochsner Neuroscience Institute, Ochsner Health System, New Orleans, LA 70433, USA
6. Department of Neurology, Tulane Center for Clinical Neurosciences, Tulane University School of Medicine, New Orleans, LA 70112, USA
7. Department of Anatomical Sciences, St. George's University, Grenada FZ 818, West Indies
8. Department of Surgery, Tulane University School of Medicine, New Orleans, LA 70112, USA
* Correspondence: maciej.radek@umed.lodz.pl
† These authors contributed equally to this work.

**Abstract:** Intramedullary spinal cord abscess (ISCA) is a rare clinical pathology of the central nervous system that usually accompanies other underlying comorbidities. Traditionally it has been associated with significant mortality and neurological morbidities because it is often difficult to diagnose promptly, owing to its nonspecific clinical and neuroimaging features. The mortality rate and the outcome of these infections have been improved by the introduction into clinical practice of antibiotics, advanced neuroimaging modalities, and immediate surgery. We report the case of a 65-year-old male patient who presented with a progressive spastic gait and lumbar pain, predominantly in the left leg. An MRI image revealed an expansile intramedullary cystic mass in the thoracic spinal cord, which was initially diagnosed as a spinal tumor. He underwent laminectomy and myelotomy, and eventually the pus was drained from the abscess. The follow-up MRI showed improvement, but the patient's paraplegia persisted. In light of his persistent hypoesthesia and paraplegic gait with developing neuropathic pain, he was readmitted, and an MRI of his lumbar spine revealed multilevel degenerative disease and tethered spinal cord syndrome with compression of the medulla at the L2–L3 level. The patient underwent central flavectomy with bilateral foraminotomy at the L2–L3 level, and the medulla was decompressed. Postoperatively, his neurological symptoms were significantly improved, and he was discharged from hospital on the third day after admission. In support of our case, we systematically reviewed the recent literature and analyzed cases published between 1949 and May 2022, including clinical features, mechanisms of infection, predisposing factors, radiological investigations, microbial etiologies, therapies and their duration, follow-ups, and outcomes. Initial clinical presentation can be misleading, and the diagnosis can be challenging, because this condition is rare and coexists with other spinal diseases. Hence, a high index of suspicion for making an accurate diagnosis and timely intervention is required to preclude mortality and unfavorable outcomes. Our case is a clear example thereof. Long-term follow-up is also essential to monitor for abscess recurrences.

**Keywords:** intramedullary spinal cord abscess (ISCA); abscess; spinal cord; laminectomy; myelotomy

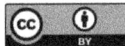

## 1. Introduction

Intramedullary spinal cord abscess (ISCA) is a rare infectious pathology of the central nervous system. The first case of a patient with ISCA was reported by Hart in 1830 [1,2]. Currently, fewer than 140 ISCA cases have been reported in the literature [3]. The mortality rate and outcome of these infections were improved when antibiotics, advanced neuroimaging modalities, and immediate surgery were accepted into clinical practice. Byrne et al. discovered that 36% of intramedullary abscesses primarily involved the cervical cord, 36% the conus medullaris, and 29% the thoracic cord; in congenital midline defects, lower thoracic and lumbar segments are the common sites [4]. In the pre-antibiotic era, 50% of ISCA cases resulted from hematogenous spreads of infection with an extraspinal focus. However, in a modern-era review of ISCA, most cases are cryptogenic and 8% are linked to hematogenous spread from an extraspinal focus [2,5]. Spinal cord tissue has exceptional resistance to infection. Additionally, the small volume of the cord compared to the brain, and the spinal cord's small lumen with an acute angle of origin of the spinal arteries have been considered protective factors, minimizing the incidence of ISCA [6]. Therefore, ISCA generally occurs together with underlying systemic conditions such as immunosuppression, diabetes mellitus, structural abnormality, adjacent spinal infection, or intravenous drug abuse. Its presentation can be divided into three types, depending on the time between initial presenting symptoms and time of diagnosis: acute, subacute, and chronic. These types have prognostic significance. The classic clinical presentation includes fever, pain, and an acute onset of neurological deficits, depending on the location. However, the ISCA triad is often absent in subacute or chronic cases [7].

During the pre-antibiotic era, Arzt reported a 90% mortality rate for ISCA cases published between 1830 and 1944 [8]. The mortality rate and prognosis were improved when antibiotics, advanced neuroimaging modalities, and immediate surgery were introduced into clinical practice. Subsequent reviews of published ISCA cases reported mortality down to 24% by 1977, while a more substantial improvement to 4% was described by Kurita et al. for cases published between 1998 and 2007 [9].

There is a bimodal age distribution among adult ISCA patients, most reported cases being diagnosed during the first and third decades of life [10]. The incidence rate is unknown, but the condition is associated with significant morbidity and mortality. Bartel et al. reported a higher incidence in women during their first four decades, whereas men had a constant incidence throughout their lifetime [11]. A high index of suspicion of ISCA is crucial for prompt diagnosis, effective clinical management, and supportive therapy, in order to prevent further neurological deterioration and to secure a favorable outcome [12].

Here, we report a case of a 65-year-old male patient who presented with a progressive spastic gait and lumbar pain and was found to have a thoracic intramedullary abscess with concomitant spinal degenerative disease. He was treated with surgical intervention and subsequent intravenous antibiotics. Following our case report, we also present a systemic review of the 70 adult cases in the current literature published between 1949 and 2022.

## 2. Case Description

A 65-year-old male patient was admitted to the Department of Neurosurgery with a progressive spastic gait and lumbar pain radiating to both lower extremities, predominantly in the left leg, without fever, following progressive paraparesis in both lower extremities. He reported difficulty in walking owing to paraparesis of grade 3/5 (Power-McCormick scale) in both lower extremities. During a neurological examination the symptoms progressed, being exacerbated by upright posture. Progressive left foot drop and claudication were also observed. Five years prior, L2/L3 discectomy was performed without any major improvement. The medical history revealed an aortic valve prosthesis implanted fifteen years previously. An MRI with contrast revealed an expansile intramedullary cystic lesion at T4 level measuring 16 mm × 11 mm × 10 mm without any enhancement (Figure 1A,B). Control lumbar MRI was comparable with a study done three years earlier.

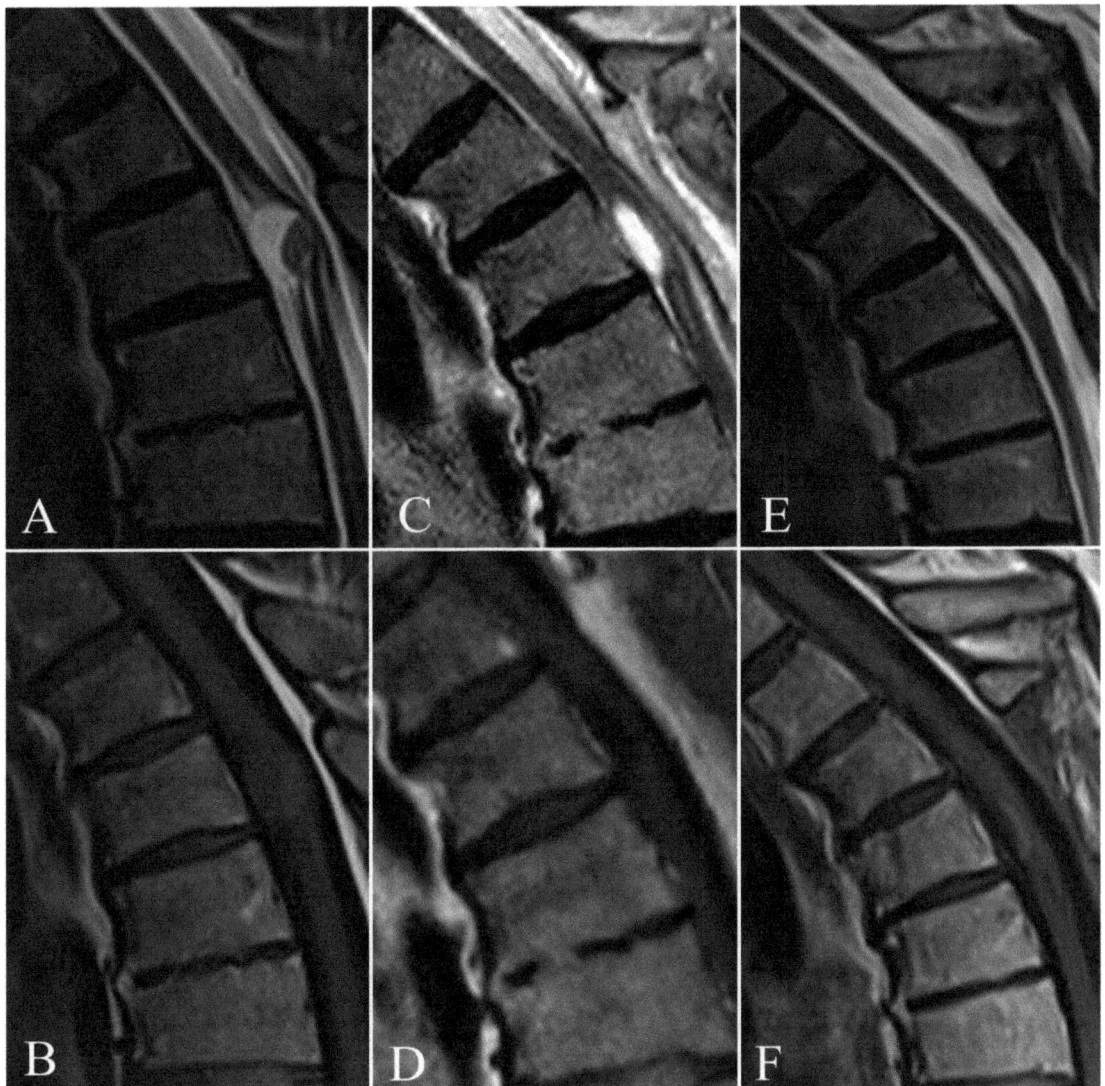

**Figure 1.** Magnetic resonance imaging (MRI) showing the sagittal scans: (**A**) T2-weighted image and (**B**) T1-weighted images of an expansile intramedullary solid-cystic lesion measuring 16 mm × 11 mm × 10 mm, without contrast enhancement, at the T4 level, with segmental widening of the spinal cord above and below the lesion. The early follow-up MRI shows no pathological mass and postoperative changes on both (**C**) T1-weighted and (**D**) T2-weighted images. The MRI performed 6 months after surgery revealed complete abscess excision in (**E**) T2-weighted and (**F**) T1-weighted sequences.

After numerous consultations over several months, he was referred to our department by a neurosurgeon, owing to persistent lumbar pain progressing to the thoracic vertebrae and the progressive spastic gait. He had hypesthesia in both lower limbs, the left foot being most affected. There was no nuchal rigidity or other meningeal signs, and he was afebrile. Laboratory tests revealed an elevated CRP level of 70 mg/L. There was no laboratory evidence of immunosuppression. The clinical picture indicated thoracic medulla lesion as the cause of the ailments. The differential diagnosis based on MRI included a neoplastic process; the lesion was presumptively diagnosed as an astrocytoma or ependymoma.

A laminectomy with intradural exploration was performed at the T4 level. When the dura was opened, the spinal cord appeared edematous and discolored. There was a yellowish ill-defined abscess capsule endophytic through the ventral side of the spinal cord, which was carefully drained through a midline myelotomy (Figure 2).

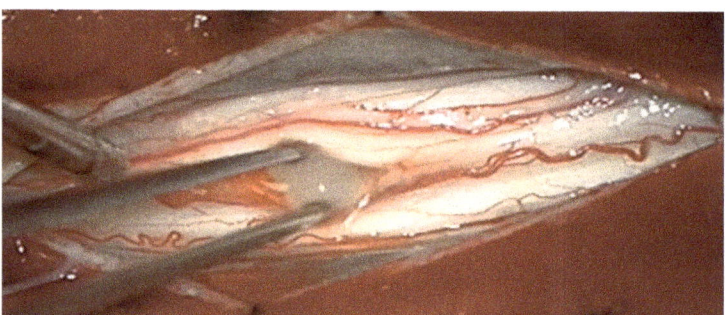

**Figure 2.** Intraoperative view of lesion showing yellowish pus after myelotomy at T4 level.

The spinal cord became lax after the abscess was drained. We encountered purulent fluid through the midline myelotomy from T3 to T4. The cavity was irrigated with saline, the dura was stitched, and the wound was closed in layers, with drainage placed. A postoperative MRI of the thoracic spine after two days and initial treatment showed complete removal of the intramedullary abscess (Figure 1C,D). A cardiovascular evaluation provided no evidence of infectious endocarditis, nor was there an oral infection. A subsequent pus culture to make a definitive diagnosis revealed Staphylococcus aureus MRSA and Staphylococcus Coagulase-negative. Blood cultures were not performed, due to good clinical state and lack of any infection, especially central nervous system infection. Subsequently, a neurogenic tumor was suspected due to MRI features. Additionally, the definitive diagnosis of degenerative lesion was difficult because no cystic features were indicated on MRI images. The culture was positive for Staphylococcus aureus, and the patient was placed on targeted antibiotics for further management. Therefore, the blood culture was deemed not essential, as it would have been difficult to extrapolate the source of infection and determine whether the infection had been spread hematogenously. We began targeted therapy, and the patient was given three weeks of postoperative intravenous vancomycin regimens.

In control laboratory tests, the infectious parameters decreased significantly, the CRP level falling to 2–3 mg/L after the antibiotic regimen. An MRI of the thoracic spine two days after the operation and initial treatment showed complete removal of the intramedullary abscess (Figure 1B,E). Nevertheless, the patient's lumbar pain and paresis remained. He was then transferred to another hospital to undergo rehabilitation therapy, and then discharged home.

Control thoracic MRI after six months showed complete removal of the abscess (Figure 1E,F). Progression of paraplegic gait was improved and controlled. However, persistent lumbar pain, hypesthesia, and paraplegic gait were reported, with developing neuropathic pain described as a burning sensation. Another MRI of his lumbar spine confirmed multilevel degenerative disease and tethered spinal cord syndrome, with the medulla compressed by L2–L3 (Figure 3A–C). However, the images were very similar, and a slight progression of L2/L3 stenosis was detected. The elective surgery was scheduled, and three months later, the patient was admitted to the award. Then, a central flavectomy with bilateral foraminotomy was performed at the L2–L3 level, with decompression of the medulla.

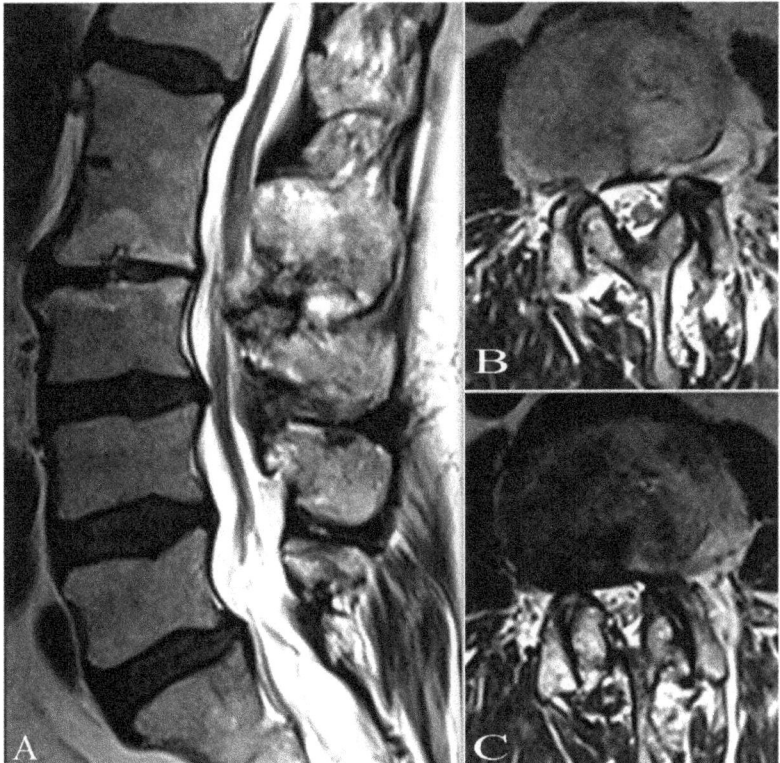

**Figure 3.** Lumbar multilevel spinal degenerative disease on MRT2-weighted images: (**A**,**B**) sagittal and (**C**) axial view at L2–L3 level; severe stenosis with compression of the conus medullaris.

Postoperatively, the patient's neurological symptoms, lumbar pain, and gait were significantly improved, and he was discharged from hospital on the second day.

## 3. Systematic Literature Review

PubMed was searched for English-language case studies and case series published from January 1949 to February 2022. The key words ((intramedullary), AND (spinal cord)) AND (abscess) were used in the search. Only English language case studies/series pertaining to ISCA in adults were taken into consideration. We also reviewed secondary articles from the references cited in previous research studies (see Section 4: Results, for further information). To facilitate the systematic feature of our work we have added a PRISMA flowchart (see Figure 4).

The demographics and clinical features of patients, mechanisms of infection, predisposing factors, radiological investigations, therapies and their duration, follow-ups, and outcomes were checked for every case. An ISCA case was defined by the following: a culture and a positive/negative Gram staining of a spinal cord aspirate, both revealing a bacterial pathogen; MRI imaging revealing an abscess associated with a specimen from a normally sterile site yielding bacteria; or a positive immunological test for a specific bacterial pathogen. Cases of culture-negative ISCA in which a spinal cord aspirate contained polymorphonuclear leukocytes, and cases where Gram staining and culture of the aspirate were negative, were also included in our study.

The clinical presentation was divided into acute (symptoms lasting less than one week), subacute (symptoms lasting 1–6 weeks), and chronic (symptoms lasting more than six weeks). The mechanism of infection was typically: (1) hematogenous spread of an extraspinal infection; (2) contiguous spread of an adjacent infection; (3) direct inoculation (i.e., penetrating trauma, post-neurosurgery); or (4) cryptogenic (infection source unknown). Outcomes were graded on the basis of ambulatory status, since all patients had motor symptoms in both the upper and lower extremities. The outcomes were grouped as follows: Complete neurological recovery, Residual neurological deficits, Persistent neurological deficits, and Death.

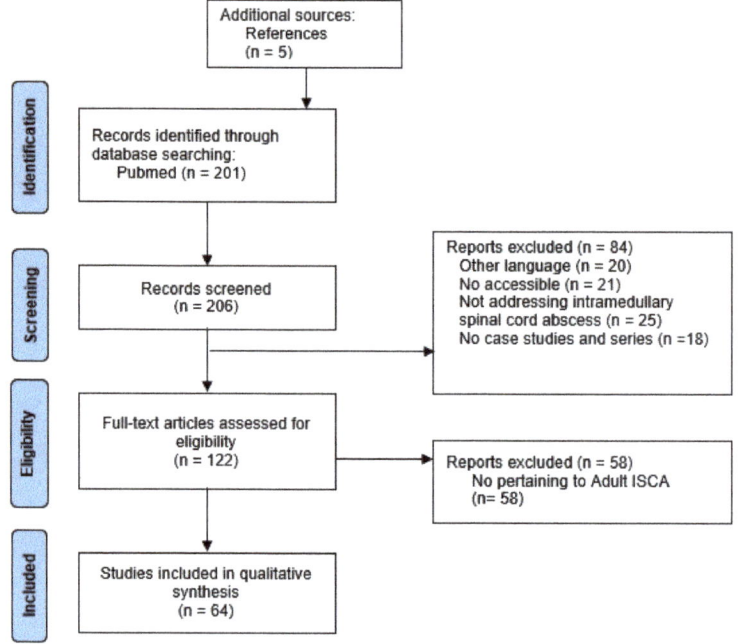

**Figure 4.** The flow-chart of publications included process.

## 4. Results

We found a total of two hundred and six (including five from references) papers on ISCA in literature published from January 1949 to May 2022. We included 122 articles that were full-text papers in English presenting a case study or case series. We identified 137 ISCA cases from 64 papers. Seventy (50.03%) adult cases and 64 (45.99%) pediatric cases were abstracted from the database. Of the 70 cases, 55 (78.5%) were males and 15 (21.4%) females. The median age at presentation was 52 (IQR: 38.5–66.5) years.

*4.1. Clinical Manifestation and Onset*

The clinical features varied, and depended on the abscess's location. Symptoms upon admission were fever, back pain, neurological deficits including motor and sensory disturbances, and urinary incontinence, amongst others, often originating from concomitant diseases such as meningitis, encephalitis, and other systemic infections (Figure 5).

Fever and neurological deficits were the most common symptoms, along with pain, and urinary incontinence was present initially in 25 cases (35.7%).

The typical clinical features are summarized in Figure 4. The patients were divided into three clinical groups depending on their clinical presentation and its duration from the onset of symptoms until hospital admission: acute (less than a week) in twenty-six (37%) patients, subacute (1–6 weeks) in twenty (28.5%), chronic (more than six weeks) in fourteen (20%), and not mentioned in six (8.5%). The most common complaint at the time of presentation was motor impairment, found in 69 cases (98.5%), followed by sensory loss in 61 cases (87.1%), pain in 39 (55.7%), and urinary involvement in 35 (50%).

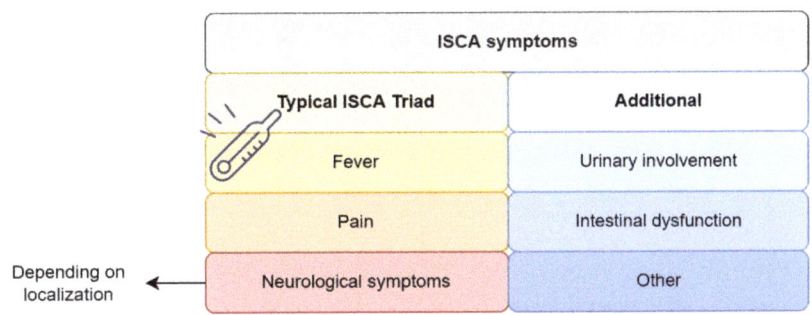

**Figure 5.** The typical clinical features of intramedullary spinal cord abscesses. Legend: ISCA—intramedullary spinal cord abscess.

Concerning concomitant diseases, the following comorbidities were reported (see Table S3): diabetes and concomitant systemic infection (n = 5), urinary tract infection (n = 4), chronic kidney diseases (n = 1), pulmonary diseases (n = 2), tuberculosis (n = 2), chronic sinusitis (n = 1), oral infection (n = 2), infective endocarditis (n = 2), sepsis and septic emboli (n = 3), systemic lupus erythematosus (n = 1), sickle cell disease (n = 1), pulmonary arteriovenous fistula (n = 1), spinal dural arteriovenous fistula (n = 1), vertebral infection (osteomyelitis, discitis and spondylodiscitis, arthritis) (n = 4), spinal anatomical abnormalities (n = 3), CNS histoplasmosis (n = 1), disseminated coccidioidomycosis (n = 2), ulcerative colitis (n = 1), and heroin/alcohol addiction (n = 5).

*4.2. Microbiology*

A bacterial pathogen was found in 64% of cases (Table 1). Four infections were polymicrobial [13–16]. The diagnosis was confirmed by positive culture of a spinal cord aspirate and biopsy in 14 (20%) cases, with additional isolation of Escherichia coli from urine culture (case 38). In four cases [4,17–19], the diagnosis was based on the identification of Gram-negative bacilli on a Gram stain of an aspirate. For 30 other patients, the diagnosis was based on a CSF culture, and *Escherichia coli* and *Enterococcus fecalis* were isolated from the patient's urine culture in three cases [17,20,21] and a blood culture in three [22–24], needle aspiration and abscess culture [6,14,25,26], and histopathology [1,20,27]. The remaining four cases [28–31] were classified as culture-negative ISCA. Two cases [25,32] had previously received antimicrobial therapy. Two others were diagnosed via blood culture [21,24], and the others were identified via urine culture [33] and histopathology [34]. There were elevated white blood cells and leucocytes in the remaining 11 (15.71%), and the diagnostic tool was not mentioned in four.

The most common causative organisms isolated in culture were *Streptococcus* spp. in 14 cases (20%) followed by *Staphylococcus* spp. in 10 (14.28%). The other organisms identified were *K. pneumoniae*, *C. albicans*, *M. tuberculosis*, *Nocardia* spp., *Actinomyces*, *Aspergillus*, *Bacteroid* spp., *Brucella* spp., MRSA, *E. coli*, *Pseudomonas* spp., *L. monocytogenes*, *H. capsulatum*, *Hemophilus* spp., and *E. fecalis*. The culture of pus in the present case revealed *Staphylococcus aureus*.

Table 1. Recovery group—summary of the clinical data, patient demographics, clinical manifestations, duration, microbiology, interventions and therapies, and outcomes of contemporary case reports on intramedullary spinal cord abscess (ISCA) in the current literature: systemic review of literature (1949–2022).

| No. | Age | Sex | Onset | Location | Infl. | Symptoms Name | Symptoms Duration | Symptoms to Treatment | Neurosurgical Management | Antibiotics Name | Antibiotics Duration | Pathogen | MOA | Follow-Up | Outcome | Ref. |
|---|---|---|---|---|---|---|---|---|---|---|---|---|---|---|---|---|
| 1 | 64 | M | Acute | N/D | + | ND (M + S) | N/D | N/D | N/D | Flucytosine Amphotericin B IV | 10 d | *C. albicans* | Cryptogenic | 1 y | Recovery | [35] |
| 2 | 27 | M | Acute | C5 | + | ND (M) | ND | N/D | Stereotactic needle aspiration | Ampicillin IV, Metronidazole IV, Trimethoprim-Sulfamethoxazole IV, Ampicillin PO | 3 w | *H. aphrophilus, A. meyeri* | Cryptogenic (Intrapulmonary AVF causing a right-to-left shunt) | N/D | Recovery | [16] |
| 3 | 80 | F | Acute | T8 | + | ND (M) | 3 d | 3 d | N/D | Ceftriaxone, Dexamethasone Metronidazole | 6 w | *St. intermedius* | Cryptogenic | 11 w | Recovery | [36] |
| 4 | 57 | M | Acute | C6-T1 | + | ND (M + S) | Sd | N/D | Myelotomy, DR | Vancomycin | 6 w | MRSA | Cryptogenic | N/D | Recovery | [37] |
| 5 | 53 | M | Acute | CM | + | ND (M + S) | 5 d | Urgent | N/D | N/D | N/D | *St. milleri, S. intermedius.* | Cryptogenic | 4 m | Recovery | [13] |
| 6 | 42 | M | Acute | C7 | + | ND (M) | 5 d | N/D | Laminectomy, DR | Linezolid | 2 w | MRSA | Hematogenous (IE) | N/D | Recovery | [22] |
| 7 | 21 | M | Subacute | T12-L2 | + | ND (M + S) | N/D | N/D | Myelotomy, EBC, IAC (Penicillin & Gentamicin | Penicillin IV, Flucloxacillin IV, Gentamicin IV | N/D | *S. epidermidis* | Contiguous (Epidermoid tumor) | 4 m | Recovery | [38] |
| 8 | 52 | M | Subacute | L1 | N/D | ND (M + S) | N/D | N/D | DR | Trimethoprim Sulfamethoxazole Imipenem-Cilastin (After Antibiogram: Trimethoprim-Sulfamethoxazole Minocycline | 1 Y | *Nocardia sp.* | Cryptogenic | 16 m | Recovery | [39] |
| 9 | 25 | F | Subacute | C5-C6 | + | ND (M + S) | 3 w | N/D | Myelotomy, DR | Isoniazid, Rifampin, Myambutol Pyrazinamide | 7 w | *M. tuberculosis* | Hematogenous (Brown Sequard syndrome; Tuberculosis & SLE) | 40 d (posthospital adm) | Recovery | [40] |
| 10 | 56 | M | Subacute | C3-C4 | + | ND (M + S) | 5 d | N/D | N/D | Amikacin, Ceftazidime, Ciprofloxacin | 3 m | *E. coli* | Hematogenous | 34 m | Recovery | [41] |

**Table 1.** Cont.

| No. | Age | Sex | Onset | Location | Infl. | Symptoms Name | Symptoms Duration | Symptoms to Treatment | Neurosurgical Management | Antibiotics Name | Antibiotics Duration | Pathogen | MOA | Follow-Up | Outcome | Ref. |
|---|---|---|---|---|---|---|---|---|---|---|---|---|---|---|---|---|
| 11 | 70 | M | Subacute | C4–C5 | + | ND (M + S) | 3 | N/D | Yes (N/S) | Ceftriaxone, Gentamicin, Amoxicillin PO | 6 w, 2 w, 3 m | *Viridans group Streptococcus* | Hematogenous (IE, radiotherapy) | 3 m | Recovery | [23] |
| 12 | 59 | M | Subacute | C7–T1 | + | ND (M + S) | 1 w | 9 d | N/D | Ampicillin, Ceftriaxone, Cefpirome, Ampicillin PO | 2 m | Sterile | Cryptogenic (Chronic sinusitis) | 2 m | Recovery | [9] |
| 13 | 51 | M | Subacute | T2–MO | + | ND (M + S) | 1 w | Urgent | N/D | Meropenem, Vancomycin, Steroid-Pulse Therapy & Immunoglobulin IV | 4 w, 3 d, 3 d | *St. viridans* | Hematogenous (Dental procedure) | 3 m | Recovery | [42] |
| 14 | 22 | M | Chronic | T12–L1 | + | ND (M + S) | >2 m | Urgent | Myelotomy, DU, DR | Yes (N.S.) | N/D | *S. aureus* | Contiguous (spinal anesthesia) | 40 d | Recovery | [43] |
| 15 | 82 | M | Chronic | T6–T7 | + | ND (M + S) | 4 m | N/D | N/D | Steroids, Gentamicin, Ciprofloxacin IV, Ciprofloxacin IM | 10 w, 4 w, 2 m | *E. coli* | Hematogenous (UTI—diabetes) | 3 m | Recovery | [33] |
| 16 | 28 | M | Chronic | T11 | + | ND (M + S) | 6 m | N/D | Y (N/S) | N/D | N/D | N/A | Cryptogenic (Infection) | N/D | Recovery | [34] |
| 17 | 67 | M | Chronic | T10–T11 | + | ND (M + S) | 1 Y | 1 Y | SDAVF embolization | Dexamethasone Meropenem IV, Moxifloxacin PO (Alone from day 71) | 4 d, 112 d | *E. faecalis* | Hematogenous (SDAVF) | N/D | Recovery | [44] |
| 18 | 44 | M | Chronic | T3 | + | ND (M + S) | 3 m | N/D | N/D | Amphotericin B Itraconazole | N/D, 3 m | *H. capsulatum* | Hematogenous (CNS histoplasmosis) | 1 m | Recovery | [45] |
| 19 | 52 | M | N/D | C4–C5 | + | ND (M + S) | N/D | N/D | DR | Oxacillin | N/D | *S. epidermidis* | Direct inoculation (penetrating trauma) Wooden Foreign Body (WBS) | 8 w | Recovery | [46] |
| 20 | 55 | M | N/D | Cervical | + | ND (M) | 5w | Urgent | Laminectomy | N/D—(Steroids, Amphotericin) | N/D | *C. immitis* | Hematogenous (Disseminated coccidioidomycosis) | 2 m | Recovery | [47] |

**Legend**: sex: F—female, M—male; location: C—cervical, T—thoracic, L—lumbar, S—sacral; infl.—inflammation; symptoms: M—motor, ND—neurological deficits, S—sensory; duration: D—day, M—months, Y—years, SW—several weeks; others: CM—conus medullaris, DR—drainage, DU—durotomy, EST—excision sinus tract, EAC—excision of abscess cavity, EEC—excision of epidermoid cyst, IAC—irrigation of abscess cavity, N/D—no data, N/S—not specified.

### 4.3. Mechanism of Infection and Predisposing Factors

Thirty-two patients (45.7%) had cryptogenic sources, including our case. Seven (10%) resulted from a spread of infection through contagious lesions, such as spinal anesthesia [43], dermal sinus tracts [38], epidural abscesses [48], epidural anesthesia [40], intrathecal morphine pump [49], spondylodiscitis [50], vertebral osteomyelitis [47], vertebral discitis, and osteomyelitis [51]. Patients with anatomical abnormalities of the spinal cord and/or vertebral column were found in four cases (5.7%). Three (4.2%) had congenital midline neuroectodermal defects (spinal dysraphism). One patient (1.4%) with congenital midline defects had related dorsal midline skin lesions, namely a dermal sinus tract opening with prior discharge from a sinus tract, accompanied by meningitis. Four other cases (5.7%) had direct penetrating trauma to the spinal cord through stab wounds, by wooden foreign bodies and surgical excision of spinal epidermoid and ependymoma [13,15]. In two other cases, spinal abscesses were secondary to postoperative complications following resection of a spinal cord dermoid cyst [38] and spinal cord ependymoma [25]. Case [29] had a cervical spinal stenosis, extrinsically compressing the spinal cord. Twenty-two cases (31.4%) had extraspinal hematogenous spreads: urinary tract infection [6,21,27], pyelonephritis [19], bronchopneumonia [52], bronchiectasis [53], tuberculosis and SLE [26,39], brucellosis [32], oral infections and dental procedures [54,55], chronic kidney diseases [17], infective endocarditis [22,23,30,51], diabetes mellitus with systemic effects [21,22,42,45], disseminated coccidioidomycosis [28], histoplasmosis [56], and neurotuberculosis [57]. Three patients (4.2%) had apparent sepsis originating from either *E. coli* [19], *S. aureus* [48], or Gram-negative bacilli [27]. One case had multiple pulmonary arteriovenous malformations [16], and another [34] had SDAVF, which are both known to be risk factors for the development of pyogenic brain abscesses.

### 4.4. Neuroimaging Features

Neuroimaging studies such as plain radiography, myelography, computed tomography scans (CT) and MRI were carried out for all but five of the patients involved in the reports. MRI was performed with contrast material in 50 cases. The findings were ring-enhancing margins, segmental widening and swelling of the spinal cord, partial or total obstruction of the cerebrospinal fluid, and tethered spinal cord in some cases [25,58,59]. The radiological features are reported in Table 2.

**Table 2.** Radiological features (myelography, CT, MRI) of intramedullary spinal cord abscess (ISCA).

| Myelography (n = 8) |
| --- |
| Spinal cord widening and swelling |
| CSF flow obstruction |
| Tethering of conus |
| **CT with myelography or MRI (n = 7)** |
| Segmental widening and swelling of cord |
| Complete or partial obstruction of CSF flow |
| **MRI (n = 50)** |
| Segmental widening and swelling of spinal cord |
| Ring-enhancing margin (abscess) |
| Cystic lesion with ring enhancement |
| CSF flow obstruction |

### 4.5. Management and Clinical Outcomes

Thirteen patients (18.6%) required urgent treatment and 11 (15.7%) were treated within a day to three weeks from onset. One (1.4%) was treated within a year; there were no data on duration for the rest of the cases. Surgery, including drainage procedures (laminectomy and myelotomy in 41 cases (58.5%) and stereotactic needle aspiration in one), was performed in

44 cases (62.8%). A second open-drainage procedure was required in case [18] following deterioration of neurological functions. Additional surgical procedures included excision of the abscess cavity (EAC) in four cases (5.7%), excision of a sinus tract (EST) in two (2.8%), excision of an epidermoid cyst (EEC) in one (1.4%), marsupialization of the abscess cavity in one (1.4%), and a biopsy in two (2.8%). Surgical intervention was not mentioned in 18 cases (25.7%). Antimicrobial therapy was administered for durations of nearly two weeks to nine months in 59 (84.2%) cases; for eight patients (11.4%) its use was not mentioned, and only one patient (1.4%) continued therapy for one year.

The clinical outcomes were recorded after follow-ups ranging from nearly two weeks to one year for all but one patient. We categorized the other cases into four groups on the basis of their prognoses: recovery in 20% of cases (Table 1), residual ND in 12 (17.1%) (Table 3), persistent ND in 28 (40%) (Table 4), and death in 10 (14.2%) (Table 5). All but two (2.8%) in the recovery group had received antimicrobial therapy, 11 (15.7%) underwent surgery, and the time frame between onset and first treatment (surgery or antibiotics) was urgent (IQR: urgent—six days). Among the 60 patients (85.7%) who survived, residual neurological deficits such as paraparesis and paraplegia persisted in 40 (57.1%). Among these, 59 (84.2%) received antibiotics and 44 (62.8%) underwent surgery. The median duration from onset to first treatment for the persistent group was 1.5 days (IQR: urgent-4.74), while for the residual group it was two days (IQR: 0.5—4.25). However, there were too few data in the death group about time from symptoms to treatment; information was only available in one case (10%). Ten patients (14.2%) died postoperatively: as a result of septic embolus with concomitant pyelonephritis in [19], UTI [6,33], chronic alcoholism and bronchopneumonia in case [52], disseminated coccidioidomycosis [28], multiple cerebral abscesses complicated by progressive hydrocephalus [53], abscess rupture inducing meningitis and brain abscess [53], Listeria meningoencephalitis [12], central nervous system nocardiosis involving the bilateral hemisphere, cerebellum, and upper cervical spinal cord due to diabetes mellitus (despite a two-stage operation) [20], cardiac arrest [51], intracranial extension of her spinal aspergillosis resulting in rapid progression of ventriculitis and cerebral vasculitis with diffuse vascular occlusion and widespread cerebral infarction [51], and refractory septic shock [60]. There were no significant differences in the time until treatment among the recovery, persistent, residual and death prognosis groups ($p = 0.613$).

**Table 3.** Residual group—summary of the clinical data, patient demographics, clinical manifestations, duration, microbiology, interventions and therapies, and outcomes of contemporary case reports on intramedullary spinal cord abscess (ISCA) in the current literature: systemic review of literature (1949–2022).

| No. | Age | Sex | Onset | Location | Infl. | Symptoms Name | Symptoms Duration | Symptoms to Treatment | Neurosurgical Management | Antibiotics Name | Antibiotics Duration | Pathogen | MOA | Follow-Up | Outcome | Ref. |
|---|---|---|---|---|---|---|---|---|---|---|---|---|---|---|---|---|
| 1 | 72 | M | Acute | C6-T2 | + | ND (M + S) | 5 d | Urgent | Myelotomy, EAC | Penicillin | 6 w | *St. viridans* | Cryptogenic (spinal cord ependymoma) | 6 w | Survived; residual ND | [25] |
| 2 | 59 | M | Acute | C3-C7 | + | ND (M + S) | 6 d | N/D | Myelotomy, DR | Cefepime IV | 6 w | *St. viridans* | Cryptogenic (Plausible infection & long immobility) | N/D | Survived; residual ND | [24] |
| 3 | 44 | F | Acute | C2-C5 | N/D | ND (M + S) | 4 d | 5 d | Myelotomy, DU | Meropenem, Vancomycin, Ceftriaxone | N/D | *S. milleri* | Cryptogenic | 1 m | Survived; residual ND | [27] |
| 4 | 35 | M | Acute | C2-C5 | + | ND (M + S) | 2 d | 2 d | Myelotomy, DR | Azithromycin, Ceftriaxone, Vancomycin, | 1 m | *St. pneumoniae* | Hematogenous (Sickle cell disease) | 12 d | Survived; residual ND | [61] |
| 5 | 47 | M | Subacute | T11 | N/D | ND (M + S) | 3 w | Urgent | Myelotomy, DU, DR, IAC | N/D | N/D | *St. anginosus* | Contiguous (Intrathecal morphine pump) | 20 m | Survived; residual ND | [50] |
| 6 | 82 | F | Subacute | T12-L1 | + | ND (M + S) | 3 w | N/D | Laminectomy | Meropenem IV, Trimethoprim-Sulfamethoxazole IV | 6 w | *N. cyriacigeorgica* | Cryptogenic | 7 w | Survived; residual ND | [54] |
| 7 | 77 | M | Subacute | L5-S1 | + | ND (M) | 10 d | 11 d | Laminectomy, drainage | Oxacillin, Clindamycin | N/D | *S. aureus* | Cryptogenic (Possibly arthritis) | 3 m | Survived; residual ND | [56] |
| 8 | 42 | F | Chronic | T12 | + | ND (M + S) | 3.5 m | 2 d | Laminectomy | Sulphonamides, N.S. | 4 m | *S. aureus* | Hematogenous spread (Urinary tract infection) | 9 m | Survived; residual ND | [6] |
| 9 | 40 | F | Chronic | T12-L2 | + | ND (M + S) | 6 m | N/D | Myelotomy, DU, DR | Streptomycin, Doxycycline, Rifampicin | 2 m | *B. melitensis* | Hematogenous (Consumption: unpasteurized goat's milk (Brucellosis risk factors) | 2 y | Survived; residual ND | [49] |
| 10 | 65 | M | Chronic | T11-CA | + | ND (M + S) | 2 m | N/D | N/D | Linezolid | 2 w | MRSA | Hematogenous (IE) | 1 y | Survived; residual ND | [51] |

**Table 3.** Cont.

| No. | Age | Sex | Onset | Location | Infl. | Symptoms Name | Symptoms Duration | Symptoms to Treatment | Neurosurgical Management | Antibiotics Name | Antibiotics Duration | Pathogen | MOA | Follow-Up | Outcome | Ref. |
|---|---|---|---|---|---|---|---|---|---|---|---|---|---|---|---|---|
| 11 | 66 | M | N/D | T5-T6 | + | ND (M + S) | N/D | N/D | N/D | Metronidazole Clindamycin | 6 w | *B. fragilis* | Hematogenous (?) (spondylodiscitis) | 6 w | Survived; residual ND | [55] |
| 12 | 45 | F | Acute | C2-C6 | + | ND (M + S) | 2 w | N/D | N/D | Cefuroxime | 6 w | *E. coli* | Hematogenous (Sepsis, UTI) | N/D | Survived; residual ND | [28] |

Legend: sex: F—female, M—male; location: C—cervical, T—thoracic, L—lumbar, S—sacral; infl.—inflammation; symptoms: M—motor, ND—neurological deficits, S—sensory; duration: D—day, W—weeks, M—months, Y—years, SW—several weeks; others: CM—conus medullaris, DR—drainage, DU—durotomy, EAC—excision of abscess cavity, IAC—irrigation of abscess cavity, N/D—no data.

**Table 4.** Persistent group—summary of the clinical data, patient demographics, clinical manifestations, duration, microbiology, interventions and therapies, and outcomes of contemporary case reports on intramedullary spinal cord abscess (ISCA) in the current literature: systematic review of literature (1949–2022).

| No. | Age | Sex | Onset | Location | Infl. | Symptoms Name | Symptoms Duration | Symptoms to Treatment | Neurosurgical Management | Antibiotics Name | Antibiotics Duration | Pathogen | MOA | Follow-Up | Outcome | Ref. |
|---|---|---|---|---|---|---|---|---|---|---|---|---|---|---|---|---|
| 1 | 71 | M | Acute | C3-C6 | + | ND (M + S) | 5 d | N/D | IAC | Penicillin IV Chloramphenicol IV, Penicillin PO | 5 w | *H. influenzae*, Viridans Streptococci | Cryptogenic | 3 m | Survived; persistent ND | [14] |
| 2 | 50 | M | Acute | C4-C7 | + | ND (M + S) | N/D | N/D | Myelotomy | Cefoperazone IV Ciprofloxacin IV | 8 w | *P. cepacia* | Cryptogenic (IV drug use) | 8 w | Survived; persistent ND | [58] |
| 3 | 72 | M | Acute | C6-T2 | + | ND (M + S) | 5 d | Urgent | Myelotomy; EAC | Penicillin | 6 w | *St. viridans* | Cryptogenic (spinal cord ependymoma) | 6 w | Survived; residual ND | [25] |
| 4 | 73 | M | Acute | T10-T11 & CM | + | ND (M) | N/D | 3 d | N/D | Ampicillin IV | 3 m | *L. monocytogenes* | Hematogenous spread (alcoholism, sepsis) | 9 m | Survived; persistent ND | [32] |
| 5 | 55 | M | Acute | T3-T7 | + | ND (M) | 2 d | 3 d | ND | Ampicillin IV | 24 d | *L. monocytogenes* | Hematogenous spread (alcoholism, sepsis) | 18 m | Survived; persistent ND | [32] |
| 6 | 37 | M | Acute | T8-T9 | + | ND (M + S) | 6 w | Urgent | Myelotomy | Antituberculosis Treatment PO & IV | N/D | Sterile | Cryptogenic | 2 m | Survived; persistent ND | [29] |

Table 4. Cont.

| No. | Age | Sex | Onset | Location | Infl. | Symptoms Name | Symptoms Duration | Symptoms to Treatment | Neurosurgical Management | Antibiotics Name | Antibiotics Duration | Pathogen | MOA | Follow-Up | Outcome | Ref. |
|---|---|---|---|---|---|---|---|---|---|---|---|---|---|---|---|---|
| 7 | 23 | F | Acute | T11-T12 | + | ND (M) | N/D | 3 w | Laminectomy, NA | Isoniazid, Rifampicin, Pyrazinamide | N/D | *M. tuberculosis* | Cryptogenic | N/D | Survived; persistent ND | [62] |
| 8 | 22 | F | Acute | Holocord | + | ND (M + S) | N/D | N/D | Myelotomy, radical debulking | N/D | N/D | *S. aureus* | Cryptogenic | 1 y | Survived; Persistent, ND | [63] |
| 9 | 47 | F | Acute | C7-T11 | N/D | ND (M + S) | 1 w | Urgent | Myelotomy | Yes (N/S) | N/D | Oral flora | Hematogenous (Oral infection) | N/D | Survived; Persistent, ND | [64] |
| 10 | 27 | M | Acute | C4-C5 | + | ND (M + S) | 1 w | N/D | Myelotomy, DR | Yes (N/S) | N/D | *E. coli* | Hematogenous (CKD, systemic infection) | N/D | Survived; Persistent, ND | [17] |
| 11 | 61 | M | Acute | T10-T11 | + | ND (M + S) | 1 m | N/D | Myelotomy, IE | N/D | 1 m | N/D | Hematogenous (Systemic infection—diabetes) | 35 d | Survived; Persistent, ND | [1] |
| 12 | 72 | M | Acute | C5, T6-T7 | + | ND (M + S) | 1 w | Urgent | Myelotomy, DR, DU | Ceftriaxone, Vancomycin, Ampicillin, Metronidazole, Penicillin G | 6 w | *St. anginosus* | Cryptogenic | 4 w | Survived, persistent ND | [12] |
| 13 | 42 | M | Subacute | C4-C5 | + | ND (M) | 15 d | 2 d | Myelotomy | Penicillin IM, Chloramphenicol | 4 w | *K. pneumoniae Streptococcus* sp. | Contiguous spread (Stab wound) | 8 m | Survived; persistent ND | [15] |
| 14 | 20 | F | Subacute | L4-L5 | + | ND (M + S) | N/D | N/D | EST | Gentamicin IV, Flucloxacillin IV, Metronidazole IV | N/D | Anaerobic *Streptococci* | Contiguous (dermal sinus tract, previous meningitis; prior resection of lumbar meningocele) | 5 m | Survived; persistent ND | [38] |
| 15 | 26 | M | Subacute | L1-L4 | + | ND (M + S) | N/D | N/D | Myelotomy, IAC | Penicillin, Chloramphenicol, Metronidazole | 5 m | Gram (-) *bacilli* | Cryptogenic (spina bifida occulta; prior excision of intradural lipoma) | 3.5 y | Survived; persistent ND | [18] |
| 16 | 42 | M | Subacute | C1-T3 | + | ND (M) | 3 w | Urgent | Myelotomy, DR | Bristopen Peflacine | N/D | *S. aureus* | Cryptogenic (IV drug use) | 5 m | Survived; persistent ND | [65] |

142

**Table 4.** Cont.

| No. | Age | Sex | Onset | Location | Infl. | Symptoms Name | Symptoms Duration | Symptoms to Treatment | Neurosurgical Management | Antibiotics Name | Antibiotics Duration | Pathogen | MOA | Follow-Up | Outcome | Ref. |
|---|---|---|---|---|---|---|---|---|---|---|---|---|---|---|---|---|
| 17 | 33 | M | Subacute | T12-L3 | + | ND (M + S) | 3 m | N/D | Biopsy | Pipellacillin-Sodium Erythromycin | 6 m | *Actinomyces* | Cryptogenic | N/D | Survived; persistent ND | [48] |
| 18 | 28 | M | Subacute | Cervical-MO | + | ND (M + S) | 3 w | Urgent | Laminectomy, DR | Broad-Spectrum Antimicrobials | N/D | *St. viridans* | Contiguous | N/D | Survived; persistent ND | [20] |
| 19 | 78 | M | Subacute | T9 | + | ND (M + S) | 14 d | 10 | Myelotomy, DU, DR | Ampicillin, Cefotaxime | N/D | *L. monocytogenes* | Cryptogenic | 2 m | Persistent, ND | [21] |
| 20 | 65 | F | Subacute | CM1-T1 | + | ND (M + S) | 2 w | Urgent | Myelotomy, DR, DU | Ceftriaxone, Vancomycin, Metronidazole, Penicillin G, Meropenem, Linezolid | 6 w | *St. anginosus* | Cryptogenic | 16 m | Survived; persistent ND | [51] |
| 21 | 69 | M | Subacute | C2-C7 | + | ND (M + S) | N/D | N/D | N/D | Ampicillin IV Gentamicin | 12 w, 14 w | *L. monocytogenes* | Cryptogenic (Spinal stenosis with spinal cord stenosis) | 2 m | Survived; persistent ND | [66] |
| 21 | 61 | M | Chronic | T9 | N/D | ND (M + S) | 4 m | 1 d | Myelotomy, EAC | Yes (Not Specified) | N/D | Sterile | Cryptogenic | 1 y | Survived; persistent ND | [67] |
| 22 | 55 | F | Chronic | T1-T2 | + | ND (M + S) | N/D | N/D | Myelotomy, IAC | Vancomycin IV, Ceftazidime IV Clindamycin PO Ciprofloxacin PO | 2/6 w | Sterile | Cryptogenic | N/D | Survived; persistent ND | [4] |
| 23 | 68 | M | Chronic | T1-T2 | + | ND (M + S) | N/S | N/S | N/D | Cefotaxime IV | 6 w | *Gam (-) bacilli* | Cryptogenic | 3 y | Survived; persistent ND | [4] |
| 24 | 19 | M | Chronic | CM | N/D | ND (M + S) | 3 m | N/D | Myelotomy | N/D | N/D | *Gram (+) cocci* | Cryptogenic | 1 y | Persistent, ND | [17] |
| 25 | 72 | M | Chronic | Thoracic-Lumbar | + | ND (M + S) | 5 d | N/D | Laminectomy, DR | Tazobactam/Piperacillin (Hospitalization Onset, No More Info About Drugs) | ~1 Y | *K. pneumoniae* | Hematogenous (Diabetes mellitus, recurrent liver abscess) | ~1 y | Persistent ND | [57] |
| 26 | 32 | M | N/D | C3-C6 | + | ND (M + S) | N/D | 14 d | Myelotomy | Ampicillin IV, Chloramphenicol IV Ampicillin PO | 4 w | *L. monocytogenes* | Hematogenous spread (Alcoholism, sepsis) | 18 m | Survived; persistent ND | [59] |

**Table 4.** Cont.

| No. | Age | Sex | Onset | Location | Infl. | Symptoms Name | Symptoms Duration | Symptoms to Treatment | Neurosurgical Management | Antibiotics Name | Antibiotics Duration | Pathogen | MOA | Follow-Up | Outcome | Ref. |
|---|---|---|---|---|---|---|---|---|---|---|---|---|---|---|---|---|
| 27 | 50 | M | N/D | C5–C7 | + | ND (M) | N/D | N/D | Laminectomy, myelotomy, DR | Gentamicin, Fucidin Pefloxacin | N/D | S. aureus | Contagious (Epidural abscess induced septic thrombophlebitis of the veins of the spinal cord—leading to venous infarction & abscess of the spinal cord) | N/D | Survived; persistent ND | [68] |
| 28 | 30 | F | Subacute | T3–T7 | − | ND (M + S) | 1 m | N/D | Laminectomy, myelotomy, EAC | ATT therapy | >6 m | M. tuberculosis | Hematogenous (Pulmonary Tuberculosis) | 7 m | Survived, persistent ND | [69] |

**Legend:** sex: F—female, M—male; location: C—cervical, T—thoracic, L—lumbar, S—sacral; infl.—inflammation; symptoms: M—motor, ND—neurological deficits, S—sensory; duration: D—day, M—months, Y—years, SW—several weeks; others: CM—conus medullaris, CMJ—craniocervical junction, DR—drainage, DU—durotomy, EST—excision sinus tract, EAC—excision of abscess cavity, IAC—irrigation of abscess cavity, N/D—no data, N/S—not specified.

**Table 5.** Death group—summary of the clinical data, patient demographics, clinical manifestations, duration, microbiology, interventions and therapies, and outcomes of contemporary case reports on intramedullary spinal cord abscess (ISCA) in the current literature: systemic review of literature (1949–2022).

| No. | Age | Sex | Onset | Location | Infl. | Symptoms Name | Symptoms Duration | Symptoms to Treatment | Neurosurgical Management | Antibiotics Name | Antibiotics Duration | Pathogen | MOA | Follow-Up | Outcome | Ref. |
|---|---|---|---|---|---|---|---|---|---|---|---|---|---|---|---|---|
| 1 | 76 | M | Acute | T3–T12 | + | ND (M + S) | N/D | N/D | N/D | Yes (Not Specified) | 3 w | Gram (−) bacilli | Hematogenous spread (Septic embolus, pyelonephritis) | 3 w | Died | [19] |
| 2 | 51 | M | Acute | Cervical | + | ND (M + S) | N/D | N/D | N/D | N/D | N/D | Staphylococcus | Hematogenous spread (Alcoholism, bronchopneumonia) | N/D | Died | [52] |
| 3 | 59 | M | Acute | C4–C6 | + | ND (M + S) | N/D | N/D | Myelotomy | Chloramphenicol IV Ceftazidime IV Metronidazole | 31 d | B. disiens | Hematogenous spread (bronchiectasis) | 31 d | Died | [53] |

Table 5. Cont.

| No. | Age | Sex | Onset | Location | Infl. | Symptoms Name | Symptoms Duration | Symptoms to Treatment | Neurosurgical Management | Antibiotics Name | Antibiotics Duration | Pathogen | MOA | Follow-Up | Outcome | Ref. |
|---|---|---|---|---|---|---|---|---|---|---|---|---|---|---|---|---|
| 4 | 59 | M | Subacute | C3-T1 | + | ND (M + S) | 2 w | Urgent | Laminectomy, DR | Amikacin, Ceftriaxone Trimethoprim Sulfamethoxazole | 12 d | N. asteroides | Hematogenous spread (Cerebral abscess, diabetes) | N/D | Died | [70] |
| 5 | 79 | M | Acute | C3-C4 | + | ND (M + S) | 5 d | N/D | N/D | IV Trimethoprim-Sulfamethoxazole, Dexamethasone | 10 | N. farcinica | Hematogenous spread | N/D | Died | [30] |
| 6 | 45 | F | Acute | C2-C6 | + | ND (M + S) | 2 w | N/D | N/D | Cefuroxime | 6 w | E. coli | Hematogenous spread (Sepsis, UTI) | N/D | Died | [28] |
| 7 | 19 | M | N/D | T12-L1 | N/D | ND (M + S) | 5w | N/D | Laminectomy, USG-guided aspiration | Voriconazole | N/D | Aspergillus | Contagious (Vertebral discitis, osteomyelitis) | N/D | Died | [26] |
| 8 | 69 | M | Subacute | T7-CM | + | ND (M + S) | 17 d | N/D | N/D | Ceftriaxone, Metronidazole—On the 3rd day of admission. Meropenem—On the 5th day. | 1 w | B. pseudomallei | Cryptogenic (suspicion of hematogenous, Diabetes mellitus) | N/D | Died | [71] |
| 9 | 50 | M | | C2-C6 | | ND (S) | | | myelotomy | N/D | N/D | L. monocytogenes | Hematogenous spread (sepsis) | N/D | Died | [72] |
| 10 | 44 | F | Chronic | T10-T11 | + | ND (M + S) | >1 Y | N/D | Laminectomy, DR | N/D | N/D | C. albicans | Hematogenous spread (History of CNS fungal infection and neurotuberculosis) | N/D | N/D | [60] |

**Legend:** sex: F—female, M—male; location: C—cervical, T—thoracic, L—lumbar, S—sacral; infl.—inflammation; Symptoms: M—motor, ND—neurological deficits, S—sensory; duration: D—day, M—months, Y—years, SW—several weeks; others: CM—conus medullaris, DR—drainage, EEC—excision of epidermoid cyst, IAC—irrigation of abscess cavity, N/D—no data, N/S—not specified.

## 5. Discussion

ISCA is rare neurological entity in spinal cord infection, fewer than 140 cases having been reported since its first description by Hart in 1830. These infections traditionally correlate with high morbidity and mortality [37]. Furthermore, they can be located throughout the spinal cord, and multiple abscesses occurred in 26% of cases [73]. Byrne et al. discovered that 36% of intramedullary abscesses primarily involved the cervical cord, 36% the conus, and 29% the thoracic cord, whereas lower thoracic and lumbar segments are the common sites in congenital midline defects [4]. In previous studies, intramedullary spinal cord abscesses mostly involved the cervical and upper segments of the thoracic cord [74]. In our review, twenty-five abscesses (35.71%) primarily involved the cervical cord, nineteen (27.14%) the thoracic cord, three (4.2%) the lumbar cord, eight (11.42%) cervical to thoracic, eight (11.42) thoracic to lumbar, one (1.42%) lumbar to sacral and holocord, and two (2.85%) the conus; four cases had multiple abscesses (see Figure 6). In the cases between 1944 and 1975, the average spinal cord abscess length was six levels, and the abscesses grew preferentially along fiber tracts longitudinally [75]. The reduction in the size and number of spinal cord abscesses in recent cases can be attributed to improved early detection, surgical intervention, and antibiotics (Byrne). Two-thirds occur during the fourth decade of life, predominantly in males (M:F ratio 5:3) [73]. A bimodal age distribution among adult patients has been described; most patients were diagnosed with ISCA during the first and third decades of life. The incidence rate in women was higher during the first four decades, whereas in men it was constant throughout their lifetime [11,24,63].

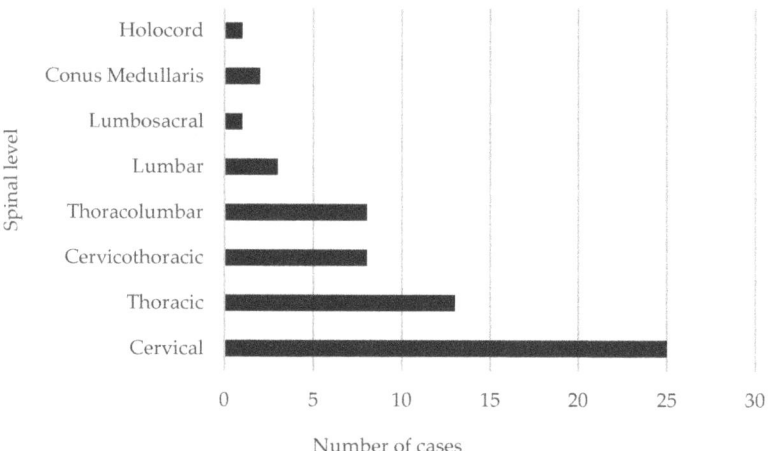

**Figure 6.** The typical localization of spinal cord abscess in 61 patients with intramedullary spinal cord abscess.

### 5.1. Etiology and Pathogenesis

According to the available literature, spinal abscesses begin in the central gray matter and extend peripherally into the white matter. The suppurative infiltrate causes inflammation with a predominance of polymorphonuclear cells and liquefactive necrosis-producing enzymes. The necrotic area is encapsuled by fibroblasts and the abscess then extends caudad and cephalad, separating the fiber tracts without compression until the later stages of the disease. Fibrous proliferation and gliosis, both rostral and caudal to the abscess cavity and surrounding the adjacent areas of necrosis, are found on histopathological examination and could cause the signal changes on the MRI [65]. Polymorphonuclear leukocytes and lymphocytes often thicken and infiltrate the meninges, with frequent venous thromboses transversing the areas of abscess [37]. ISCA is a suppurative infection with abscesses that develop similarly to pyogenic brain abscesses, normally concomitant with other pathologies.

Normal spinal cord tissue has an exceptional resistance to infection [61]. ISCA generally occurs together with underlying systemic conditions such as immunosuppression, diabetes mellitus, or intravenous drug abuse [76].

Several risk factors (especially for cervical spinal abscess) including dermoid cysts, ependymoma, meningomyelocele, osteomyelitis, pre-existing spinal pathologies including spinal tumors, dural arteriovenous malformations or fistulas, previous surgeries and iatrogenic or stab wounds, penetrating or iatrogenic injuries to the spine, intravenous drug use and alcoholism, genitourinary infections, infective endocarditis, pulmonary disease, septic embolism, and bacterial meningitis can precipitate intramedullary infections [17,22,24,44,46,51,61,65,77–79]. Other predisposing factors for intradural infection and ISCA in children are congenital midline defects such as anatomical abnormalities of the spinal cord or congenital dermal sinus [7]. According to our literature search and review, we can categorize these conditions into four groups: bacterial and fungal infections, penetrating trauma to the spinal cord, congenital dural sinuses, and chronic tuberculosis. Intramedullary abscess formations have rarely been associated with acute bacterial meningitis [61]. Bartel et al. found the primary focus of infection in 7.5% of cases. An immunocompromised state associated with diabetes, HIV infection, prolonged steroid therapy, and drug addiction also appear to be important [11]. However, our patient was neither immunocompromised nor apparently subject to any of those predisposing conditions.

## 5.2. Classification

### 5.2.1. Mechanism of Infection and Predisposing Factors

Classifying ISCA according to infection mechanisms enables us to predict the organism(s) most likely to be causal. The causative factors of ISCA development can be grouped as follows: hematogenous spread (i.e., extraspinal focus of infection), contiguous spread (i.e., adjacent focus of infection), and direct inoculation (e.g., via penetrating trauma, neurosurgery, or a cryptogenic mechanism). Hematogenous spread appears to be most common; we thought this was the case with our patient, but we could not identify the source of the infection. The patient's prior surgery and aortic prosthetic valve were assumed to be the only important predisposing factors; therefore, the infection mechanism remains cryptogenic [2,80,81].

During the pre-antibiotic era, 50% of cases were due to hematogenous spreads of infection with an extraspinal focus; nearly 20% had an underlying infectious lung disease. Other main sites of infection included soft-tissue infections and infective endocarditis [2]. In a modern-era review of ISCA, Chan and Gold et al. found that 44% of cases were linked to anatomical spinal cord or vertebral column abnormalities. Twenty-four percent (24%) of cases resulted from a contiguous infection spread through sinus tract openings, 8% from hematogenous spread with an extraspinal focus, and 64% were cryptogenic. A bacterial pathogen was identified in 64% of cases, while the remaining cases were classified as culture-negative ISCA [2,37].

Organisms typically found in cryptogenic cases were Listeria monocytogenes, Streptococci viridans, Hemophilus spp., Enterobacteriaceae, anaerobes, anaerobic streptococci, and oral anaerobic Gram-negative bacilli. Therefore, careful examination of the skin of a patient exhibiting neurological symptoms suggestive of a spinal cord syndrome can provide an early clue to the diagnosis of ISCA. In these cases, the causative organisms that reflect skin-colonizing species such as *S. epidermides*, *S. aureus*, Enterobacteriaceae, and anaerobes including Bacteroides fragilis are related to ISCA cases in the dermal sinus tract. Additionally, in the lumbar region, pathogens commonly include enteric Gram-negative rods and anaerobes as well as Staphylococcus species [37].

Although ISCA can result from hematogenous spread from an extraspinal source, Hoche demonstrated that the introduction of microorganisms into the CSF of animals did not cause ISCA unless thrombi were also introduced. This led to the discovery that ISCA is rare without pre-existing spinal cord abnormalities. The major sources of hematogenous spread (42%) are from the urogenital tract (e.g., vulvovaginitis, urinary tract infection, pyelonephritis, or perinephric abscess), followed by pneumonia, endocarditis, middle ear infection, and sagittal sinus thrombosis. Schistosomiasis and brucellosis are also possible hematogenous sources. Direct spread of the microorganism from adjacent structures is not as frequent, but if this occurs it is typically after spinal procedures, the administration of epidural anesthesia, or vertebral osteomyelitis [2,76,80].

ISCA during the pre-antibiotic and modern eras resulted in similar proportions of contagious cases (38% vs. 24%). Only around 10% of infections in the pre-antibiotic era were found in congenital dermal sinuses [2]. In contrast, several infections resulted from the direct extension of local, deep-seated infections [82].

Most recent ISCA cases are cryptogenic, probably arising from transient bacteremia of mucosal surfaces or clinically unknown extraspinal sites of infection. Several lines of evidence support the hypothesis that this transient bacteremia can seed areas of subclinical spinal cord injury or microinfarction. In the present review, nearly 20% of cases of cryptogenic ISCA were in patients with structural abnormalities in their spinal cord and/or vertebral bodies (spinal cord ependymoma, previous resection of a spinal cord lipoma, or spinal stenosis). Furthermore, cryptogenic cases were mainly located in the cervical and upper thoracic segments of the spinal cord [2]. Additionally, around 25% of cases were from contiguous spread of infection from dermal sinus tracts. Predisposing factors in pediatric ISCA include congenital midline defects and anatomical abnormalities of the spinal cord or vertebral column [74]. This shift in pathogenesis is likely to be related to the wide availability of effective antimicrobial agents to treat the primary sites of infection. Moreover, advances in non-invasive imaging could recognize the primary sites of infection earlier.

Sterile culture was the most common finding in earlier reports. This also applies in our review, especially in chronic cases. In one chronic case the culture was probably sterile because of prior administration of antibiotics. Although 30% of spinal abscesses are microbiologically sterile, a diverse range of organisms have been identified amongst the remaining 70% such as Staphylococcus (the most frequently reported cause at 25%), Streptococcus, Escherichia coli, Proteus, Listeria, Bacteroides, Pseudomonas, Brucella, Hemophilus, Histoplasma, Actinomyces, and Mycobacterium [83]. Anaerobes are uncommon, but many types of microorganisms have often been found in spinal abscesses in patients with ISCA [79]. Common causes of intramedullary abscesses include Gram-positive cocci, especially those native to oral or skin flora [13,14,20,27,30,37,56,64,84]. Implications for the selection of an empirical antimicrobial regimen in this population have arisen because opportunistic pathogens such as *Fusarium* spp. or *Aspergillus* spp. have been reported as causing intramedullary abscesses in immunocompromised patients. This further emphasizes the importance of obtaining culture data for direct therapy. When broad empirical coverage is started, clinicians should consider not only the wide array of pathogens that can cause intramedullary abscesses but also the patient's risk for tuberculosis and fungal infections, and their immune status [26,85]. The outcomes of these infections have apparently improved since antibiotics were introduced into clinical practice. The first review of ISCA cases 1830 and 1994 reported a mortality rate of 90%. A review between 1994 and 1997 reported a mortality rate of only 8%. Kurita et al. described a case of cervical ISCA treated with antibiotics alone, but whether this suffices is a matter of debate [2,8,9]. Despite the improvement of survival rates since the pre-antibiotic era, neurological deficits persist in most patients who survive. In our patient, the mechanism of infection appeared to be hematogenous spread, though we could not identify the origin of infection. We assume that the prior neurosurgical procedure and aortic valve implantation were the important predisposing factors, which could have caused bacteria to seed to the intramedullary space of the thoracic spinal cord. Thus, the mechanism of infection remains cryptogenic in this case. His wound culture from the ISCA was positive for *S. aureus*, which is part of the oral flora and is consistent with our proposed etiology.

### 5.2.2. Onset and Clinical Presentation

According to Foley, the time between initial presenting symptoms and time of diagnosis has prognostic indications. The presentation of ISCA can be divided into three clinical groups: acute, subacute, and chronic [6]. Acute symptoms last less than a week, and patients are more likely to have a fever and leucocytosis. In the subacute and chronic groups, the symptoms persist, respectively, from 1–6 weeks and for more than six weeks. These two groups are unlikely to present with fever and leucocytosis.

Acute spinal cord abscesses often follow the same clinical course as transverse myelitis, whereas chronic abscesses resemble an expanding spinal cord tumor. Our patient had an acute onset with neurological worsening. Menezes et al. observed that acute presentations had worse outcomes; patients with symptoms for less than four days had a 90% mortality rate, while those with symptoms lasting more than a week had a 60% mortality rate [86].

Motor and sensory deficits (68%), pain (60%), bladder dysfunction (56%), fever (less than 50%), meningmus (12%), and brainstem dysfunctions (4%) were the most common presenting complaints [9,87]. The triad of ISCA is fever, pain and neurological deficits, but not all patients show all three; the ISCA triad is commonly absent in subacute or chronic cases [7]. Signs and symptoms suggesting a structural lesion of the spinal cord, as opposed to features that suggest infection, are most common. Spinal epidural abscess presentations show the same pattern, so epidural abscesses should always be included in the differential diagnosis. Without concomitant vertebral osteomyelitis, primary spinal epidural abscesses are rare. This correlation could assist in a differential diagnosis of subdural and epidural spinal abscesses [2,88]. As was observed in our patient, the presentation of intramedullary abscesses is frequently marked by progressive dorsal pain followed by neurological deficits. Our patient's onset was acute, and four of the main clinical signs were present. The clinical presentation can be insidious and can imitate a spinal tumor or other chronic myelopathy-inducing condition. The multifocality of abscesses causes further complications within an already complex clinical picture [89]. Finally, meningitis can recur as a result of abscesses rupturing into the subarachnoid space [67,79]. For the purpose of management, it is crucial to differentiate ISCA from other tumorous pathologies so that adequate medical and surgical treatment can be initiated promptly.

### 5.3. Evaluation and Management

Laboratory data can help in making a definitive diagnosis when there is clinical suspicion of a spinal cord abscess. Clinical findings of ISCA are nonspecific and do not lead to a final diagnosis. Leucocytosis and elevated inflammatory markers (e.g., increased platelets, C-reactive protein, and/or erythrocyte sedimentation rate) are common. There is abnormal CSF in 78% of patients, and tests can indicate elevated leucocytosis, decreased glucose, increased protein, and/or a positive Gram stain. Nonetheless, CSF test results can be normal in spinal abscess cases [76].

### 5.4. Neuroimaging Features

The main route to diagnosing patients with spinal abscesses has traditionally been radiological. Conventional radiographs and myelography were the only imaging modalities used for diagnosing spinal abscesses, and the only diagnostic approaches mentioned in literature, until 1980. This was prior to the widespread availability of computed tomography (CT) scans and magnetic resonance imaging (MRI) [90].

A spinal intramedullary ring-enhancing mass is a nonspecific imaging feature in various non-inflammatory benign and neoplastic processes, but rarely in ISCA [36]. Because ISCA is very rare, MRI features have only been described in single case reports and seem to resemble changes in brain abscesses [91]. Extended hyperintensity of the spinal cord on T2-weighted images with a circular enhancement on T1-weighted images were included after intravenous application of gadolinium chelates [36]. Edema has a range of severities and the grade of contrast enhancement depends on the lesion stage. MRI is mostly performed in a later capsular stage, since clinical manifestations are often nonspecific and only 40–50%

of patients are febrile upon examination [36]. In our study, a hypointense abscess capsule was seen on MRI T2-weighted images, which we assumed to be caused by the susceptibility effects of free radicals and extended edema of the thoracic cord.

Features that suggest a structural lesion rather than signs of infection are more often found in ISCA presentation. MRI with contrast is the gold standard for accurate identification of the location and extent of an abscess and for identifying any predisposing structural abnormalities of the spinal cord [80]. The MRI features of ISCA include enlargement of the spinal cord with increased signal intensity on T2-weighted images and marginal enhancement with central low signal intensity on T1-weighted images with gadolinium administration. Several non-inflammatory benign and neoplastic processes have a similar ring-enhancing appearance, so this is a nonspecific imaging finding for abscesses. Enhancement can occasionally show extension to an adjacent dura or epidural space [2,7,36,87,88,91,92]. Spinal cord tumors (necrotic glioma, metastases), resolving hematoma, infarction, granulomatous disease, and demyelinating disease (multiple sclerosis) can be included in the radiographic differential diagnosis of a ring-enhancing mass [36,91]. Hyperintensity on T2-weighted images tends to resolve markedly as infections are suppressed by treatment [12,92]. An ISCA that could require immediate surgery should always be considered, although MRI features can resemble those of a tumor, which would not necessarily be considered for immediate resection.

In recent years, diffusion-weighted imaging (DWI) has been added to the list of diagnostic imaging techniques and has been recommended as a more sensitive and specific method for differential diagnosis of abscesses and cystic or necrotic tumors, since the latter present with low signal intensity and show increased values of ADC [40,93,94]. Pus in an abscess cavity is a thick mucoid fluid containing inflammatory cells, bacteria, necrotic tissue and high viscosity proteinaceous exudates. Water mobility and the microscopic diffusional motion of water molecules are heavily impeded, leading to a decreased ADC in the abscess center [40,95]. Necrotic tumor-tissue debris, fewer inflammatory cells than in an abscess, and clearer serous fluid than pus are the usual contents of the cystic and necrotic cavities of tumors. However, an abscess cavity can have variable hyperintense signal intensity on DWI and low ADC values because of a difference in the concentration of inflammatory cells and particularly in abscess fluid viscosity [36]. This reflects decreased diffusion, which can help to distinguish ISCA from cystic spinal cord tumors. DWI signal intensity is higher in abscess cavities than in normal brain parenchyma, indicating restricted diffusion, whereas the signal intensity is generally hypointense in tumor cysts and necrosis, indicating more isotropic diffusion, as in CSF [91]. Previously described precipitation or drop signs characterized by an accumulation of pus at the conus medullaris could be more specific for spinal abscesses [96]. In clinically atypical acute myelopathies, a DWI can also help to distinguish spinal cord infarction from inflammatory myelopathies such as multiple sclerosis, ADEM, neuromyelitis optica, and parainfectious myelopathy [93]. The viscosity depends on the age of the abscess, the etiological organism, and the host's immune response [36].

*5.5. Management and Therapy*

Prognosis is affected by the extension and aggressiveness of the infective agent and the treatment applied. There is no significant difference between surgically and non-surgically treated patients in the frequency of residual neurological injury. Antibiotic treatment alone can be as effective as surgery plus antibiotic therapy [22].

Prompt diagnosis and intervention are essential for a prognosis and to prevent morbidity and mortality [9,87]. Ages under 25 correlates with good or full recovery, while poor outcomes are more likely after an acute presentation of spinal cord abscess [5,87]. As in the treatment of pyogenic brain abscesses, which are often polymicrobial, a combination of antimicrobial and surgical therapies is recommended for treating ISCA [21].

An interdisciplinary approach involving specialists in neurosurgery, neuroradiology, and infectious diseases is recommended for managing ISCA. Effective prompt surgical evacuation through limited laminectomy and myelotomy, with copious irrigation with normal saline followed by antibiotics according to culture and sensitivity, is the treatment of choice since significant tissue injury can result from the space-occupying nature of lesions. This can limit the extent of neurological injury [16,97].

An open surgical approach (laminectomy and myelotomy) or stereotactic needle aspiration of the lesions under CT guidance can achieve diagnostic and therapeutic drainage of the abscess [2]. There are reported cases of non-surgically treated patients in whom the abscess did not extend more than 2.2 vertebral bodies [7].

Bartels et al. reported that 63% of cases were treated with surgery and 37% without. In the surgical group, 13.6% died, 75% of whom had not received antibiotics. Among those who survived with surgery, 22% recovered completely, 56% improved neurologically, 7% remained unchanged, and one deteriorated. The non-surgical group had 100% mortality. Only 3% of the non-surgically managed patients were treated with antibiotics because 82% of those cases occurred during the pre-antibiotic era. The mortality rate decreased significantly from 90% in the pre-antibiotic era to 8% more recently, which can be attributed to both the development of powerful antibiotics and earlier diagnosis through modern imaging modalities. However, neurological deficits remained in more than 70% of surviving patients [11,24].

The presumed mechanism of infection and the results of Gram staining of aspirate should be the basis for empirical antimicrobial therapy. Since a wide range of microbes can be isolated from an ISCA culture, early treatment with antibiotic combinations effective against *Staphylococcus* spp., *Streptococcus* spp., enteric Gram-negative bacilli, and anaerobes should be used until the causative organisms in each individual case are identified. Chan and Gold recommend including ampicillin in the initial treatment regime for all cases of cryptogenic ISCA to combat L. monocytogenes [2]. Although the optimal duration of antimicrobial therapy is still debatable, a minimum of 4–6 weeks of parenteral antibiotic treatment is recommended, while some authors have proposed the use of intravenous antibiotic therapy for more than nine weeks. Two to three months of additional oral antimicrobial therapy is worth considering [76,97–100]. Park et al. suggest adjusting the duration of treatment according to the level of ISCA resorption, as indicated by MRI. Using steroids as an adjuvant therapy to decrease edema was recommended in a previous study [101]. Our patient underwent surgery because of his afebrile back pain and persistent neurological deficits. We performed a laminectomy, a myelotomy, and drainage of pus followed by irrigation with saline. The culture yielded *S. aureus*, but his paraplegia did not improve. Accordingly, the patient underwent rehabilitation but his gait impairment persisted and the pain symptoms exacerbated. Another control MRI comparable with previous control MRIs, revealed slight progression of L2–L3 stenosis.

In the view of patient's progressive stenosis and lumbar pain, an elective surgery was planned. We avoid a major intervention with selective minimal invasive L2/L3 surgery. Postoperatively, patient experienced a dramatic improvement in pain and neurological symptoms. These findings were accidental as the degenerative changes were present before paraplegic gait, with concomitant tethered spinal cord syndrome (medulla to the L3 level) and conus medullaris compression by the L2–L3 stenosis.

Thorough history taking and clinical investigation is fundamental to establish the and differentiate the concomitant diseases that might cause similar clinical symptoms. This can be misleading in establishing definitive diagnosis and tailoring the best therapeutic strategies in cases with similar clinical presentation.

*5.6. Outcome and Follow-Up*

Evaluation of the patient's response to therapy should be based on follow-up neurological assessments and the results of serial CT or MRI scans to document the resolution of the lesions. Regular follow-up via clinical examinations and MRI during the first year following surgery is highly recommended because intramedullary spinal abscesses recur in 25% of cases. Kurita et al. reported a successfully treated case with the use of antibiotics alone, while Gupta et al. reported a bad outcome from medical treatment alone and emphasized the need for early surgical drainage. There were poor outcomes for ISCA in the pre-antibiotic era, but favorable outcomes can be reached through prompt diagnosis, early and adequate surgical intervention, and antibiotics [1,9].

We were delayed in treating our ISCA case accurately because of the initial misdiagnosis and the patient's severe paraplegia, which showed no neurological recovery after first surgery. This initial failure to improve was probably caused by a neurological insult incurred from infarction of the cervico-dorsal cord and the delay in surgical treatment. After 11 months the patient underwent the second surgery, after which his neurological deficits improved, and he was able to walk with support after three days.

In general, a good prognosis can be achieved by early drainage and antibiotic infusion [1]. The only significant factors influencing the outcome for ISCA patients are the administration of antibiotics and the time between the onset of symptoms and surgery. Simon et al. reported the deaths of 20% of ISCA patients, residual neurological deficits in 60%, and a 20% recovery rate without sequelae. Patients who did not develop neurological sequelae continued with surgical drainage at a median time from surgery of 1.5 days (range 1–8 days) after hospitalization. Patients who developed neurological sequelae continued with surgical drainage for a median time from surgery of four days (range 1–78 days) after hospitalization. The median time from the onset of symptoms to surgery for those without neurological sequelae was seven days; it was 22 days (range 2–1088 days) for those who developed neurological sequelae. Moreover, a patient's outcome can be related to the pace of onset of symptoms. Patients developing symptoms in under four days have a mortality rate of 90%, while those whose symptoms last more than seven days have a mortality rate of 67% [76]. Recently, Kurita et al. found no significant difference between surgically and non-surgically treated patients in the frequency of neurological sequelae, but the number of cases in their study was small and the surgically treated group had significantly more extensive abscesses. Thus, patients should receive an appropriate treatment strategy according to their clinical state. A number of patients still experience marked functional neurological impairment, including paraplegia, because of recurrent or chronic abscess formation or spinal cord infarction, despite better prognoses today thanks to advanced surgical techniques and effective antibiotic treatment [1,9]. Our review also revealed that the recovery group received earlier treatment than the persistent, residual, and death groups, though the difference was not significant. Early diagnosis and surgical evacuation, along with broad-spectrum antibiotics, can result in a favorable neurological outcome, as evidenced by our case.

The present case is unique due to its preoperative neuroradiological definitive diagnosis and atypical neuroimaging features, as the findings of MRI were not pertinent for diagnosis of spinal cord abscess. The MRI images did not reveal the characteristic findings of intramedullary spinal cord abscess, including expansion of spinal cord by a ring-enhancing lesion and surrounding edema, which resulted in difficulties in preoperative neuroradiological definitive, and initial diagnosis of neurogenic tumor with abscess. Therefore, we believe that this unusual case will be useful in the diagnostic and patient-specific treatment planning for clinicians and neurosurgeons encountering similar cases of ISCA.

## 6. Conclusions

ISCA is rare and may be associated with underlying pathological conditions that can lead to the formation of a spinal intramedullary abscess. Initial symptoms can be misleading, so a thorough history with precise localization and early diagnosis is valuable. Serious consequences, including risks of severe sequelae and mortality, can result from intramedullary abscesses. A high index of suspicion for proper diagnosis and timely intervention is required to prevent mortality and neurological injury. Contrast-enhanced MRI and novel application of DWI at appropriate levels is the ideal investigation for accurate diagnosis. Any misdiagnosis or delay in adequate treatment can lead to unfavorable outcomes, though the diagnosis is likely to be challenging because the condition is rare. Our case is a clear example thereof. Long-term follow-up is also essential in order to monitor for abscess recurrences.

**Supplementary Materials:** The following supporting information can be downloaded at: https://www.mdpi.com/article/10.3390/jcm11175148/s1, Table S1: The mechanism behind the development of intramedullary spinal cord abscess in adults; Table S2: The predisposing factors of intramedullary spinal cord abscess in adults (see Tables 1–3 for additional information); Table S3: Concomitant diseases.

**Author Contributions:** Conceptualization, R.J. and B.S.; investigation, R.J., B.S. and W.L.; writing—original draft preparation, R.J.; writing—review and editing, B.S., J.J., A.P., G.W., J.I., R.S.T. and M.R.; funding acquisition, M.R. All authors have read and agreed to the published version of the manuscript.

**Funding:** This research received no external funding.

**Institutional Review Board Statement:** Not applicable.

**Informed Consent Statement:** Patient consent for publication was waived because details that could identify our patient were not reported.

**Data Availability Statement:** Not applicable.

**Acknowledgments:** We would like to extend our sincere gratitude to all the authors who reported their intramedullary spinal cord abscess cases. Without their efforts, this publication would never have become possible. We would like to thank our patient for motivation and his trust in our specialists.

**Conflicts of Interest:** The authors declare no conflict of interest.

# References

1. Iwasaki, M.; Yano, S.; Aoyama, T.; Hida, K.; Iwasaki, Y. Acute onset intramedullary spinal cord abscess with spinal artery occlusion: A case report and review. *Eur. Spine J.* **2011**, *20*, 294–301. [CrossRef] [PubMed]
2. Chan, C.T.; Gold, W.L. Intramedullary abscess of the spinal cord in the antibiotic era: Clinical features, microbial etiologies, trends in pathogenesis, and outcomes. *Clin. Infect. Dis.* **1998**, *27*, 619–626. [CrossRef] [PubMed]
3. Szmyd, B.; Jabbar, R.; Lusa, W.; Karuga, F.F.; Pawełczyk, A.; Błaszczyk, M.; Jankowski, J.; Sołek, J.; Wysiadecki, G.; Tubbs, R.S.; et al. What Is Currently Known about Intramedullary Spinal Cord Abscess among Children? A Concise Review. *J. Clin. Med.* **2022**, *11*, 4549. [CrossRef] [PubMed]
4. Byrne, R.W.; Von Roenn, K.A.; Whisler, W.W. Intramedullary abscess: A report of two cases and a review of the literature. *Neurosurgery* **1994**, *35*, 321–326. [CrossRef] [PubMed]
5. Rogers, A.P.; Lerner, A.; Metting, S.; Sahai-Srivastava, S. Cervical intramedullary spinal cord abscess: A case report. *Radiol. Infect. Dis.* **2017**, *4*, 113–116. [CrossRef]
6. Foley, J. Intramedullary Abscess of the Spinal Cord. *Lancet* **1949**, *254*, 193–195. [CrossRef]
7. Lim, H.Y.; Choi, H.J.; Kim, S.J.; Kuh, S.U. Chronic spinal subdural abscess mimicking an intradural-extramedullary tumor. *Eur. Spine J.* **2013**, *22*, 497–500. [CrossRef]
8. Arzt, P.K. Abscess Within the Spinal Cord: Review of the Literature and Report of Three Cases. *Arch. Neurol. Psychiatry* **1944**, *51*, 533–543. [CrossRef]
9. Kurita, N.; Sakurai, Y.; Taniguchi, M.; Terao, T.; Takahashi, H.; Mannen, T. Intramedullary spinal cord abscess treated with antibiotic therapy–case report and review. *Neurol. Med. Chir.* **2009**, *49*, 262–268. [CrossRef]
10. Keefe, P.; Das, J.M.; Al-Dhahir, M.A. Spinal Cord Abscess. In *StatPearls*; StatPearls Publishing: Tampa, FL, USA.
11. Bartels, R.H.M.A.; Gonera, E.G.; Van Der Spek, J.A.N.; Thijssen, H.O.M.; Mullaart, R.A.; Gabreels, F.J.M. Intramedullary spinal cord abscess. A case report. *Spine* **1995**, *20*, 1199–1204. [CrossRef] [PubMed]
12. Cerecedo-Lopez, C.D.; Bernstock, J.D.; Dmytriw, A.A.; Chen, J.A.; Chalif, J.I.; Gupta, S.; Driver, J.; Huang, K.; Stanley, S.E.; Li, J.Z.; et al. Spontaneous intramedullary abscesses caused by Streptococcus anginosus: Two case reports and review of the literature. *BMC Infect. Dis.* **2022**, *22*, 141. [CrossRef]
13. Hassan, M.F.; Mohamed, M.B.; Kalsi, P.; Sinar, E.J.; Bradey, N. Intramedullary pyogenic abscess in the conus medullaris. *Br. J. Neurosurg.* **2012**, *26*, 118–119. [CrossRef]
14. Blacklock, J.B.; Hood, T.W.; Maxwell, R.E. Intramedullary cervical spinal cord abscess. Case report. *J. Neurosurg.* **1982**, *57*, 270–273. [CrossRef]
15. Wright, R.L. Intramedullary spinal cord abscess. Report of a case secondary to stab wound with good recovery following operation. *J. Neurosurg.* **1965**, *23*, 208–210. [CrossRef]

16. David, C.; Brasme, L.; Peruzzi, P.; Bertault, R.; Vinsonneau, M.; Ingrand, D. Intramedullary abscess of the spinal cord in a patient with a right-to-left shunt: Case report. *Clin. Infect. Dis.* **1997**, *24*, 89–90. [CrossRef]
17. Mohindra, S.; Gupta, R.; Mathuriya, S.N.; Radotra, B.D. Intramedullary abscess in association with tumor at the conus medullaris: Report of two cases. *J. Neurosurg. Spine* **2007**, *6*, 350–353. [CrossRef]
18. Hardwidge, C.; Palsingh, J.; Williams, B. Pyomyelia: An intramedullary spinal abscess complicating lumbar lipoma with spina bifida. *Br. J. Neurosurg.* **1993**, *7*, 419–422. [CrossRef]
19. Davey, P.W.; Berry, N.E. Intramedullary spinal abscess co-incident with spinal anaesthesia. *Can. Med. Assoc. J.* **1951**, *65*, 375.
20. Weng, T.I.; Shih, F.Y.; Chen, W.J.; Lin, F.Y. Intramedullary abscess of the spinal cord. *Am. J. Emerg. Med.* **2001**, *19*, 177–178. [CrossRef]
21. Roh, J.E.; Lee, S.Y.; Cha, S.H.; Cho, B.S.; Jeon, M.H.; Kang, M.H. Sequential magnetic resonance imaging finding of intramedullary spinal abscess including diffusion weighted image: A Case Report. *Korean J. Radiol.* **2011**, *12*, 241–246. [CrossRef]
22. Arnáiz-García, M.E.; González-Santos, J.M.; López-Rodriguez, J.; Dalmau-Sorli, M.J.; Bueno-Codoñer, M.; Arévalo-Abascal, A. Intramedullary cervical abscess in the setting of aortic valve endocarditis. *Asian Cardiovasc. Thorac. Ann.* **2015**, *23*, 64–66. [CrossRef] [PubMed]
23. Fernández-Ruiz, M.; López-Medrano, F.; García-Montero, M.; Hornedo-Muguiro, J.; Aguado, J.M. Intramedullary cervical spinal cord abscess by viridans group Streptococcus secondary to infective endocarditis and facilitated by previous local radiotherapy. *Intern. Med.* **2009**, *48*, 61–64. [CrossRef] [PubMed]
24. Terterov, S.; Taghva, A.; Khalessi, A.A.; Kim, P.E.; Liu, C. Intramedullary abscess of the spinal cord in the setting of patent foramen ovale. *World Neurosurg.* **2011**, *76*, 361.e11–361.e14. [CrossRef]
25. Babu, R.; Jafar, J.J.; Huang, P.P.; Budzilovich, G.N.; Ransohoff, J. Intramedullary abscess associated with a spinal cord ependymoma: Case report. *Neurosurgery* **1992**, *30*, 121–123. [CrossRef] [PubMed]
26. McCaslin, A.F.; Lall, R.R.; Wong, A.P.; Lall, R.R.; Sugrue, P.A.; Koski, T.R. Thoracic spinal cord intramedullary aspergillus invasion and abscess. *J. Clin. Neurosci.* **2015**, *22*, 404–406. [CrossRef] [PubMed]
27. Sinha, P.; Parekh, T.; Pal, D. Intramedullary abscess of the upper cervical spinal cord. Unusual presentation and dilemmas of management: Case report. *Clin. Neurol. Neurosurg.* **2013**, *115*, 1845–1850. [CrossRef] [PubMed]
28. Thakar, S.; Rao, A.; Mohan, D.; Hegde, A. Metachronous occurrence of an intramedullary abscess following radical excision of a cervical intramedullary pilocytic astrocytoma. *Neurol. India* **2013**, *61*, 322. [CrossRef] [PubMed]
29. Tacconi, L.; Arulampalam, T.; Johnston, F.G.; Thomas, D.G.T. Intramedullary spinal cord abscess: Case report. *Neurosurgery* **1995**, *37*, 817–819. [CrossRef]
30. Samkoff, L.M.; Monajati, A.; Shapiro, J.L. Teaching NeuroImage: Nocardial intramedullary spinal cord abscess. *Neurology* **2008**, *71*, e5. [CrossRef]
31. Menezes Penetrative Injury to the Face Resulting in Delayed Death After Rupture of a Cavernous Sinus Aneurysm on the Contralateral Side. *Am. J. Forensic Med. Pathol.* **2015**, *36*, 271–273. [CrossRef]
32. Pfadenhauer, K.; Rossmanith, T. Spinal manifestation of neurolisteriosis. *J. Neurol.* **1995**, *242*, 153–156. [CrossRef]
33. Akhaddar, A.; Boulahroud, O.; Boucetta, M. Chronic spinal cord abscess in an elderly patient. *Surg. Infect.* **2011**, *12*, 333–334. [CrossRef]
34. Liu, J.; Zhang, H.; He, B.; Wang, B.; Niu, X.; Hao, D. Intramedullary Tuberculoma Combined with Abscess: Case Report and Literature Review. *World Neurosurg.* **2016**, *89*, 726.e1–726.e4. [CrossRef]
35. Lindner, A.; Becker, G.; Warmuth-Metz, M.; Schalke, B.C.G.; Bogdahn, U.; Toyka, K.V. Magnetic resonance image findings of spinal intramedullary abscess caused by candida albicans: Case report. *Neurosurgery* **1995**, *36*, 411–412. [CrossRef]
36. Dörflinger-Hejlek, E.; Kirsch, E.C.; Reiter, H.; Opravil, M.; Kaim, A.H. Diffusion-weighted MR imaging of intramedullary spinal cord abscess. *Am. J. Neuroradiol.* **2010**, *31*, 1651–1652. [CrossRef]
37. Hood, B.; Wolfe, S.Q.; Trivedi, R.A.; Rajadhyaksha, C.; Green, B. Intramedullary Abscess of the Cervical Spinal Cord in an Otherwise Healthy Man. *World Neurosurg.* **2011**, *76*, 361.e15–361.e19. [CrossRef]
38. Maurice-Williams, R.S.; Pamphilon, D.; Coakham, H.B. Intramedullary abscess- A rare complication of spinal dysraphism. *J. Neurol. Neurosurg. Psychiatry* **1980**, *43*, 1045–1048. [CrossRef]
39. Mukunda, B.N.; Shekar, R.; Bass, S. Solitary spinal intramedullary abscess caused by Nocardia asteroides. *South. Med. J.* **1999**, *92*, 1223–1224. [CrossRef] [PubMed]
40. Kim, Y.J.; Chang, K.H.; Song, I.C.; Kim, H.D.; Seong, S.O.; Kim, Y.H.; Han, M.H. Brain abscess and necrotic or cystic brain tumor: Discrimination with signal intensity on diffusion-weighted MR imaging. *Am. J. Roentgenol.* **1998**, *171*, 1487–1490. [CrossRef]
41. Lascaux, A.S.; Chevalier, X.; Brugières, P.; Levy, Y. Painful neck stiffness secondary to an intra-medullary abscess of the spinal cord in a hiv infected patient: A case report. *J. Neurol.* **2002**, *249*, 229. [CrossRef]
42. Higuchi, K.; Ishihara, H.; Okuda, S.; Kanda, F. A 51-year-old man with intramedullary spinal cord abscess having a patent foramen ovale. *BMJ Case Rep.* **2011**, *2011*, bcr1120103512. [CrossRef] [PubMed]
43. Rifaat, M.; El Shafei, I.; Samra, K.; Sorour, O. Intramedullary spinal abscess following spinal puncture: Case report. *J. Neurosurg.* **1973**, *38*, 366–367. [CrossRef]
44. Ueno, T.; Nishijima, H.; Funamizu, Y.; Kon, T.; Haga, R.; Arai, A.; Suzuki, C.; Nunomura, J.I.; Baba, M.; Midorikawa, H.; et al. Intramedullary spinal cord abscess associated with spinal dural arteriovenous fistula. *J. Neurol. Sci.* **2016**, *368*, 94–96. [CrossRef] [PubMed]

45. Recker, M.J.; Housley, S.B.; Lipinski, L.J. Indolent nonendemic central nervous system histoplasmosis presenting as an isolated intramedullary enhancing spinal cord lesion. *Surg. Neurol. Int.* **2021**, *12*, 392. [CrossRef]
46. De Silva, R.T.; de Souza, H.C.; de Amoreira Gepp, R.; Batista, G.R.; Horan, T.A.; Oliveira, P.C.R. Penetrating cervical spine injury and spinal cord intramedullary abscess. *Arq. Neuropsiquiatr.* **2012**, *70*, 308–309. [CrossRef] [PubMed]
47. Tan, L.A.; Kasliwal, M.K.; Nag, S.; O'Toole, J.E.; Traynelis, V.C. Rapidly progressive quadriparesis heralding disseminated coccidioidomycosis in an immunocompetent patient. *J. Clin. Neurosci.* **2014**, *21*, 1049–1051. [CrossRef]
48. Ushikoshi, S.; Koyanagi, I.; Hida, K.; Iwasaki, Y.; Abe, H. Spinal intrathecal actinomycosis: A case report. *Surg. Neurol.* **1998**, *50*, 221–225. [CrossRef]
49. Vajramani, G.V.; Nagmoti, M.B.; Patil, C.S. Neurobrucellosis presenting as an intra-medullary spinal cord abscess. *Ann. Clin. Microbiol. Antimicrob.* **2005**, *4*, 14. [CrossRef]
50. Vadera, S.; Harrop, J.S.; Sharan, A.D. Intrathecal granuloma and intramedullary abscess associated with an intrathecal morphine pump. *Neuromodulation* **2007**, *10*, 6–11. [CrossRef]
51. Takebe, N.; Iwasaki, K.; Hashikata, H.; Toda, H. Intramedullary spinal cord abscess and subsequent granuloma formation: A rare complication of vertebral osteomyelitis detected by diffusion-weighted magnetic resonance imaging. *Neurosurg. Focus* **2014**, *37*, E12. [CrossRef]
52. Parker, R.L.; Collins, G.H. Intramedullary abscess of the brain stem and spinal cord. *South. Med. J.* **1970**, *63*, 495–497. [CrossRef]
53. Erlich, J.H.; Rosenfeld, J.V.; Fuller, A.; Brown, G.V.; Wodak, J.; Tress, B.P. Acute intramedullary spinal cord abscess: Case report. *Surg. Neurol.* **1992**, *38*, 287–290. [CrossRef]
54. Lee, J.; Whitby, M.; Hall, B.I. Nocardia cyriacigeorgica abscess of the conus medullaris in an immunocompetent host. *J. Clin. Neurosci.* **2010**, *17*, 1194–1195. [CrossRef]
55. Crema, M.D.; Pradel, C.; Marra, M.D.; Arrivé, L.; Tubiana, J.M. Intramedullary spinal cord abscess complicating thoracic spondylodiscitis caused by Bacteroides fragilis. *Skeletal Radiol.* **2007**, *36*, 681–683. [CrossRef]
56. Damaskos, D.; Jumeau, H.; Lens, F.-X.; Lechien, P. Intramedullary Abscess by Staphylococcus aureus Presenting as Cauda Equina Syndrome to the Emergency Department. *Case Rep. Emerg. Med.* **2016**, *2016*, 9546827. [CrossRef]
57. Matsumoto, K.; Sawada, H.; Saito, S.; Hirata, K.; Ozaki, R.; Ohni, S.; Nishimaki, H.; Nakanishi, K. A case of spinal cord transection for an intramedullary abscess containing gas. *J. Orthop. Sci.* **2021**. [CrossRef]
58. Koppel, B.S.; Daras, M.; Duffy, K.R. Intramedullary spinal cord abscess. *Neurosurgery* **1990**, *26*, 145–146. [CrossRef]
59. Morrison, L.C.R.E.; Brown, C.J.; Gooding, M.R.S. Spinal cord abscess caused by Listeria monocytogenes. *Arch. Neurol.* **1980**, *37*, 243–244. [CrossRef]
60. Zito Raffa, P.E.A.; Vencio, R.C.C.; Corral Ponce, A.C.; Malamud, B.P.; Vencio, I.C.; Pacheco, C.C.; D'Almeida Costa, F.; Franceschini, P.R.; Medeiros, R.T.R.; Pires Aguiar, P.H. Spinal intramedullary abscess due to Candida albicans in an immunocompetent patient: A rare case report. *Surg. Neurol. Int.* **2021**, *12*, 275. [CrossRef]
61. Vo, D.T.; Cravens, G.F.; Germann, R.E. Streptococcus pneumoniae meningitis complicated by an intramedullary abscess: A case report and review of the literature. *J. Med. Case Rep.* **2016**, *10*, 290. [CrossRef]
62. Cheng, K.M.; Ma, M.W.; Chan, C.M.; Leung, C.L. Tuberculous intramedullary spinal cord abscess. *Acta Neurochir.* **1997**, *139*, 1189–1190. [CrossRef] [PubMed]
63. Desai, K.I.; Muzumdar, D.P.; Goel, A. Holocord intramedullary abscess: An unusual case with review of literature. *Spinal Cord* **1999**, *37*, 866–870. [CrossRef] [PubMed]
64. Applebee, A.; Ramundo, M.; Kirkpatrick, B.D.; Fries, T.J.; Panitch, H. Intramedullary spinal cord abscess in a healthy woman. *Neurology* **2007**, *68*, 1230. [CrossRef] [PubMed]
65. Sverzut, J.M.; Laval, C.; Smadja, P.; Gigaud, M.; Sevely, A.; Manelfe, C. Spinal cord abscess in a heroin addict: Case report. *Neuroradiology* **1998**, *40*, 455–458. [CrossRef]
66. Chu, J.Y.; Montanera, W.; Willinsky, R.A. Listeria spinal cord abscess–clinical and MRI findings. *Can. J. Neurol. Sci.* **1996**, *23*, 220–223. [CrossRef]
67. Miranda Carus, M.E.; Ancicones, B.; Castro, A.; Lara, M.; Isla, A. Intramedullary spinal cord abscess. *J. Neurol. Neurosurg. Psychiatry* **1992**, *55*, 225–226. [CrossRef]
68. Derkinderen, P.; Duval, X.; Bruneel, F.; Laissy, J.P.; Regnier, B. Intramedullary spinal cord abscess associated with cervical spondylodiskitis and epidural abscess. *Scand. J. Infect. Dis.* **1998**, *30*, 618–619. [CrossRef]
69. Singh, J.; Agrawal, Y.; Agrawal, R.; Sharma, B.S. Spinal Intramedullary Tubercular Abscess. *J. Mahatma Gandhi Univ. Med. Sci. Technol.* **2017**, *2*, 102–105. [CrossRef]
70. Durmaz, R.; Atasoy, M.A.; Durmaz, G.; Adapinar, B.; Arslantaş, A.; Aydinli, A.; Tel, E. Multiple nocardial abscesses of cerebrum, cerebellum and spinal cord, causing quadriplegia. *Clin. Neurol. Neurosurg.* **2001**, *103*, 59–62. [CrossRef]
71. Rudrabhatla, P.; Nair, S.S.; George, J.; Sekar, S.; Ponnambath, D.K. Isolated Myelitis and Intramedullary Spinal Cord Abscess in Melioidosis—A Case Report. *Neurohospitalist* **2022**, *12*, 131–136. [CrossRef]
72. King, S.J.; Jeffree, M.A. MRI of an abscess of the cervical spinal cord in a case of Listeria meningoencephalomyelitis. *Neuroradiology* **1993**, *35*, 495–496. [CrossRef]
73. Menezes, A.H.; Graf, C.J.; Perret, G.E. Spinal cord abscess: A review. *Surg. Neurol.* **1977**, *8*, 461–467.
74. Chandran, R.S.; Bhanuprabhakar, R.; Sumukhan, S. Intramedullary Spinal Cord Abscess: Illustration of Two Cases and Review of Literature. *Indian J. Neurosurg.* **2017**, *6*, 31–35. [CrossRef]

75. Keener, E.B. Abscess formation in the spinal cord. *Brain* **1955**, *78*, 394–400. [CrossRef]
76. Simon, J.K.; Lazareff, J.A.; Diament, M.J.; Kennedy, W.A. Intramedullary abscess of the spinal cord in children: A case report and review of the literature. *Pediatr. Infect. Dis. J.* **2003**, *22*, 186–192. [CrossRef]
77. Ameli, N.O. A Case of Intramedullary Abscess: Recovery After Operation. *Br. Med. J.* **1948**, *2*, 138. [CrossRef]
78. Baradaran, N.; Ahmadi, H.; Nejat, F.; Khashab, M.; Mahdavi, A.; Rahbarimanesh, A.A. Recurrent meningitis caused by cervicomedullary abscess, a rare presentation. *Child's. Nerv. Syst.* **2008**, *24*, 767–771. [CrossRef]
79. Da Silva, P.S.L.; de Souza Loduca, R.D. Intramedullary spinal cord abscess as complication of lumbar puncture: A case-based update. *Child's Nerv. Syst.* **2013**, *29*, 1061–1068. [CrossRef]
80. Kalia, V.; Vibhuti; Aggarwal, T. Holocord intramedullary abscess. *Indian J. Pediatr.* **2007**, *74*, 589–591. [CrossRef]
81. Hart, J. Case of Encysted Abscess in the Spinal Cord. *Med. Chir. Rev.* **1831**, *14*, 284–286. [CrossRef]
82. Hung, P.C.; Wang, H.S.; Wu, C.T.; Lui, T.N.; Wong, A.M.C. Spinal intramedullary abscess with an epidermoid secondary to a dermal sinus. *Pediatr. Neurol.* **2007**, *37*, 144–147. [CrossRef] [PubMed]
83. Chidambaram, B.; Balasubramaniam, V. Intramedullary Abscess of the Spinal Cord. *Pediatr. Neurosurg.* **2001**, *34*, 43–44. [CrossRef] [PubMed]
84. Agyei, J.O.; Qiu, J.; Fabiano, A.J. Fusarium species intramedullary spinal cord fungus ball: Case report. *J. Neurosurg. Spine* **2019**, *31*, 440–446. [CrossRef] [PubMed]
85. Menezes Intra-arterial digital subtraction angiography. *Radiol. Clin. N. Am.* **1985**, *23*, 293–319. [CrossRef]
86. Al Barbarawi, M.; Khriesat, W.; Qudsieh, S.; Qudsieh, H.; Loai, A.A. Management of intramedullary spinal cord abscess: Experience with four cases, pathophysiology and outcomes. *Eur. Spine J.* **2009**, *18*, 710–717. [CrossRef]
87. Tsiodras, S.; Falagas, M.E. Clinical assessment and medical treatment of spine infections. *Clin. Orthop. Relat. Res.* **2006**, *444*, 38–50. [CrossRef]
88. Bajema, K.L.; Dalesandro, M.F.; Fredricks, D.N.; Ramchandani, M. Disseminated coccidioidomycosis presenting with intramedullary spinal cord abscesses: Management challenges. *Med. Mycol. Case Rep.* **2016**, *15*, 1–4. [CrossRef]
89. Reihsaus, E.; Waldbaur, H.; Seeling, W. Spinal epidural abscess: A meta-analysis of 915 patients. *Neurosurg. Rev.* **2000**, *23*, 175–204. [CrossRef]
90. Reiche, W.; Schuchardt, V.; Hagen, T.; Il'yasov, K.A.; Billmann, P.; Weber, J. Differential diagnosis of intracranial ring enhancing cystic mass lesions-Role of diffusion-weighted imaging (DWI) and diffusion-tensor imaging (DTI). *Clin. Neurol. Neurosurg.* **2010**, *112*, 218–225. [CrossRef]
91. Murphy, K.J.; Brunberg, J.A.; Quint, D.J.; Kazanjian, P.H. Spinal cord infection: Myelitis and abscess formation. *Am. J. Neuroradiol.* **1998**, *19*, 341–348.
92. Marcel, C.; Kremer, S.; Jeantroux, J.; Blanc, F.; Dietemann, J.L.; De Sèze, J. Diffusion-weighted imaging in noncompressive myelopathies: A 33-patient prospective study. *J. Neurol.* **2010**, *257*, 1438–1445. [CrossRef]
93. Noguchi, K.; Watanabe, N.; Nagayoshi, T.; Kanazawa, T.; Toyoshima, S.; Shimizu, M.; Seto, H. Role of diffusion-weighted echo-planar MRI in distinguishing between brain abscess and tumour: A preliminary report. *Neuroradiology* **1999**, *41*, 171–174. [CrossRef] [PubMed]
94. Guo, A.C.; Provenzale, J.M.; Cruz, L.C.H.; Petrella, J.R. Cerebral abscesses: Investigation using apparent diffusion coefficient maps. *Neuroradiology* **2001**, *43*, 370–374. [CrossRef]
95. Chittem, L.; Bommanakanti, K.; Alugolu, R. "Precipitation sign": A new radiological sign for spinal intramedullary tubercular abscess. *Spinal Cord* **2014**, *52*, S1–S2. [CrossRef] [PubMed]
96. Rosenblum, M.L.; Mampalam, T.J.; Pons, V.G. Controversies in the management of brain abscesses. *Clin. Neurosurg.* **1986**, *33*, 603–632.
97. Dominguez, E.A.; Patil, A.A.; Johnson, W.M. Ventriculoperitoneal shunt infection due to listeria monocytogenes. *Clin. Infect. Dis.* **1994**, *19*, 223–224. [CrossRef]
98. Bennett, J.E.; Dolin, R.; Blaser, M.J. Mandell, Douglas, and Bennett's principles and practice of infectious diseases. *Lancet. Infect. Dis.* **2010**, *10*, 303. [CrossRef]
99. Gerlach, R.; Zimmermann, M.; Hermann, E.; Kieslich, M.; Weidauer, S.; Seifert, V. Large intramedullary abscess of the spinal cord associated with an epidermoid cyst without dermal sinus. Case report. *J. Neurosurg. Spine* **2007**, *7*, 357–361. [CrossRef]
100. Park, S.W.; Yoon, S.H.; Cho, K.H.; Shin, Y.S.; Ahn, Y.H. Infantile lumbosacral spinal subdural abscess with sacral dermal sinus tract. *Spine* **2007**, *32*, E52–E55. [CrossRef] [PubMed]
101. Mohindra, S.; Gupta, R.; Chhabra, R.; Gupta, S.K.; Pathak, A.; Bal, A.K.; Radotra, B.D. Infected intraparenchymal dermoids: An underestimated entity. *J. Child Neurol.* **2008**, *23*, 1011–1016. [CrossRef]

MDPI
St. Alban-Anlage 66
4052 Basel
Switzerland
www.mdpi.com

*Journal of Clinical Medicine* Editorial Office
E-mail: jcm@mdpi.com
www.mdpi.com/journal/jcm

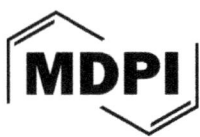

Disclaimer/Publisher's Note: The statements, opinions and data contained in all publications are solely those of the individual author(s) and contributor(s) and not of MDPI and/or the editor(s). MDPI and/or the editor(s) disclaim responsibility for any injury to people or property resulting from any ideas, methods, instructions or products referred to in the content.